Social Networks and Health

Social Networks and Health

Models, Methods, and Applications

Thomas W. Valente

OXFORD

UNIVERSITY PRESS

2010

OXFORD

UNIVERSITY PRESS

Oxford University Press, Inc., publishes works that further
Oxford University's objective of excellence
in research, scholarship, and education.

Oxford New York
Auckland Cape Town Dar es Salaam Hong Kong Karachi
Kuala Lumpur Madrid Melbourne Mexico City Nairobi
New Delhi Shanghai Taipei Toronto

With offices in
Argentina Austria Brazil Chile Czech Republic France Greece
Guatemala Hungary Italy Japan Poland Portugal Singapore
South Korea Switzerland Thailand Turkey Ukraine Vietnam

Copyright © 2010 by Oxford University Press, Inc.

Published by Oxford University Press, Inc.
198 Madison Avenue, New York, New York 10016
www.oup.com

Oxford is a registered trademark of Oxford University Press

Library of Congress Cataloging-in-Publication Data
CIP data on file

ISBN 978-0-19-530101-4

To
Becca, Kate, and Thomas

for being such a supportive and fun network.

Preface

This book provides an introduction to the major theories, methods, models, and findings of social network analysis research and application with attention to medical and public health topics. It is designed to be accessible to anyone interested in network analysis but also is designed for use in graduate introductory courses on social network analysis. The fundamental distinction of social network analysis research is that relationships—who is connected to whom—are of paramount importance in explaining behavior. Relationships and the pattern of relationships have a large and varied influence on individual and group action. Research on social network analysis has been conducted within the scientific community for over 70 years, although recent advances in computing and communication technology have dramatically altered the science.

This book is divided into three sections. Chapters 1 through 4 comprise Part I, "Models." Chapter 1 introduces the major areas of study and research questions with which social network analysis is concerned. Chapter 2 provides a historical review of the field and an introduction to how social network analysis complements existing behavior change theories. Chapter 3 presents a typology of the five different methods of network data collection, each of which has a general and a specific form, yielding 10 different research methodologies that constitute network data collection. Chapter 4 describes personal and ego-centric network effects and the many hypotheses tested using personal network data. Part II, "Methods," provides information on methods used to calculate concepts and metrics from network data. Centrality measures provide a means to locate the most important nodes in the network, and this is covered in Chapter 5. Chapter 6 presents methods used to define groups within a network, Chapter 7 presents methods used to identify positions within a network, and Chapter 8 presents network-level measures such as density, average path length, and clustering. Part III, "Applications," discusses the applications of social network analysis to behavior change in Chapters 9 through 11. In this section, individual behavior within the context of social network connections becomes important. Three application areas are reviewed and developed: stochastic network estimation or exponential random graph models, diffusion of innovations, and network interventions. Part III ends with a book summary in Chapter 12.

Every attempt has been made to make the text clear, concise, and comprehensible to a lay audience. Occasionally some chapters and sections will contain short mathematical formulas for some key indicators or concepts. Readers less mathematically inclined should be able to skip these equations with no loss of comprehension or flow. Readers more mathematically inclined may be a bit disappointed in the superficial treatment of these concepts. My apologies to both mathematically and non–mathematically inclined readers with this attempt to balance these sometimes competing needs.

My hope is that this book will enable researchers interested in understanding social network analysis to adopt this method in their research and/or practice. The field of network analysis offers many exciting tools and techniques useful in research and practice that can be applied to any situation ranging from organizational improvements, understanding risk behaviors, coordinating coalitions, or the delivery of health care services. The only barrier to widespread use of social network analysis has been people's understanding and training of how network analysis works. This book aims to make some progress in removing that barrier and helping us all become better networkers and network analysts.

Acknowledgments

This book has emerged from a desire to create a text useful for introducing public health researchers to the field of social network analysis. It has benefited greatly from the support of my colleagues at the University of Southern California including studies conducted with Chih-Ping Chou, Michael Cousineau, Kayo Fujimoto, Marientina Gotsis, Andy Johnson, Mary Ann Pentz, Alan Stacey, Donna Spruijt-Metz, Anamara Ritt-Olson, Steve

Sussman, and Jennifer Unger, among others. I would also like to thank the many students who have taken my social network analysis course over the years at Johns Hopkins University and the University of Southern California. I also want to thank the students who have worked with me conducting social network studies. In particular, my thanks to Kate Coronges, Heather Hether, Patty Kwan, Janet Okamoto, Lisa Prosser, and Beth Hoffman. I am also indebted to Marc Boulay (Johns Hopkins University), Jenine Harris (St. Louis University), and Charles Kadushin (Brandeis University) who read and commented on a penultimate draft. My wife, Rebecca Davis, has provided invaluable insight and counsel on almost every aspect of this volume.

Most of the network graphs in this book were drawn with NetDraw and much of the analysis conducted with UCINET.

I have also received support from several funding agencies, including National Institute on Drug Abuse (NIDA) support for the USC Transdisciplinary Drug Abuse Prevention Research Center (TPRC), particularly Project 2: TND Network (DA16094); National Cancer Institute support for the Transdisciplinary Tobacco Use Research Centers (P50-CA84735); National Institute on Drug Abuse support for Steps Toward Effective Prevention (STEP) (CA-012524, Pentz, PI); National Cancer Institute–funded Transdisciplinary Research on Energetics and Cancer (U54 CA 116848); California Endowment's support of our network studies of coalitions (HS-CG-06-000006); and Robert Wood Johnson Foundation support of our Wellness Partners study (U-64448).

Contents

Part I Models

1   Introduction   3
    Relationships Matter   *3*
    Random Sampling Is Not Enough   *6*
    Literature Overview   *7*
    Major Research Advances   *9*
    Individual- and Network-Level Measures   *21*
    Summary   *25*

2   History   26
    History Reconsidered   *28*
    Behavioral Science   *30*
    Life Span Approaches   *35*
    Public Health and Medical Applications   *36*
    Summary   *39*

3   Methods   41
    Data Collection Techniques   *43*
    Data Management   *50*
    Data Characteristics   *55*
    Network Variables   *55*
    Summary   *60*

4   Ego- and Personal-Network Effects   61
   Measures   65
   Statistical Analysis   70
   Personal Network versus Sociometric Variables   72
   Snowball/Sequenced Data   74
   Summary   77

Part II   Measures

5   Centrality   81
   Degree   82
   Closeness   83
   Distances for Unconnected Nodes   85
   Betweenness   87
   Correlation among Centrality Measures   91
   Other Centrality Measures   93
   Link or Edge Centrality   93
   Centrality versus Centralization   94
   Centrality and Behavior   95
   Characteristics of Opinion Leaders   98
   Summary   99

6   Groups   100
   Components and K-Cores   101
   Girvan-Newman Technique   105
   Groups and Behavior   108
   Group Membership and Disease   109
   Groups, Density, and Bridges   110
   Summary   113

7   Positions   114
   Network-Level Positions   115
   CONCOR   121
   Individual Positional Measures   122
   Individual Measures as Positions   123
   Positions and Behavior   124
   Network Weights   125
   Summary   126

8   Network-Level Measures   128
   Size   129
   Density   129
   Mutuality/Reciprocity   130
   Triads/Transitivity   132
   Diameter/Average Path Length   134
   Density and Cohesion   135
   Clustering   137

Centralization   *138*
Core-Periphery   *140*
Two-Mode Data   *144*
Individual Network-Level Interactions   *146*
Summary   *147*

Part III   Applications

9   Exponential Random Graph Models, P* and Actor
         Oriented Models   151
         Estimating the Link   *153*
         Vectorizing the Matrix   *153*
         Exponential Random Graph Models (ERGM)   *156*
         Simulation   *157*
         New Specifications   *160*
         Obesity Example   *161*
         Actor-Oriented Model   *163*
         WINCART   *166*
         Summary   *170*

10   Diffusion of Innovations   172
         Homogeneous Mixing   *175*
         Integration and Opinion Leadership   *179*
         Structural Models   *181*
         Dynamic Models   *184*
         Empirical Estimates Using Diffusion Network Data   *187*
         Infection and Susceptibility   *190*
         Thresholds   *191*
         Limitations to Diffusion Theory   *194*
         Summary   *194*

11   Network Interventions   196
         Opinion Leaders   *197*
         Key Players   *201*
         Groups   *202*
         Identifying Leaders and Groups   *203*
         Snowball Sampling or Network Recruitment   *205*
         Rewiring Networks   *207*
         Bridges and Potential Bridges   *208*
         Links versus Nodes   *209*
         Networks and Attributes   *212*
         Iatrogenic Effects   *214*
         A Pharmaceutical Marketing Example   *216*
         Summary   *218*

12 Summary 219
 Agent-Based Modeling 224
 Increasing the Threshold 231
 Statistical Analysis 232
 Network Scale 232
 Future Research Questions 233
 How to Get Started 237
 Limitations 237
 Conclusion 238

Appendix A: Glossary 239

Appendix B: Sample Sociometric Survey 241

Appendix C: Sample Egocentric Survey 243

Appendix D: Centrality Scores for Network in Figure 1–1 245

Appendix E: Input Files (Network and Attribute) for the
  Network in Figure 1–1 247

References 251

Author Index 269

Subject Index 273

PART I

MODELS

1

Introduction

This book presents social network models for understanding human behavior—particularly health behaviors. It provides a general introduction to the many theories, methods, and models of social networks and how researchers use social networks to understand and change human behaviors. The models show that social networks and the communication *among, within,* and *between* people and groups exert their influence and constrain behavior in myriad and complex ways. The network paradigm focuses on relationships, or connections, among people. Social networks are measured and defined as connections among people, organizations, political entities (states or nations), and/or other units. Social network analysis is a theoretical perspective and a set of techniques used to understand these relationships and how they affect behaviors.

Relationships Matter

Relationships influence a person's behavior above and beyond the influence of his or her individual attributes. Attributes such as sex, age, educational level, income, occupation, and ethnicity are very important and influence a person's attitudes, beliefs, and behaviors. These attributes also influence who people know and spend time with: Their social networks. Although individual attributes are important and can in part determine a person's social network, network analysis focuses on the types of relations people have and how these relationships influence behavior. As Borgatti (2009) notes, "One of the most potent ideas in the social sciences is the notion that individuals are embedded in thick webs of social relations and interactions" (p. 892).

Social networks are most often composed of who knows whom or who talks to whom within a community or an organization. Network models are constructed to show how these relations influence attitudes, beliefs, and behaviors. There are also networks that connect organizations and networks of computers, organic cells, streets, power stations, and just about anything one can think of. Networks are ubiquitous and varied. Networks describe relationships between people and between people and things. By studying relationships, network researchers add another dimension or set of factors that can explain human behavior. Throughout this book, many new terms will be used, and a glossary of relevant network definitions is provided in Appendix A.

Figure 1–1 shows a network based on friendships in one sixth-grade class in a California middle school. We asked students to name their closest friends

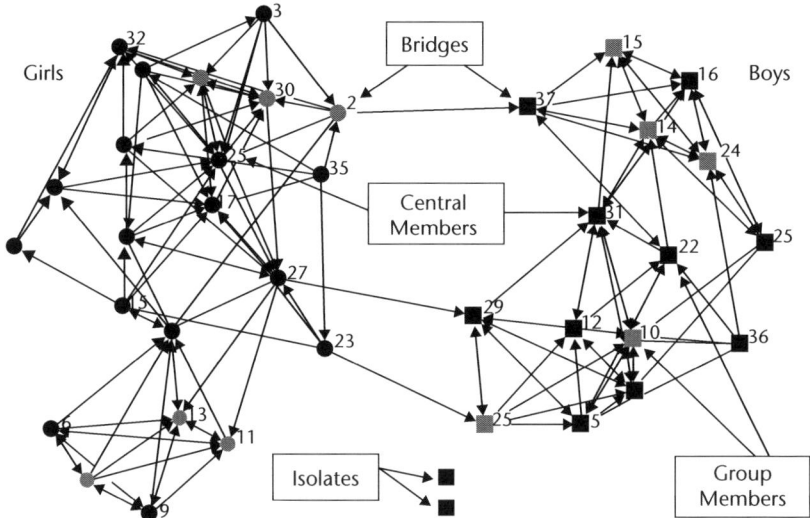

Figure 1–1. The network of friendship choices among six-grade students who named their five closest friends in the class. Girls are depicted as circles and boys as squares. The data can be used to identify positions in the network such as isolates, central members, group members, bridges, and so on. In addition, the network can be characterized as dense or sparse, centralized or decentralized, and so on. Grey shaded students are susceptible to smoking. (This graph and others were generated with Netdraw, 2006.)

by selecting them from a class roster. There was a unique identification (ID) number (1 to 34) for each student that they wrote on a form (a copy of the survey is given in Appendix B) and the form included a space for their own ID number. The list of ID numbers was entered into a spreadsheet, and the friendships then were mapped using widely available social network analysis software. Each circle or square represents a student; boys are depicted as squares and girls as circles. The ID number for each student is shown next to his or her circle or square, and lines connecting them indicate who nominated whom. In this example, the boundary of the network is the classroom, whereas in other cases it might be a grade in school or even the entire school.

The lines have arrows indicating the direction of the nomination. For example, 27 named 3 as a friend, but 3 did not name 27. The length or width of the arrows in this graph does not have meaning, although it is possible to make graphs that vary line properties (width or style) to represent strength of relation or type of relation. The graphs are usually drawn with the people who are most central in the center and then their connections are placed near them. There are many different ways to place people in the graph and many different techniques to arrange everyone in the graphing space. Colors or shapes can be used to represent different properties of the people. There are up to four attributes of the nodes that can be included in a network graph by using color (or shading), shape, labels, and size, and two attributes of the relations can be indicated using line size and style.

There are specific positions in a network and most people instinctively look to see who is at the center of a network. There are, however, deceptively numerous ways to define and hence identify central members (see Chapter 5). It might also be useful to determine isolates (people with no connections) or peripheral members (people with one or few links on the outside of the network). It should be emphasized that while many people equate being on the periphery or isolated in a network as a negative quality, often peripheral members have connections to other people and other networks in which they may occupy important positions. It is also true that peripheral members may act as bridges connecting different networks. In Figure 1–1, we can identify people (numbers 3 and 27) who occupy bridging positions within the network.

In this network, there are also two groups defined by sex (boys and girls). It is possible to categorize people as being members of specific groups, and here again there are numerous ways to define a group and hence partition a network into groups (see Chapter 6). Network analysts have also devised ways to partition a network into distinct positions. People occupy similar positions in a network to the extent they have similar relations to others in the network (see Chapter 7). Consequently, people may be in the same group but in different positions and vice versa.

This book provides the techniques and tools used to analyze social networks and to learn how ideas and behaviors spread through them. The considerations of centrality, bridging, groups, and positions in the past few paragraphs can influence how behaviors are distributed in networks.

In the network in Figure 1–1, no students were smokers in the sixth grade, but some were susceptible to smoking (indicated by refusing to state they would not smoke in the future) (Pierce et al., 1998). Susceptibility to smoking increased from three to eight of these students within 2 years. Eight students became susceptible to smoking during the study period indicated by gray shading. There is clustering in the pattern of susceptibility since everyone who became susceptible was connected to someone who already reported being susceptible.

The overall configuration or pattern of relationships can also be important. Although each person's connections may affect his or her behavior, the influence of these connections may vary depending on the overall pattern of relations in the whole network. The pattern of links in the whole network is referred to as the network structure, and structure matters. For example, this network can be described by its density (the number of links in the network expressed as a proportion of the total possible links), the amount of reciprocity, the number of subgroups, and so on. The network analysis field has created a standard set of metrics to use when describing a network (see Chapter 8). Describing networks by these metrics is interesting, but it is also possible to study whether these network properties are associated with outcomes. For example, does behavior spread more rapidly in a dense or sparse network (Valente, 1995)? Once network data are collected, researchers can extract individual- and network-level measures and study how ideas, opinion, attitudes, and behaviors are distributed in that network. This book presents the techniques to understand these considerations and more.

Random Sampling Is Not Enough

Traditional methods and approaches in the social and behavioral sciences—random sampling in particular—are *not* adequate for measuring network concepts. In fact, random sampling often limits the kind of research questions that can be asked and studied. Random sampling removes individuals from the social context that may influence their behavior. Some have called for new approaches and methods that complement existing knowledge and yet provide new ways to tackle health problems (Needle et al., 1995). Network analysis has emerged as a new paradigm useful for complementing other research methods, while at the same time offering a new set of assumptions, methods, tools, and techniques useful for addressing many social and behavioral issues.

When random sampling designs are used, it is possible to collect network data using egocentric techniques (see Chapter 4). Egocentric data collection techniques are used to measure the local or personal network environment, typically from the ego's (the respondent's) perspective. Although these data are somewhat limited in terms of network information, they provide considerable explanatory power when trying to predict individual behavior.

Literature Overview

The scientific study of social networks has been ongoing for decades, and the past few years have seen tremendous growth in its application and publicity. Increasingly, network analysis is used to study the Internet and other electronic communications. Network analysis concepts and techniques have found wide application across a number of scientific disciplines including anthropology, business, communication, computer science, economics, education, marketing, medicine, public health, political science, psychology, and sociology, to name a few. Accompanying this growth and proliferation of network studies is the need to understand the procedures and limits of network analysis studies. While networks are everywhere, there is a set of precedents, techniques, and models that constitute the network paradigm, which has grown considerably in recent years.

There are numerous introductions and reviews of network methods and theory (Boissevain, 1974; Burt, 1980; Burt & Minor, 1983; Carrington, Scott, & Wasserman, 2005; Degenne & Forsé, 1999; Harary et al., 1966; Knoke & Kuklinski, 1982; Knoke & Yang, 2008; Luke & Harris, 2007; Marsden, 1990; Marsden & Lin, 1982; Rogers & Kincaid, 1981; Scott, 2000; Valente, 2007; Wasserman & Faust, 1994; Wellman & Berkowitz, 1988). There are also texts that address social network application to specific domains such as collective action (Diani & McAdam, 2003), marketing (Van den Bulte & Wuyts, 2007), organizational behavior (Monge & Contractor, 2003; Nohria & Eccles, 1992), social influence (Friedkin, 1998), and substance abuse (Coyle et al., 1995), among others.

One primary reason social network research has grown in recent decades is that scholars have become dissatisfied with attribute theories of behavior. For example, theories that show attitudes toward a behavior are associated with the behavior often do not help us understand how to change those attitudes. In general, many attribute theories have not explained why some people do things (e.g., quit smoking) while others do not. Social network explanations have provided good explanations of behavior as seen in the example of smokers who quit when their important social ties (e.g., a spouse) exerted pressure on them to quit (Christakis & Fowler, 2008).

Every health topic can be viewed through the network perspective. Major areas of network study have been the transmission of HIV/STDs via sexual contact networks (Morris, 2004; Rothenberg et al., 1998); substance abuse (Valente et al., 2004) including injection drug use (Friedman et al., 1997; Neaigus et al., 2001); smoking (Alexander et al., 2001; Ennett & Baumman, 1993, 1994); suicide (Bearman & Moody, 2004); romantic relationships (Bearman et al., 2004); physician behavior (Gross et al., 2002); contraceptive use (Entwisle et al., 1996; Valente et al., 1997); obesity (Christakis & Fowler, 2007); and many others. In addition to individual behaviors, many have used network analysis to study interorganizational collaborations (Harris et al., 2008; Provan et al., 2003) and communication in the delivery of health services (Kwait et al., 2001).

A second reason social network analysis has grown recently is that many social activities today are inherently network activities. The spectacular growth in electronic communications, cell phones, the Internet, and email has made networks and networking a prominent part of everyday life. The availability of motorized and jet transportation and increased travel has changed social networks in profound and unforeseen ways. Social networks of most people on the planet 200 years ago were constrained to family members and others in their community. Today, most people's networks are more diverse and expansive than their ancestors of only two or three generations ago. Most of us feel that we are defined in large part by the company we keep: we have recognized that our social contacts—our networks—are an important part of our identity.

A third reason for the growth in network analysis has been that computing and graphical display software has become available in the last decade. Analysis of social networks in the past was cumbersome and lacked the convenience of graphical displays to highlight network features and properties. The advent of sophisticated computing technologies created the platforms for major analytic advances to proceed. Today, there are dozens of social network computer platforms researchers can choose from (Huisman & van Duijn, 2005).

Finally, the promise of network analysis is that it provides an in-depth understanding of how behaviors are distributed in a network and the factors associated with behavior change. Network information can be used to accelerate behavior change or reduce the negative consequences that occur when bad behaviors spread (see Chapter 11). For example, network analysis can be used to find naturally occurring opinion leaders and recruit them to be champions of a new product or idea (Valente & Davis, 1999). Network data can also be used to find bridges that might be responsible for spreading diseases between groups. Network research has grown considerably in the past decade, and while it is impossible to keep up with all the advances, there are several major research advances that have characterized and will continue to characterize the network field in the near future.

Major Research Advances

As network research has grown, a number of major research fronts have been forged in which scholars focus their energies. While there are many different types of models and researchers that occupy the scientific study of social networks, this volume focuses on how these studies, findings, and models affect human behavior. This section describes some of the major areas in which network research has advanced in recent decades.

Small World Networks

The *small world* phrase was initially coined by researchers trying to estimate how many steps it would take for strangers to relay information to one another (Box 1–1). A *small world network* is formally defined as a network in which most nodes (people) have few connections yet the overall distance between any two people in the network is shorter than expected by chance (Watts, 1999). Small world networks are characterized by local clustering, which indicates dense pockets of interconnectivity. There are, however, bridges that connected these subgroups and these bridges enable people to connect to seemingly distant others by fewer steps than would occur in a random network. Pool and Kochen (1978) formulated many of the reasons small worlds exist and what data existed in studies of human networks to postulate properties of human contact networks. Small world networks garner popular attention because the "small world" phenomenon is familiar to most people.

Box 1–1. The Milgram Small World Experiment

When two people meet for the first time, they might learn they have a place or event in common. A person might say, "I lived in such and such town" or "I used to work at such and such place or went to a particular school." If the other person happens to know someone who lived in that town or went to that school, he or she might ask "Oh, do you know so and so?" At times, people discover they have an acquaintance in common or they both know the same person. This discovery is often accompanied by the remark, "Gee, what a small world!" Many of us have our favorite small world story or a story about seeing someone we know in a strange or different place.

The small world phenomenon can be generalized as a social structural phenomenon and generalized with the following research question: What is the likelihood that two people, chosen randomly are connected by

(Continued)

Box 1–1. Continued

1, 2, 3, ... K ties? To answer this question, Stanley Milgram, a social psychologist at Harvard University,[1] conducted a study published in 1969 (Milgram, 1967; Travers & Milgram, 1969).

Milgram selected a "target" person who was a Boston stockbroker and then selected 3 random samples of about 100 people each: (1) residents in Nebraska randomly selected, (2) residents in Nebraska randomly selected who owned blue chip stocks, and (3) residents in Boston randomly selected. Study participants received a packet that they were asked to send to the target person by giving it to a friend or someone they knew who might be able to eventually get it to the target. Once people sent the packet to a friend, they were instructed to mail a postcard attached to the packet with data about themselves and who they gave the packet to.

Of the 296 packets, 217 (73.4%) were passed to at least one person. Of these, 64 (29.5%) eventually made it to the Boston stockbroker (a 21.6% completion rate). The average number of steps for the completed deliveries was 5.2. The list of names from the initial person to the target person is a chain. The average length of completed chains for those who used professional links (passing the packet to another stockbroker) was 4.6, but the chain length was 6.1 for those who passed the packet to acquaintances based on geography (getting it to someone who knew someone in Massachusetts). These data, coupled with one of Milgram's earlier studies, led to the popular conception that only six steps separate everyone in the world—that is, "six degrees of separation."

There is some debate in the network field as to whether the small world number really is 6 and studies have been conducted to replicate the study using modern electronic communications (Liben-Nowell & Kleinberg, 2008).

Milgram is perhaps better known as the scientist who conducted experiments on how people respond to authority. He had research subjects administer electric shocks to other people they thought were also research subjects when in fact they only pretended to be shocked. Study subjects increased the dosage to near what appeared to be lethal levels. Milgram discovered that people were quite willing to cause considerable pain and suffering in others if they thought they were supposed to.

There are at least three different types of small world occurrences: (1) when two people meet for the first time and discover a common link via a third person (or place), (2) when a third person discovers a link between two of his or her contacts, and (3) when two people who know one another meet unexpectedly somewhere (e.g., at an airport). Most people have a favorite small world story; mine occurred in Los Angeles, where we live. Once we threw a large house-warming party at our house to which we invited many guests, including some work colleagues. One guest at the party is a first cousin of mine who also happens to live in Los Angeles even though our families are based on the East Coast of the United States (approximately 2,500 miles away). One of my close colleagues who was also at the party has a daughter who played soccer. To my surprise, my work colleague knew my cousin as "Coach Jordan." "Small world," huh? Yes, we are all connected. I would never have known my colleague knew my cousin, even though he had talked about his daughter on numerous occasions in the past, and of course I have known my cousin for a lifetime.

There are countless stories of two strangers who meet and discover a friend or acquaintance in common or, as in my case, a party or dinner conversation at which people discover mutual acquaintances or even close friends in common. Regardless of the type of small world phenomenon experienced, we are often surprised (and reassured, and sometimes even relieved) when it occurs. The small world effect occurs for two reasons: (1) networks are not random but in fact are structured by the social position and choices people make and (2) people know their friends but do not have much information about the friends of their friends, or the friends of their friends' friends. Networks are clustered and yet each of us only has vague ideas of their friends' friends and the subsequent global network structure to which we are all connected. In other words: *we can only see so far into a network.* Small world networks are important and interesting, but they leave unanswered the question, How do networks become small world networks? Attempts to answer this question have led to the discovery of scale-free networks.

Scale-Free Networks

If networks have a noticeable structure, how do they get that way? Another way to ask this question is: *Do individuals (or nodes) have preferences for certain others they link to when joining an existing network?* Barabási (2003) studied a number of different types of networks and discovered what he called their *scale-free property.* By "scale free," Barabási (2003) meant that there is a predictable distribution in the number of connections to and from each person and this distribution is not normal but instead is highly skewed. Many people will have one link, predictably fewer will have two, still fewer will have three, and so on, so that there will be one person with hundreds of connections, or in some cases thousands of them.

Barabási (2003) hypothesized that the scale-free distribution occurred because people prefer to connect to the network at its most central locations. This is particularly true with Internet growth. If someone creates a new web-site and wants lots of people to visit that site, the best strategy is to link the site to the most central site that is relevant. Thus, as the network grows, sites that are most central retain their central position and those on the periphery continue to struggle to increase their popularity. This is sometimes referred to as "the rich get richer," network speaking.

Social networks are also likely to show preferential attachment. When a new adolescent joins a school, he or she can quickly determine who is the most popular person in the school. The new student may attempt to become friends with that person to enhance his or her own popularity. The leader's reaction to the new person may determine the new student's position in the social hierarchy. Scale-free networks and preferential attachment suggest that networks will—to some extent—be rigid, thus having predictable and stable structures. But to what extent do networks remain stable, and to what extent do they change?

Network Dynamics

The field of network analysis has begun investigating the dynamic properties of social networks, at both the individual and the network level (Banks & Carley, 1997; Doreian & Stokman, 1997). New members can join a network, and people can leave it. Within a given network, links can be added or deleted, and the nature of relationships can change, for example, from being close friends to acquaintances. These dynamics create formidable analytic challenges because the set of people involved in the relationship may change. Given the inherent problem with comparing apples and oranges, changes in people, most social network dynamic research compares the same people or the same organizations over time.

In networks, change occurs at two levels: the individual and the network. Individuals add and lose connections, and individual indicators of centrality, personal network density, and reciprocity (as well as other indicators) change over time. At the network level, the overall network density, centralization, and transitivity (as well as other indicators) change over time. Researchers often need to choose whether they will study changes in individual indicators over time or study network evolution. Network dynamics have been important because research has shown that networks can provide access to resources and information.

Social Capital

Traditionally, economic or material success was thought to be a product of one's intellect (aka human capital) and existing wealth (aka material capital) (Borgatti et al., 1998; Coleman, 1990). Lately, scholars have realized what every businessman knows: *It is not what you know, but who you know.* And further, it is not just who you know, but how well one uses his or her social resources. These social resources are referred to by some as *social capital,* which is the quality and quantity of resources available in a person's social network (Lin, 2001). A person with high social capital has an impressive Rolodex.

Social capital provides access to job opportunities (Granovetter, 1973, 1974) and information on the job that provides advantage. Social capital also can be used to provide access to health information or access to better or more appropriate health care. It has also been defined as the trust and/or the desire and ability to join civic groups. Putnam (2000), credited with popularizing the social capital concept, argued that social capital has been in decline in the United States because people are less inclined to join civic organizations, such as the Rotary Club, and more likely to spend their leisure time watching television.

Many have measured social capital as the trust they have in their neighborhood (Moore et al., 2005). This has lead to research on how to define and identify social capital and to considerations of its application to improving individual and community health. By trying to identify and strengthen available assets, social capital provides the opportunity to put a positive spin on the dire situation facing many underserved and deprived neighborhoods. Even the poorest have social capital manifested as knowledge about who has power and resources in the neighborhood. If this social capital can be mobilized, then perhaps some of the neighborhood's problems can be ameliorated. Conversely, focusing on social capital puts the burden on the community without acknowledging the institutional and historical causes that may have put communities in this disadvantaged position in the first place.

Homophily

Small worlds, scale-free networks, and social capital are concepts that describe mostly networks at the macro level: the big picture network. But much of network structure and processes reside at the micro or individual level. One of the most salient features of networks is *homophily:* the tendency for people to affiliate and associate with others like themselves. People tend to choose friends, and be restricted in their choice of friends, to others of the same sex, ethnicity, socioeconomic status, religion, and, in many cases, beliefs, attitudes, and behaviors (McPherson et al., 2006). A person's social network tends to be a reflection of himself or herself because people feel more comfortable being with people like themselves rather than with people who are different. For example, in the network in Figure 1–1, boys overwhelmingly chose boys as friends and girls chose girls. Specifically, boys had an average 3.44 male friends, whereas girls had an average of 0.33

male friend; girls had an average 4.09 female friends, whereas boys had an average of 0.91 female friend.

The human tendency for homophily also explains why the small world effect occurs. Because most people have contacts of the same ethnicity, social status, and/or religion, when two people meet, they have social networks composed of people with similar characteristics. Thus, the set of people from which contacts are drawn is narrowed by these characteristics. So the probability that two people have an acquaintance in common is much higher than random chance alone would dictate.

The tendency for homophily to occur also means that new ideas and practices have difficulty getting a foothold within most social networks. Because most people talk to others like themselves, usually those others hold similar attitudes, beliefs, and practices. Thus, there is little opportunity for new ideas to enter networks because most of the time when people talk they are in agreement. Generally, people avoid others who do not share their views, slowing the spread of new ideas.

Homophily can also speed diffusion (as explained in the next section). Because people feel comfortable with others like themselves, there tends to be considerable trust in social networks. Interpersonal communication between people within homogeneous networks tends to flow easily, and once a new idea or practice infiltrates these networks, it can spread quickly. Homophily can then speed idea and behavior spread within groups but tends to create a barrier between groups because there are few ties between disparate groups.

Diffusion/Contagion

The composition and evolution of networks (whether small world or scale free) have helped us understand what social networks look like. Network properties also have implications for how ideas, attitudes, and behaviors spread. As stated previously, a person's ideas, opinions, attitudes, beliefs, and behaviors are a function of his or her social networks' ideas, opinions, attitudes, beliefs, and behaviors. Diffusion of innovations is the process via which new ideas and practices spread within and between communities (Rogers, 2003). There is considerable evidence to suggest that a person's adoption of a new idea, attitude, opinion, or practice is strongly influenced by the behavior of their social network (Valente, 1995). Although this social influence may account for the spread of new ideas and practices, it is also true that the similarity of behaviors among people who are connected to one another arises because of selection.

Selection is the tendency for people to seek out friends whose behaviors are consistent with their own. A person who smokes is likely to seek friends who smoke because this will reduce any cognitive dissonance that may emerge due to behavioral differences between the individual and his or her friends. Because smoking and perhaps other behaviors can be markers for cultural beliefs, a person might select friends based on these overt behaviors with the expectation that the friends will hold the same beliefs and values as the focal person. Teasing out how social influence spreads—how an idea spreads through a network—can be complicated because of the way networks form (i.e., their homophily). Because people choose friends who are like themselves, it is hard to know whether networks influence behavior or whether people choose friends who engage in behaviors they want to emulate (Hoffman et al., 2007).

There have been several notable studies of the diffusion of innovations through social networks. Three specific studies—medical innovation, Brazilian farmers, and Korean family planning—have become classics because they contain specific data on when people adopted a new behavior and who in the community they were connected to via advice-seeking or discussion relationships. These three studies collected time-of-adoption data so the trajectory of diffusion could be plotted (Figure 1–2). The network data in these studies permitted the investigation of how network characteristics were associated with adoption times (Valente, 1995).

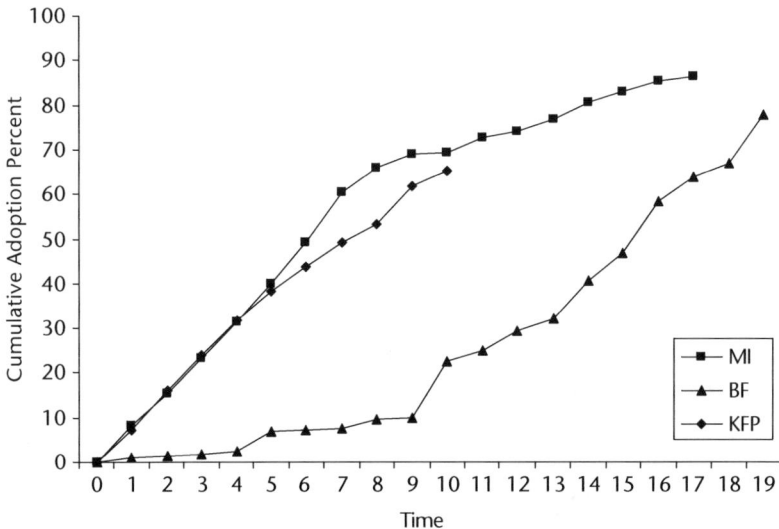

Figure 1–2. Diffusion curves for three studies: MI, medical innovation (given in months); BF, Brazilian farmers (given in years), and KFP, Korean family planning (given in years). Each line represents the cumulative percentage of adopters over time in each study.

The study of diffusion is further complicated by the long time span over which diffusion occurs. Very few new ideas and practices spread rapidly, and many adoption decisions are made by market forces beyond an individual's control. Still, networks matter, and whether by selection or influence, the behavior of one's peers seems to have a strong effect on one's behavior, but there is considerable variation in how much. It seems that individuals have varying thresholds to adoption such that some people adopt an idea when no or few others have, while other people wait until a majority of others have adopted. The distribution of thresholds governs how an idea or a practice is adopted within a network (Valente, 1995, 1996). A population composed primarily of people with high thresholds will be resistant to diffusion and hence diffusion will be slowed.

Another network factor shown to affect diffusion is one's position in the network (Becker, 1970). Several studies have found that people in the center of the network may be earlier adopters of certain ideas and behaviors (Alexander et al., 2001; Rogers & Kincaid, 1981; Valente et al., 2005). Having a central position in the network provides an advantaged viewpoint of seeing what other people do. It also provides advantage in terms of influencing others because opinion leaders, by definition, influence many others' opinions. Opinion leaders, often measured as central members in the network, both reflect and drive the diffusion process (Valente & Davis, 1999; Valente & Pumpuang, 2007).

Centrality

Because central members are so important in the network and because people instinctively want to know who is in the center and who are the leaders, network analysts have developed numerous measures of centrality (Borgatti & Everett, 2006). *Centrality* is the extent to which a person inhabits a prestigious or critical position in the network. Centrality can be measured simply as the number of choices one receives from others in the network. Other centrality measures include *betweenness,* the extent to which a person lies on the shortest path connecting others in the network, and *closeness,* the average distance that a person is located from everyone else in the network (Freeman, 1979). Chapter 5 explains the many ways that centrality is calculated and how to decide which centrality measure one might use to answer various research questions.

Centrality is related to all of the concepts we have discussed so far. Central people are the ones to whom newcomers attach when they join a network, giving rise to the scale-free phenomenon. These central members often provide bridges between different parts of a network to make them small world networks, having a short overall path length for a network of a given size. Centrality thus tends to be a central concept in the study of social networks because the pattern of central nodes and the behavior of those nodes provide the keys to network structure, evolution, and influences on behavior. And central members can have a significant influence on the speed of behavior change (diffusion). Given the tendency for homophily, however, *why do some people become more popular than others?*

There is little evidence to show whether popularity and opinion leadership are innate or learned characteristics. Most networks have some central members while the vast majority are regular members—having neither a large nor a small number of contacts. In many interorganizational networks, there will be a group of organizations sharing a central position and many other organizations on the periphery. Core-periphery analysis can be conducted to determine which organizations are in the central core and which are on the periphery and how well a core-periphery describes the pattern of links in the network (Borgatti & Everett, 1999). Yet being in the periphery may be a function of the network boundary: people on the periphery of one network can be integrated or central members of another network.

To some extent, organizations or people choose these positions by aspiring to be involved or popular, while others choose to be on the periphery. On the other hand, these positions may be derived from innate characteristics of the organizations, individuals, or cultural norms of the community. Social network analysis involves understanding the factors that determine the extent of core-peripheriness and who is in the core or periphery, as well as the consequences of these network patterns for interorganizational effectiveness or performance.

Small worlds, scale-free networks, core-periphery structures, and other models have thus far been postulated to influence the ability of ideas and behaviors to spread within these networks. At the same time, central members of the networks have been postulated as influential regardless of network structure and, indeed, as covered in this book, many network factors influence behavior change. A question often posed then is: *Can optimal or efficient network forms be discovered and created?*

Efficient Network Forms

As scholars have discovered so many important properties of networks and their importance in everyday life, a reoccurring question has emerged in some circles: *What is the most efficient network structure for reaching group goals?* A naïve view might propose that the more communication there is—as in greater network density—the more efficient is the network. Research on diffusion of innovations has argued that innovations diffuse more quickly in dense rather than in sparse networks (Valente, 1995). But empirical evidence suggests that this may not always be the case. Too much density creates redundant communications and reduces the ability of people in the network to access outside sources of information and influence (Valente et al., 2007). As Granovetter (1973) noted in his strength of weak ties argument, connections to outside sources of information and resources can be very valuable. So the optimal density level for an organization to achieve certain outcomes might be difficult to determine.

The association between performance (e.g., overall productivity) and network density is likely to be curvilinear with a certain density threshold being necessary to achieve certain outcomes and too much density being redundant or even harmful. *Optimal* density is also likely to vary over time, with *higher* levels of density being necessary early in a network's development but *lower* levels of density needed as the network matures. Of course, the optimal level of density is also highly dependent on the nature of the task being attempted and abilities of the persons involved.

Linking network structure to organizational performance has clear appeal in terms of profitability or function. Other outcomes, however, are also important to study. For example, certain network forms may be more sustainable or more robust than others. For example, Krebs (2002) notes that terrorist networks are characterized by little centralization so that they are less vulnerable to attack. A decentralized network cannot be easily crippled because one would have to remove many links to cripple communications. On the other hand, a centralized information network can be disabled by removing the most central nodes.

A simple answer to the question of what is the optimal level of density for an organization or group will be elusive. Network researchers are beginning to compile a set of results indicating how the association between network measures and performance varies with these and other characteristics. Other network characteristics such as *centralization* (see Chapters 5 and 8) may also be investigated in terms of their relation to performance and optimal configurations.

Interventions

One of the challenges facing the new science of networks is whether and to what degree networks can be changed and optimized for performance. *If optimal network forms are discovered, can they be created?* Cross and Parker (2004) conducted a number of studies using network data to discover gaps in organizational communication structure and then creating interventions to close those gaps. Results have shown that once organizational managers are presented with network data, they are keen to implement such changes. The outcome of such efforts can be measured by observing changes in communication structure or, ultimately, changes in performance.

There are several approaches to applying network data to organizational or health promotion interventions (Valente & Fosados, 2006). The most common approach has been to identify opinion leaders using social network methodology and to have these opinion leaders act as change agents (Lomas et al., 1991). Another approach is to identify subgroups in the network and approach them with behavior change promotions, or locate the leaders within the subgroups and enlist their assistance (Buller et al., 1999). Valente and Davis (1999) proposed identifying leaders first and forming groups around those leaders based on the social network nominations. To date, evidence indicates that network data can be quite helpful in behavior change efforts (Valente et al., 2003, 2006, 2007). Network data can also be used to identify groups and positional hierarchies and change efforts directed or tailored to these groups.

It is also possible to deliberately change networks so that bridges are created or strengthened. Network data in organizations can be collected so holes or gaps in the network can be spanned or divisions that become revealed can be mended together via deliberate relationship building. It might also be the case that network analysis reveals one person or a set of people who are overly taxed and burdened with requests or communications, which makes the organization vulnerable should that person or persons leave or become ill. These diagnostic tools provide many ways for managers and employees to become empowered about organizational change. Network data may also be collected at the community or market level to identify appropriate change agents.

One of the challenges for network interventions is to incorporate network and behavioral data. It may not be sufficient to find opinion leaders; rather, it may be necessary to find opinion leaders who hold appropriate opinions about the behaviors being promoted. For example, getting employees to adopt a new billing system may require using network data to find the appropriate change agents in the organization, and it may be necessary for these change agents to be both critical and supportive of the new system.

Agent-Based Modeling and Simulation

The growth in network applications has been fueled in part by the availability of sophisticated computer technology and programs that can simulate how networks function (Epstein, 2006). Early research on the flow of ideas and behaviors in networks was simulated using a cellular automoton model in which people were linked as in a grid to four neighbors (Bak, 1996). The researcher would then vary the conditions under which ideas and practices can spread in that grid by varying the number of initial adopters, the percentage of adopters in one's neighborhood necessary to trigger adoption (individual thresholds), and how well adopters persuade nonadopters to adopt.

Lately, scholars have been able to increase considerably the typologies of networks modeled, allowing for variation in the reciprocity of ties, the amount of centrality, whether the network is a small world network, and so on. These models are also quite useful for contingency planning to explore "what if" scenarios. For example, bioterrorism and influenza (flu) epidemic preparedness dictates that action plans are needed to prepare for population-level threats such as virulent flu strains. Agent-based model programs can establish parameters on what level of flu virulence under what conditions of population connectivity will give rise to epidemic conditions. Other models can be run to determine who should be vaccinated first and the effects of vaccination sequences on epidemic spread.

Computer simulations can also be used to explore theoretical developments in hypothetical network analysis. For example, Figure 1–3 shows a hypothetical network diffusion simulation comparing differences in diffusion in an empirical network compared with hypothetical diffusion in a random network. In the network condition, we assumed 5% of the population adopted a new idea, and we assumed new adopters would adopt it when 15% of their personal network did so. The random condition used randomly generated networks of the same size and density as the empirical one, but with ties distributed randomly. The simulation in the network condition shows

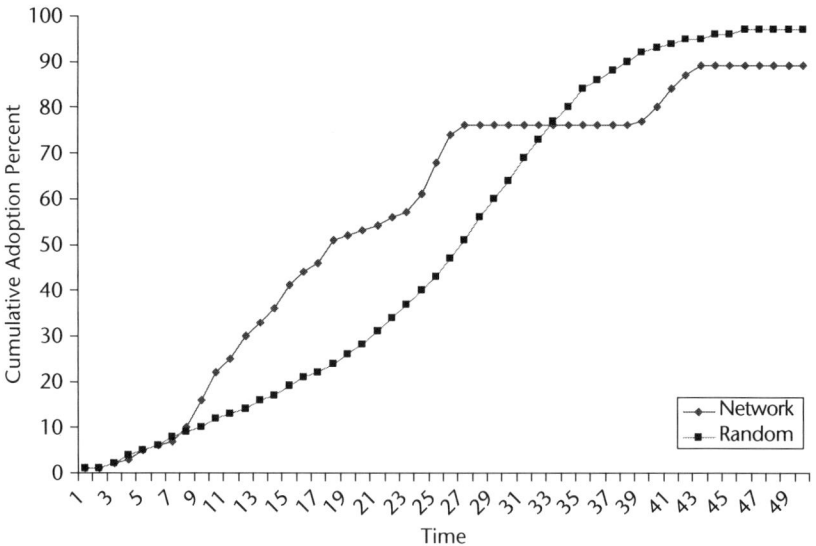

Figure 1–3. Hypothetical network diffusion simulation comparing differences in diffusion in an empirical network compared with hypothetical diffusion in a random network. In the random network, the process is smooth and continuous; in the empirical network, pockets of interconnectivity accelerate diffusion.

unevenness in the diffusion process, with the adoption rate accelerating within pockets of interconnectivity in the network. The diffusion rate levels off from time periods 27 to 41 as the innovation attempts to travel from one pocket of interconnectivity to another (Valente, 2005). The diffusion rate is smooth in the random condition, indicating that network structure does not affect the rate of diffusion.

Algorithms and Measures

While research continues on many scientific fronts, many network researchers continue to refine and expand on algorithms and measures of core constructs in the field. For example, to date at least eight centrality measures have been published and used in network research, but scholars continue to develop more efficient algorithms to calculate these measures (Brandes & Erlebach, 2005; Newman et al., 2006) and to expand discussion of existing centrality algorithms (Koschützki et al., 2005). Since the basis of network theory is mathematics, these developments are likely to continue unabated for decades.

In addition to new algorithms, network scholars devote energy to calculating validity and reliability statistics for measures (Marsden, 2005; White & Watkins, 2000) and determine how robust network measures are under conditions of missing data (Costenbader & Valente, 2003; Borgatti, et al., 2004). Understanding validity, reliability, and missing data issues is critical to the science of social network analysis as they lay the foundation for expanded use of social network concepts in many other scientific fields. In addition, there are at least a few commonly used social network software platforms, creating a robustly competitive environment for tool development (Huisman & van Duijn, 2005).

Perhaps the most significant development in the network field has been the advent of exponential random graph modeling (ERGM) and the actor-oriented co-evolution model discussed in Chapter 9. Statisticians have developed the underlying distributions of network properties well enough to create computer programs that permit statistical testing of network dynamics and evolution. This is analogous to the developments that occurred in the 1950s and 1960s in terms of understanding the basics of probability so that inferential statistics could be developed.

Individual- and Network-Level Measures

The previously outlined major research advances in understanding homophily, small world networks, scale-free networks, and other network properties have implications for understanding how innovations diffuse through networks. To explain this process, however, requires an understanding of network measures and the complex interaction between individual- and network-level measures.

Individual-level measures provide information about each person in the network based on the relationships reported by the members of the network. For example, each person can be categorized as being an isolate in the network or as being connected to the network. Measures of centrality can be calculated that indicate the extent to which each person is in the center or the periphery of the network. Individuals can be classified as bridges between subgroups or as members of such groups. In short, everyone, in response to a survey, indicates to whom they are connected, and the pooling of these responses enables the researchers to classify every person according to his or her position in the network. Moreover, once behaviors are included, individual exposures to behavior can be calculated.

Network-level measures provide information about overall properties of the network. For example, the network can be described as dense or sparse. Dense networks have many links sparse ones few. There are other network-level measures such as centralization which is the degree links are concentrated among one or a few nodes. Reciprocity, the proportion of reciprocated ties, and transitivity, proportion of transitive triangles are also commonly used network-level indicators. These terms—*density, centralization, reciprocity, transitivity,* and many others—will be given precise definitions in later chapters. Network-level measures provide indicators for the overall structure of a network. Network diagrams provide a visual sense of the overall network structure, but diagrams have their limitations. Large networks are hard to examine pictorially, and it is hard to compare different networks using only graphs.

When a network is measured, three types of information can be calculated: (1) individual measures of local relations are used to characterize a person's social network (e.g., how many friends are female), (2) individual measures of social network position (e.g., how central is each respondent in the network), and (3) network-level measures of the overall structure of the network (e.g., whether the network is dense or sparse).

Behavior

This rich tapestry of models and research questions has been applied to social behavior, organizations, power grids, traffic systems, earthworms, food webs, and many other diverse arenas of life (Watts & Strogatz, 1998). Everything is connected, and the science of this connectedness has become a popular field of research (Barabasi, 2003). *But how do these models apply to human behavior, specifically the health and well-being of individuals and populations?* For starters, small world properties provide pathways for disease, ideas, and behaviors to spread more rapidly. The bridges that make networks small world networks provide pathways critical to information, disease, and behavior spread.

The small world phenomenon affects global–macro/network structure, which creates a changed environment at the micro/individual level. If bridges did not exist, then people in a small town on one continent would not be at risk for diseases that originate in another continent. Bridges provide the pathways for diseases to spread to new populations, yet also create diffusion of modern technology and new cultural ideas. The advent of modern jet travel, trade flows, and political interconnectedness means that no population can isolate itself from health threats that emerge elsewhere. A contagious disease can spread globally almost as easily as it can spread locally.

Isolation from global threats would not be desirable because it would make the community vulnerable later. It is best to allow communities to be exposed to disease threats and develop appropriate prophylactic protections rather than attempt isolation. Further, while exposure to diseases or other threats may feel risky, in exchange, communities and their populations are also exposed to many beneficial ideas and opportunities, making them more resilient to other threats. Because we cannot isolate ourselves and because connectedness is a necessary condition of life in the modern age, it is best to find ways to maximize the advantages accrued to being connected.

As scale-free research has shown, most people and most communities do not have control over their position in a network. For most people, the likely sets of connections that are developed derive from the familial, socioeconomic, geographic, and cultural contexts into which they are born. Choose your parents wisely, we are told, because they are likely to provide the context within which you will first begin developing your social networks. Throughout the life course, these social networks provide primary socializing agents and, during adolescence and young adulthood, the context for health risk networks as well as opportunities for career and life growth.

Adolescents increasingly turn to peers as sources of information and influence as they attempt to separate from their parents and establish their own identities. Adolescent social networks play an important role in young people's lives as they form deep bonds and engage in making independent decisions for the first time, which sometimes entail risk taking. Popular students are often seen as those most likely to succeed, and their superior socializing ability puts them at an advantage for career success. In some settings, however, popularity is a risk factor for higher rates of tobacco and substance use, as popular students attempt to emulate the perceived norms of their communities (Valente et al., 2005).

During young adulthood, social contacts provide companionship and are the source for early career decisions and contacts. Success at finding gainful and productive early career employment can often depend on having contacts that allow one to get "a foot in the door" at a prestigious or profitable organization. The "old boy" network is alive and well and increasingly is being seen as simply the "network." The importance of networking has never been stronger as more and more people fight for white collar, information industry jobs.

Thus, social capital—the resources available in one's network—has become as critical as human or material capital. Having friends in high places provides early exposure to the "ins and outs" of how a business works. It is no surprise that the offspring of Hollywood stars have a better chance of becoming stars than do others. They have seen from an early age how the industry works and have the contacts to gain auditions and screenings not available to the aspiring actor. Wall Street tends to reproduce itself, and the names of Washington politicians are eerily repetitive.

Can we change our social capital? It is not easy. Young men and women born into poverty in underprivileged households have few opportunities to build contacts and networks that will provide access to high-paying jobs. But networks provide the key to untangling this predicament by encouraging the development of positive social capital. Communities can identify the contacts and connections they possess collectively to change their neighborhoods. Policies and programs designed to improve the lives of people living in underserved communities can succeed only if the social capital inherent in these communities is identified and strengthened through programs designed to create positive network environments. Communities that can identify the assets within their own communities increase the likelihood they can transition to healthier neighborhoods.

Because networks are so often governed by homophilous ties, they tend to be closed. As mentioned, getting new ideas and behaviors to spread through these networks is difficult unless one finds the right bridge to connect communities and engages opinion leaders to be drivers for change. Adoption of new behaviors, whether they be risky or protective, tends to occur within the context of close strong ties. It is weak ties at the macro level, however, that affect globally whether the new ideas can penetrate closed core groups.

The promise of social network research is that it will provide a deeper understanding of human behavior on several levels. First, by modeling human relations, researchers can measure people's strong and weak ties and show how they influence behavior. Second, social network analysis can be used to model explicitly the contact networks through which diseases are transmitted. Third, social network analysis can link macro- and micro-level structural influences by, for example, investigating whether personal network characteristics are differentially important based on network-level characteristics. Fourth, by understanding how diffusion occurs, network interventions can be created to accelerate diffusion or curtail disease spread. Fifth, social networking technology has made the management and maintenance of social networks easier and more multimediated than ever before. Finally, interesting questions about how and with whom people interact and communicate can be posed and answered. There are many fundamental properties of social interaction just now beginning to be addressed in the network paradigm. This book will provide the background necessary to conduct research on social network influences on behavior and performance.

Summary

This chapter has outlined some of the major research fronts and principles under study in the network analysis field. Although the research topics are diverse and have been applied to a diverse set of phenomenon, they have all been fundamentally interested in *connectedness* and how the set of social relations can be studied. These various research topics shed some light on how these diverse areas of investigation have implications for studying human behavior, how people gain access to resources and jobs, and how social networks influence individual and system behavior. This book will delve deeper into social network models and how they influence human behavior. In particular, we will be interested in how health risks and protective behaviors spread, to answer the following question: *How does an understanding of social networks help us understand the spread of disease and risk behaviors at the individual and population levels?*

2

History

This chapter provides a brief introduction to the history of social network analysis research and notes that network research development was delayed in part by an overemphasis on inferential statistics within the social science community. The chapter then reviews how major behavioral science theories have used social network concepts. The chapter closes with a brief literature review section on the public health and medical applications of network analysis.

Freeman (2004) wrote an informative history of the social network analysis field, in which he acknowledged that some early sociological research was social network research. For Freeman, social network research consists of research with at least the following four qualities: (1) considers the whole network structure, (2) makes arguments about how network structure influences individual action, (3) uses graphical displays, and (4) uses mathematical formalism. Research with these four qualities can be considered social network analysis.

Freeman discussed the work and lives of many of the early social network analysts. Particular attention was paid to Jacob Moreno (1934), who was one of the first to develop a program of research studying social networks and outcomes. Moreno developed a methodology in which he asked youth (usually elementary school students, ages 6–12 years) to write down the names of other students who would be ideal in various roles such as leader, friend, enemy, and so on. Moreno could then classify students in the class based on the pattern of sociometric ties in the data. Students who received many nominations as leader or friend were often thought to be socially popular and mentally and socially healthy. Developmental psychologists still use these techniques today to measure social well-being among children (e.g., Cairns et al., 1988).

By the 1950s, various research groups had begun to create a field called *social network analysis* or *sociometry*. There was a group dynamics center at the University of Michigan that is credited with training excellent scholars on the early uses of graph theory to understand social networks. Several noted social psychologists such as Heider, Cartwright, Homans, and Festinger, as well as many others, conducted studies on social networks in the workplace and in communities.

Scott's (2000) history identifies two different social network analysis communities that had developed centers of network research by the beginning of the 1960s. The first community was the Manchester Anthropologists (from Manchester, United Kingdom) consisting of Barnes, Bott, Boissevain, and Mitchell, who conducted a series of studies in Africa on the network structure of communities in small villages. Several classic books and studies emerged from this group showing that there existed patterned structures of interaction that affected everyday life in these villages. The second community was centered around sociologist Harrison White, in the 1960s, then at Harvard University. White began training a series of graduate students in sociology who later became the leaders of the social network field. These scholars included Bonacich, Boorman, Breiger, Carley, Granovetter, Wellman, and others who were defined as *structuralists* because they studied network structure. The Harvard structuralists became the foundation for establishing a network paradigm in the United States that spanned several disciplines.

By the mid-1970s, two meetings were held in Hawaii in an attempt to bring together the various disparate scholars interested in studying social networks. These meetings culminated in the launch of the International Network for Social Network Analysis (INSNA) and a commitment to hold an annual meeting starting in 1981. The journal *Social Networks* was launched, as was the bulletin/journal *Connections*. Thus, a professional community of scholars was born. INSNA provided a venue to develop social network analysis methods, theories, and applications and to support the growth of network scholarship. In the 1980s, there was concern over how to keep a professional academic discipline alive when there were few academic departments that openly supported the field.

According to Knoke and Kuklinski (1982), the two central insights of network analysis are that connections (networks) are nonrandom and that the pattern of connections in a network can often be reduced to a set of functionally equivalent positions (see Chapter 7). These two insights provided a basis for the burgeoning science of networks and a preoccupation with finding mathematical descriptions for network properties and analysis. By the mid-to-late 1980s, network analysis scholars had begun to develop a library of social network algorithms for measuring key constructs and a culture of scientific exchange, collegiality, and cooperation. UCINET was first released in the mid-1980s, which provided a platform for social network analysis.

The advent of the AIDS epidemic and influx of public health researchers eager to use these tools for investigating important public health issues helped bolster the viability of the network community in the early 1990s. Now no longer a nascent community, the network field began to develop more powerful and user-friendly computer tools and programs. The explosive growth of the World Wide Web, Internet, and computer communications made networks and networking both explicit and ubiquitous. Thus, the network field suddenly discovered it was relevant and central to investigations in a number of disparate disciplines.

As we entered the twenty-first century, network analysis seemed to be relevant to many disciplines. Disciplines such as computer science, physics, and biology discovered the importance of connectedness, relationships, and networks. One discipline that stormed the network field in force was physics. Networks are inherently mathematical, and a number of physicists revisited old network questions and raised new ones (Bonacich, 2004). Suddenly, network analysis was being discussed in science publications, periodicals, and the popular press with surprising frequency. New companies were created to store and use social networks, and social networking was a hot new pastime. At the same time, network analysis began to become accepted as a legitimate and necessary tool to answer research questions posed in many fields.

History Reconsidered

While this received view of the history of network analysis is largely accepted, a few caveats and notes are warranted. First, the reason social network analysis did not become more widely adopted as a scientific method in the 1950s and 1960s is perhaps attributed to the ascendance of computer statistical packages such as SAS (SAS Institute, Cary, NC) and SPSS (SPSS Inc., Chicago, IL). These programs were created to make population parameter estimates from a randomly selected sample of respondents. Precision in predicting polling data was considered more important than understanding how social interaction and networks influenced those opinions. Regression became the tool of choice to understand whether one variable caused another, and the social scientific enterprise became a study of people's attitudes and behaviors measured by Likert-type scales. Virtually all social science research consisted of recruiting random samples and interviewing respondents, with little consideration of their social context.

Social scientists wanted legitimacy, and the best way to achieve it was to assume a mantel of scientific investigation. The statistics of populations and inference were the tools being promulgated to "even the playing field" between the social and physical sciences. Social scientists were trained to collect random samples and administer population surveys. The surveys typically included questions to assess knowledge, attitudes, and practices, and because the measures were drawn from a randomly generated sample, inferences to the population could be made. Scientists overwhelmingly were trained in the importance of random sampling and inferential statistics. Few social scientists were trained in linear algebra or matrix manipulation, the techniques needed to understand the procedures being used in a network study. The study of human behavior then typically became one in which people were removed from their social and interpersonal contexts.

A further barrier to wider use of network analysis in the 1960s occurred within the study of the diffusion of innovations. By the late 1950s, hundreds of studies of diffusion had been conducted and a general paradigm emerged that underscored the importance of interpersonal communication and social networks in the diffusion process (Valente & Rogers, 1995). In a convergence of politics and science, the mid-1960s witnessed a backlash against unchecked diffusion of innovations in farming practices that were having an adverse affect on the environment. Many scholars had used diffusion theory to show how new pesticides and farming practices were being adopted, but now advocates wanted this diffusion to stop. So diffusion theory was implicated in the success of the diffusion of new technology and its subsequent negative environmental impacts. The study of diffusion became synonymous with cultural imperialism and was largely abandoned (Valente & Rogers, 1995). The study and application of diffusion theory, which would have generated considerable network research, was somewhat curtailed as a result of these developments, so the opportunity for network research to flourish at an earlier time was missed.

Finally, because the social network study of diffusion was not a methodology available to most scholars, diffusion theory seemed moribund as an area of scientific investigation. To most scientists, it probably seemed as if the interesting diffusion questions had already been answered without realizing that an entirely alternative set of tools, in the form of social network analysis, was needed to answer the many unanswered diffusion questions.

Recent developments in statistical analysis have now come to appreciate the importance of context and the nonindependence of most human data.

Statisticians realize that the truly random independent sample is a rarity and they have developed statistical tools to account for the nonindependence of observations. Two survey interviews conducted at households in the same zip code are likely to elicit responses that are more alike than those from two different zip codes. Thus, individual respondents are not independent but rather are often clustered based on geography or some other criteria (Murray, 1998). The extensive attention to clustered designs in statistical analysis is now converging with the importance of social network analysis in terms of understanding the importance of context and nonindependence. So while network analysis has become widely accepted as part of social and behavioral theory today, it has had a slow and contentious adolescence.

In sum, the use of application of social network analysis was slowed by an overemphasis on individual explanations of behavior and disenchantment with diffusion of innovations of theory for political and cultural reasons. The gradual appreciation of nonindependence of most human data, however, has led to a convergence of social and behavioral research that underscores the importance of environment and particularly interpersonal relationships as an influence on behavior. Today it "appears then that social network analysis is finally succeeding in providing an alternative to the traditional individualism of most mainstream social research" (Freeman, 2004, p. 167).

Behavioral Science

Theories serve many functions, including how they define and channel the types of research questions that get asked and the kinds of research methods used to answer them. Theories guide our thinking about how the world works and how humans interact and behave. It guides our choices of data collection, what questions we ask, and how we ask them. The following section discusses how networks have been incorporated into behavioral theories and studies, providing a general review of the literature.

Homophily and Selection

Birds of a feather flock together. This simple conception is not much more than an observation that people tend to cluster together based on shared outcomes or beliefs. Most researchers agree that people who engage in a particular behavior are often surrounded by friends, family members, and associates who also engage in the behavior or approve of doing so. There are numerous empirical examples (Hoffman et al., 2006). Studies have shown that an individual adolescent's substance use is associated with, and perhaps causally linked with, substance use by their friends. In the case of smoking, for example, having a best friend who smokes (Urberg et al., 1997) and having friends who smoke (Alexander et al., 2001; Aloise-Young et al., 1994; Botvin et al., 1993; Bauman & Ennett, 1994; Ennett et al., 2006, 2008; Flay et al., 1994; Kirke, 2004, 2005; Urberg et al., 1997) is associated with smoking. There is cross-sectional evidence that suggests that among high school adolescents, peer involvement in illicit drug use (Rai et al., 2003; Windle, 2000) and alcohol use (Windle, 2000) are associated with one's own involvement in these behaviors.

Longitudinal evidence linking peer and individual use also exists (Ennett et al., 2008; Pearson & West, 2005; Rice et al., 2003). Other studies have examined the association between the number of friends who use substances and the individual's substance use (Donato et al., 1994; Meijer et al., 1996; Wang et al., 1997). There is evidence that the number of friends who use illicit drugs (Jenkins & Zunguze, 1998) and smoke cigarettes (Wang et al., 1997) is positively associated with one's own illicit drug use and smoking, respectively. Unger and Chen (1999) provide longitudinal evidence that suggests that individuals who have friends who smoke are more likely to start smoking themselves. Ennett and Bauman (1994) found that membership in a friendship group was associated with smoking. Nonsmokers who associated with people in cliques composed of smokers were more likely to become smokers than were those who associated with people in nonsmoking cliques. Friedman and others (1997) showed that being connected to a large group of people who use drugs is associated with drug use.

Alexander and others (2001) found that adolescents with a majority of friends who smoke were almost twice as likely to smoke themselves. Studies have also found a positive association between smoking and the proportion of friends who smoke (Botvin et al., 1993; Urberg et al., 1997). Sieving and others (2000) examined adolescent friendships longitudinally for 3 years and demonstrated that, over time, higher levels of friends' drug use led to increased alcohol use. Estimates are that a personal network change from no adopters or users to one completely filled with adopters or users (0% versus 100% exposure) increases the likelihood of the focal person being an adopter or user by 200%. How does this homophily occur?

Social Learning Theory

The "birds of a feather flock together" notion is simplistic. One would want to understand the mechanisms underlying this network clustering. One theory that might be invoked to provide an explanation of this clustering is social learning theory. Social learning theory (Bandura, 1986) posits that involvement in a behavior is the result of modeling significant others' behaviors and the social reinforcement that comes from that. Social learning theory suggests that people gain an interest in behaviors by watching others get rewarded for those behaviors. For example, a child who sees a peer get a present by screaming for it will mimic that behavior. This vicarious exposure and reward might consist of exposure to behaviors via the mass media such as movies, TV, DVDs, and magazines. Vicarious exposure can also come from others one observes at a distance in the neighborhood, community, school, or organization. Finally, much of that vicarious exposure is likely to come from close friends and trusted colleagues and associates. Behaviors are observed, and in some cases overt instruction and pressure can incline a person to try the new behavior.

Selection

Both diffusion of innovations and social learning theory assume that people engage in behaviors because they are influenced by their peers. However, there may be a different explanation: People may select friends based on the similarity of attitudes and behaviors between the focal person and a potential friend. For example, Donohew and others (1999) posit that individuals who are high on sensation-seeking tend to select friends who are also high on sensation-seeking and more likely to experiment with alcohol, marijuana, and other substances. Consistent with this assertion, Pearson and West (2005) used Markov models to show that people who became substance users transitioned from belonging to non–risk-taking groups to risk-taking groups.

Ennett and Baumann (1994) conducted a study to determine whether the homogeneity of smoking behavior within groups was caused by social influence or friendship selection based on smoking behavior. This study was motivated, in part, by the need to understand how much of the correlation between adolescent smoking and that of their peers is due to influence and how much is due to selection. They conclude, "Although our findings contradict the popular wisdom that peer group influence is largely responsible for adolescent smoking, they substantiate previous research that found that both influence and selection processes contribute to smoking homogeneity among peers" (Ennett & Baumann, 1994, p. 660). Kandel's (1985) longitudinal study of high school students also found that models that included both selection and peer influence explained initiation into marijuana use more fully than did either factor alone.

Other studies have also attempted to disentangle influence from selection (Engels et al., 1997; Fisher & Bauman, 1988). Fisher and Bauman (1988) looked at stable dyadic friendships and showed that the two persons became similar in their smoking behavior, suggesting influence. On the other hand, dynamic friendship dyads also showed similarity, indicating an effect of selection. Engels and others (1997) also found support for both influence and selection. In a more recent study, Urberg and others (1997) included assessments of the peer group behavior and friend's smoking reports. They found that "the amount of influence over the school year was very modest in magnitude and came from the closest friend for initiation of use" (Urberg et al., 1997, p. 840). Michell and Amos (1997) showed that girls who belonged to groups where smoking was common were more likely to smoke. Indeed, the authors showed that girls began smoking to enhance their prestige in the community. Many girls initiated smoking early to demonstrate their status as being more mature. In sum, both social influence and peer selection are responsible for the similarity of smoking behavior among friends, and each suggests different causal mechanisms for how peers contribute to smoking onset and maintenance.

Hall and Valente (2007) suggested that influence and selection could be measured based on the direction of the relationship. They suggested that ties emanating from a person (out-degree) represent selection as it indicates whom they select as friends, whereas ties going to a person (in-degree) indicated influence as that is who might try to influence a person. Hall and Valente (2007) showed that selecting smokers as friends in the sixth grade predicted both smoking and smoking susceptibility in the seventh grade. It is also clear that separating influence from selection may not be possible given the dynamics of friendships and relationships. As it is, most studies find selection and influence to be approximately equal as explanations for the similarity of individual behaviors and those of their peers.

Norms

From the earliest days of behavioral science, studies have shown that perceptions of what others believe and do affect individual choices. Solomon Asch (1956) conducted influential experiments in which subjects were shown three lines on a wall and asked to indicate their relative length (e.g., whether they were the same size, shorter, longer, etc.). Asch (1956) showed that study participants would bias their reports of line length to be consistent with other participants in the study.

The Theory of Reasoned Action in its simplest form posits that one's perceptions of (peer) social norms, one's willingness to comply with those norms, and one's expectations regarding the cost and benefits of engaging in the behavior will influence one's own intentions to act. These intentions often lead to behaviors (see Fishbein & Ajzen, 1981). This constellation of normative beliefs is strongly influenced by interaction with peers. Like social learning theory, norms are learned from observing peers' behaviors and/ or hearing what their friends tell them. In some cases, the pervasive influence of peers leads to gross inaccuracies in one's social perceptions of what is normative for different reference groups. For example, a person whose friends use certain substances may believe it is normative for everyone to use these substances even though only a small percentage does.

Theory of reasoned action states that behavior is influenced in part by perceived peer norms (Fishbein & Ajzen, 1981). One finding from research on adolescents has been that youth often misuse substances because they incorrectly believe that it is normative to use them. Adolescents often overestimate the prevalence of smoking, drinking, and drug consumption in their schools. For example, Sussman and others (1988) found that regardless of smoking status, eighth- and ninth-graders overestimated weekly use of cigarettes among youth their age. However, nonsmokers made gross underestimations and regular smokers made overestimations of smoking among their age group. This finding has been used in substance use prevention programs to "re-norm" these perceptions. In an intervention study, MacKinnon and others (1991) found that change in perceptions of friends' tolerance of drug use was the most substantial mediator of program effects on drug use.

One potential research question is whether youth overstate drug use in general or base their general inaccurate judgments of use on accurate perceptions of use by significant others. If youth overestimate drug use in general, then one might confront youth with actual use rates among persons they know or others in their physical environment to instruct and correct the overestimate (and, hence, reduce perceptions that one should use drugs because "everybody else does"). However, if overestimates of friends are accurate, one would need to expose these youth to wider social use norms and perhaps counteract deviant influences among friends. Ianotti and Bush (1992) asked students to name their three closest friends and to state whether they thought each smoked, drank alcohol, or used marijuana. They found that respondent reports of their friends use did not correlate well with those friends' self-reports. Ianotti and Bush (1992) found that perceptions of friends' use was more highly associated with one's self-reports of use. Similarly, Rice and others (2003) found that high school student reports to a general question regarding friends' use did not correlate with the self-reports of their friends. Perceptions of friends' use may reflect projection and implicit cognitions (Stacy et al., 2004) rather than environmental influence.

In a related study, Valente and others (1997) found that women in voluntary organizations in Cameroon misjudged their friends' contraceptive use. They found however, that perceived friends' use was associated with one's own use, regardless of those perceptions' accuracy. There is a need to determine factors that are associated with discrepancies between peer reports and self-reports of health risk behaviors. The data suggest that people do not accurately know their friends' behaviors, with errors of estimation in a direction consistent with their own behavior, such as smokers overstating that their friends smoke.

Perceived Social Consequences

There is also a need to distinguish between peer use and perceptions of peer approval of use. Many adolescents believe that desirable social consequences, such as peer acceptance or peer support, will occur as a result of using substances and therefore are motivated to initiate substance use. For example, Jenkins (2001) found that among non–substance-using high school students, peer pressure was the most frequently cited reason why refusing beer, marijuana, and drug use offers was difficult. Among continuation (alternative) high school students, Sussman and others (1995) also found that perceived peer pressure was a reason why at-risk students use drugs other than tobacco.

Furthermore, other studies have shown that among high school boys, drug use (Luthar & D'Avanzo, 1999) and cigarette smoking (Alexander et al., 2001; Vega et al., 1996) are associated with peer acceptance of such use.

Life Span Approaches

It should be noted that the effects of peer influence, peer selection, perceived peer norms, and perceived social consequences may differ among people at different ages, due to changes in the structure and importance of peer relationships during the life span. In a longitudinal study, Feiring and Lewis (1991) found that peer networks were larger by age 13, and the number of same-sex friends increased. By high school age, youth spend more time away from adults and their lives become less dominated by social interactions with small groups of same-sexe peer groups. Concomitantly, they become exposed to a wider range of unsupervised social gatherings, which consist more of interactions with crowds, more dyadic relationships such as dating, and more "weak" ties (liaisons) than in earlier years (e.g., Dunphy, 1963; Gavin & Furman, 1989; Shrum & Cheek, 1987). Of course, social-situational factors, including same-sex peer group relationships, remain quite important predictors of behavior during middle and late adolescence (Sussman et al., 1995).

However, other findings suggest that the influence of specific friends may become attenuated during adolescence, due to the development of one's self-concept. For example, Clark-Lempers, and others (1991) suggest that the importance of various people, including one's same-sex best friend, decreases from early to late adolescence. Hence, intervention studies on adolescents should also target individual characteristics, such as motivation to resist substance use and social skills to resist substance use offers (Sussman et al., 2006). In sum, network analysis has been a component of social and behavior theories and explanations for human behavior, and network analysis has enjoyed extensive application in public health, particularly adolescent risk behaviors.

Public Health and Medical Applications

In addition to these studies on adolescent substance use, applications of network analysis to health issues can be divided into at least five areas:

(1) Social support and its influence on mortality and morbidity represent the largest area of application (Albrecht & Adelman, 1987; Gottlieb, 1985; House, 1981; Knowlton, 2003; Sarason et al., 1983).

(2) AIDS/STDs and family planning research have benefited from network theory and modeling (Aral, 1999; Klovdahl, 1985; Kohler, 1997).

(3) Community health projects have used network analysis to improve message dissemination and program implementation (Stoebenau & Valente, 2003).

(4) Interorganizational collaboration, cooperation, and exchange studies have been conducted to improve understanding of health service provision (Harris et al., 2008; Kwait et al., 2001; Wickizer et al., 1993; Valente et al., 2007a).

(5) Understanding and improving health care provider performance (Lomas et al., 1991; Soumerai et al., 1998).

Social Support

Social support consists of an objective appraisal of an individual's set of network contacts and the functions these contacts perform. Social support also consists of a subjective appraisal of the resources and reactions an individual's network provides to him or her. Social support represents one type of affect that is transmitted through social networks and represents an important means in which social networks influence health (Albrecht & Adelman, 1987; Berkman & Syme, 1979; Cassel, 1976; Cohen & Syme, 1985; Gottlieb, 1985; Hammer, 1983; House, 1981; Knowlton, 2003; Orth-Gomer & Unden, 1987; Sarason, et al., 1983; Turner & Marino, 1994; Vaux, 1988). Many social support studies have been conducted on the relationship between social support and stress and coping, and there have been a number of studies on the relationship between social support and general health and well-being. There are at least four types of social support: (1) emotional, (2) instrumental, (3) informational, and (4) appraisal (Barrera, 1983; Barrera & Ainlay, 1983; Cutrona & Suhr, 1992; House, 1981). *Emotional* support is provided by friends and family who express sympathy, concern, care, and empathy with the focal individual. *Instrumental* support is the provision of aid, resources, money, goods, equipment, and services at a time of need. *Informational* support is the provision of advice, knowledge, suggestions, and tools useful to the individual. *Appraisal* support is the feedback and analysis that allow the focal individual to evaluate his or her situation.

HIV/STDs

HIV/STD network research represents an important area of application because HIV/STDs are transmitted by sexual contact (Klovdahl, 1985; Morris, 1995, 2004). Klovdahl (1985) analyzed sexual contact data collected by the Centers for Disease Control and Prevention (CDC) to demonstrate that HIV was transmitted via sexual networks. Klovdahl further argued that improved travel technology creates the possibility of global epidemics and showed how understanding network structure improves the understanding of epidemics. Other studies have been conducted to demonstrate how networks channel the spread of HIV/STD infection (Fisher et al., 1988; Friedman et al., 1995, 2001; Havanon et al., 1993; Klovdahl et al., 1994; Obbo, 1993; Treboux & Busch-Rossnagel, 1990; Rothenberg et al., 1998). For example, Bettinger and others (2004) showed that core and bridge adolescents perceived themselves at lower STD risk than isolates and, as a result, they were less likely to use condoms. Some scholars rely on mathematical models and computer simulations to understand how HIV/STDs spread (Anderson & May, 1992; Wallace, 1994).

Recently, network analysis of factors associated with contracting sexually transmitted infections (STIs), tuberculosis (TB), malaria, and many other infectious diseases has begun (e.g., Aral et al., 1999; Klovdahl et al., 2001). Because contagion occurs via person-to-person contact, it makes sense to use network methodology to analyze the spread of these communicable diseases. Health departments have used contact tracing methods for decades to treat infected individuals and to find core groups. These methods and ideas are now being combined with network graphing and analytic tools to combat the spread of infectious diseases.

Intravenous drug users (IDUs) have been a focus of numerous studies that show that drug users form networks to support drug acquisition (Neaigus et al., 1994) and to establish community norms and a sense of belonging (Needle et al., 1995). For example, Latkin and others (1998) found that IDUs with dense and multiplex personal networks were more likely to share needles than were IDUs in nondense and nonmultiplex networks.

Family Planning and Reproductive Health

Family planning (FP) programs have benefited from network models and analysis techniques. Interpersonal communication is an important channel for FP information and influence (Bhatia et al., 1980; Rosenfield et al., 1973; Valente et al., 1994, 1997). An early study of networks and family planning was conducted by Rogers and Kincaid (1981; Park et al., 1974) in Korea in 1973 that analyzed data collected in 24 Korean villages among women of childbearing age. The network questions solicited the names of up to five other women in each village with whom the respondents discussed general information, child's education, consumer goods, health, family planning, and abortion. These data continue to be extensively reanalyzed (Granovetter, 1978; Montgomery & Chung, 1999; Valente, 1995) as they represent the best data available on networks and family planning use. Scholars have studied the diffusion of the idea of fertility regulation as well as the adoption of specific methods of contraception.

Community Health

Community health interventions benefit from network tools to the extent that community interventions rely on opinion leaders and other network structure characteristics for message dissemination. For example, Kelly and others (1991) used key informants to locate opinion leaders who acted as information disseminators. Kelner and Wellman (1991) showed how individuals use their networks to obtain information concerning medical treatment alternatives with regard to back pain. Information flow within a community is often dependent on both individual and group network properties. Risk behaviors occur within a sociocultural context, and public health programs can be made more effective by understanding the characteristics of this context (Trotter et al., 1995).

Information seeking, giving, and referral represent a nice overlap between networks and health. Information seeking has been investigated in areas such as back pain (Kelner & Wellman, 1991) and family planning (Rosenfield et al., 1973). These network studies have shown that individuals rely on others from similar backgrounds yet slightly higher socioeconomic status for information regarding appropriate care. They also show that physicians are considered as credible sources of information, yet trust is more likely to be found in their peer networks.

While most community interventions focus on behavior change among individuals, other studies have focused on behavior change among physicians and other health care providers. Because physicians and other health care providers have a significant impact on health, it is sometimes important to understand how provider networks influence the type of care given. For example, Coleman, Katz, and Menzel (1966) studied the networks of physicians in four Illinois communities to show how interpersonal networks influenced these physicians' adoption of a new drug. They found that physicians who were more integrated into the medical community were earlier adopters of a new drug (tetracycline). They also found that early adopters were influenced by physicians in their advice and discussion networks, while those who adopted later were influenced by physicians in their friendship networks.

Interorganizational Relations

There have been many studies of how health, health care, and other agencies are connected via formal agreements, client referrals, collaboration, and cooperation (Galaskiewicz, 1985). Some have studied how clients are passed through the health system in a type of exchange (e.g., Beniger, 1984), while others have used these data as measures of collaboration and interconnectedness between these service organizations. Wickizer and others (1993) used network indices to show how an intervention may increase interorganizational collaboration and cooperation (also see Provan et al., 2005). The flow of resources, materials, personnel, and information between health sector organizations is still further complicated by the presence of government and policy issues, third party payers, and technological change.

Chapter 11 discusses how network analysis can be used to identify key players and opinion leaders to act as change agents to improve provider performance. For example, Lomas and others (1991) used network analysis to identify physicians in selected hospitals. These leaders were then trained in the promotion of a vaginal birth after a first cesarean (VBAC) birth, which was a practice recommended by guidelines released at that time. This study showed that, compared with control hospitals, using opinion leaders as change agents was an effective way to increase VBAC rates. Network analysis can be conducted in many types of health care settings to identify key players and network characteristics that can be used to change provider and organizational performance.

Summary

This chapter provided a brief review of the history of social network analysis. The field has its roots in the social sciences, particularly anthropology, sociology, and psychology. The field was generally developed by scientists in these fields who favored mathematical and computational approaches to studying human behavior within these disciplines. Like most fields, fissures occasionally develop that separated scientists along substantive or methodological lines.

One unique aspect to the social network story is how its development was stymied in the 1950s and 1960s, in part by paradigmatic and political reasons. The development of advanced computing and the rise of polling and random sampling lead scientists to developing methods that treat people as atomized individuals divorced from their interpersonal contextual environments. Scholars did not appreciate the power of social networks and this led to a marginalization of the network approach. Ironically, the development of social networking software has created enthusiasm for the science of network analysis, perhaps more than is deserved.

Social networks have been an integral part of many social and behavioral theories and applications, and for years scholars have studied the distinction between selection and influence as explanations for the similarity between individual behavior and that of their peers. Most of the major behavior change theories include a component to represent social network influences and the role of norms. The chapter closed with a review of the many medical and public health applications of social network analysis. Studies of HIV/STD, substance use, family planning and contraceptive use, social support, and interorganizational relations have all figured prominently in the past few decades.

3

Methods

This chapter provides an overview of the five main network analysis data collection techniques. For each type, both a general and a specific version are presented. The chapter then provides an introduction to data management techniques and the distinctions between relational and structural measures, as well as the distinction between individual- and network-level variables. This chapter describes network data collection and management procedures so researchers can make informed choices regarding network data collection and management procedures. It is critical that researchers select the right method for their research questions.

Network data can be collected in various ways, each of which provides a different type of data with unique management and analysis requirements. The variety of data collection techniques, and their aspects and limitations, can cause confusion in how to apply network analysis to various substantive areas and how to understand the network paradigm. Figure 3–1 illustrates four different survey sampling techniques. Figure 3–1a shows a random sample, each node representing an individual who is interviewed. Notice that the nodes are clustered; they are not randomly distributed in the space. This illustrates that most survey protocols do not recruit subjects randomly but rather select clusters randomly, and then select subjects randomly within clusters. For example, a national telephone survey will select a subset of area

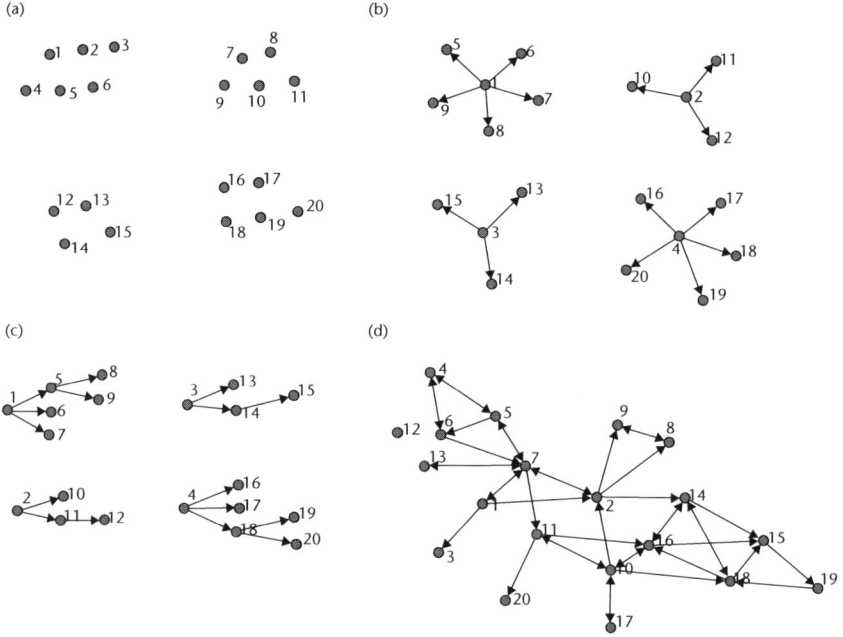

Figure 3–1. An illustration of four different survey sampling techniques: (a) random selection (although clustered), (b) egocentric, (c) sequenced or snowball, and (d) census.

codes randomly and then select random numbers within each area code (see Murray, 1998; Valente, 2002, for more on this point). Thus, most survey data are not random but are clustered. Still, data from the respondents, aside from the clustering, are presumably independent.

Figure 3–1b depicts an egocentric sample. Here, four initial respondents are selected (via random selection or other recruitment method), and during the interview they are asked to name up to five (or some other number) friends they "discuss important matters with." The respondent then provides information on each of these friends. The data provide information on each respondent's personal network from the respondent's perspective.

Figure 3–1c depicts a "snowball" or sequenced sample. Here, four initial respondents (called indexes) are selected and they provide information on a number of their contacts. The number of contacts can be few or many. In snowball sampling, the contacts, or some sample of them, are interviewed so that nodes 5, 11, 14, and 18 are also primary respondents. In sequenced sampling, the member of some random subset of the named contacts are interviewed.

Figure 3–1d depicts a sociometric sample in which all respondents are interviewed and asked about their contacts within the community of study. Here, the entire community, or as many as possible, are interviewed. Everyone

Table 3–1. Network Analysis Data Types

	General	Specific
1. Survey	Standard survey questions	Standard survey questions
2. Egocentric	Social roles (father, mother, brother, sister, etc.) Network alters are limited to social roles (e.g., Sarason et al., 1983)	Name generators and questions on the interaction between those named (e.g., Burt, 1984; Marsden, 1987; Marsden et al., 1993)
3. Sequenced	Random-walk: Index cases name alters and a random subset of those alters interviewed (Klovdahl, 1989)	Snowball: Index cases name alters and all alters are interviewed (Goodman, 1961; Palmore, 1967)
4. Census	Nominations: All members of a community are interviewed and asked one or several network questions (Valente, 1995, 1996)	Roster: All members of a community are interviewed and given a list of everyone and asked one or several network questions (Valente et al., 1997)
5. Two-mode or joint	Nominations of events attended or organizational membership (Breiger, 1974; Davis et al., 1941)	Enumeration of membership lists such as company boards of directors (Mizruchi, 1992)

is a respondent and also possibly a contact named by the respondents. It is possible to combine different types of data collection techniques in the same survey. For example, a researcher might use a sociometric design complemented with egocentric techniques to measure contacts within and outside the network boundary.

Table 3–1 reports the five network data collection techniques: (1) survey, (2) egocentric, (3) sequenced, (4) census, and (5) two-mode. These five techniques usually represent studies with increasing levels in their ability to measure social structure and decreasing levels in their generalizability. Each of these five measurement techniques has a (a) general and a (b) specific version in terms of the level of specificity required by the respondent. The remainder of this section describes each of these 10 data collection techniques.

Data Collection Techniques

Survey Data

Survey network data consist of asking individuals whether they talked to or consulted anyone about some topic. For example, general survey questions may be asked such as "Have you spoken to anyone about prenatal care?" For such questions, usually a list of social roles are presented as the response categories, such as mother, father, teacher, doctor, etc. More specific questions such as "Have you spoken to your spouse about prenatal care?" or "Have you consulted Dr. Smith about prenatal care?" Although not typically referred to as network questions, these types of survey questions represent the most rudimentary indicators of network concepts.

Egocentric Data

Egocentric data (also referred to as local network) consist of asking individuals to name others with whom they talk to about important matters or whom they talk to most frequently about a topic (McCarty et al., 1997). The specific question asked is called a *name generator,* because it is the question used to generate names (Campbell & Lee, 1991). An example of an egocentric questionnaire is presented in Appendix C. These data provide relational information in terms of the kinds of people individuals interact with most frequently. General egocentric questions ask that the respondent provide information on social roles, such as, "How often do you talk to your father?" With general egocentric questions, a list of social roles is usually presented as the response categories, for example, mother, father, brother, sister, and so on, and the respondent provides information on how often he or she talks to each.

Specific egocentric questions ask for specific names, nicknames, first names, or initials, and then ask the respondent to provide further information on each specific person. Demographic information, such as sex, age, occupation, religion, and type of relation, is collected for each tie. It is also advisable, when possible, to ask the respondent whether the persons named know one another, in order to measure personal network density.

The difference between egocentric data and simple survey questions (level 1) is that egocentric questionnaires collect data on the characteristics of the persons named, on the respondent's personal network. The additional network information is collected on the relations between the respondent and the persons nominated, and also on the relationships between the persons nominated. This additional information provides some insight into personal network characteristics and their potential influence on behavior. The most well-known study of this type is the set of egocentric questions included the 1985 version of the annual General Social Survey questionnaire administered by National Opinion Research Corporation (Burt, 1984; Marsden, 1987; McPherson et al., 2001).

Researchers can use egocentric survey techniques in any study. For example, in the evaluation of a Bolivian mass media campaign to promote contraceptive use, egocentric survey questions were used to determine if the effects of the campaign were contingent on respondents' personal networks (Valente & Saba, 1998). The campaign was more effective for those who had a minority of contraceptive users in the personal network (so-called low-threshold adopters). Measuring personal networks enabled a test of the so-called two-step flow hypothesis, which states that some people pay attention to the mass media or other sources of information and then pass on information from those media channels to others through their personal networks (see Chapter 10).

Egocentric data provide measures of an individual's personal network in terms of the kind of people each respondent interacts with or is related to. These data, however, do not provide connected groups of respondents that can be mapped. Because the respondents are chosen randomly and no exact names are elicited, there is no way to link specific individuals named with others that may be interviewed in the same study.

It is conceivable that a researcher could construct a virtual or imaginary network from the egocentric reports. For example, one could create archetypical alters based on an average from the types of alters named by the respondents. These archetypes then become cases to which multiple respondents link. If the archetypes matched respondents, then they could also have links coming from them. To date, no studies have attempted to create imaginary alters or nodes from egocentric data, but it might make an interesting study.

The next three types of data collection techniques collect data in which the persons named are also respondents and so can be linked to one another.

Sequenced Data

Sequenced data (also referred to as partial network) consist of interviewing either all or some portion of the people nominated by a respondent (Klovdahl, 1989; Klovdahl et al., 1994). Snowball sampling represents the most common type of sequenced data collection, in which all the nominees of a given respondent are included in the sample (Bogue, 1967). Snowball sampling entails interviewing all the people whom the index person nominated and is the specific version of sequenced data. Some researchers have used sequencing to develop respondent driven sampling (RDS) methodologies, useful for recruiting subjects into health promotion programs (Heckathorn, 1997). Research has shown that the respondent-driven approach provides a more diverse and more cost-effective means of reaching "hard to reach" populations than traditional outreach methods (Salganik & Heckathorn, 2004).

General sequenced data consist of taking some random sample of those nominated and interviewing only that sample (Klovdahl, 1989; Klovdahl et al., 1994). The advantages of general sequenced data over snowball sampling are that general sequenced data (Klovdahl et al., 1994) (1) are less likely to end in a social cul-de-sac; (2) provide more points of entry into the community or society; and (3) provide better population parameter estimates of social structure. Sequenced sampling is a method of cluster sampling in which the researcher samples social clusters rather than geographic ones (Klovdahl et al., 1994). A study using general sequenced data could be conducted to measure how quickly and to whom a rumor was spread.

These first three types of data collection techniques (survey, egocentric, and sequenced) are amenable to random sampling selection procedures. The researcher starts with a sample (preferably random) of respondents selected from a given population and the results are then generalizable to the population. One shortcoming with sequenced data, however, is that network indices are highly dependent on the persons initially selected to generate the names. The two final data collection techniques are less frequently used with random sample data but instead are often used to provide more in-depth understanding of network and community structure. Census data are the type most people refer to when they discuss network analysis methods.

Census Data

Census (or saturation) sampling consist of interviews conducted with all (or almost all) members of a community or population. Census sampling is also referred to as *complete network data*. Organizations, schools, and rural communities represent the most common sampling frames used in this type of data collection (Rogers & Kincaid, 1981; Valente, 1995; 1996). Census sampling is preferred when the researcher can enumerate all members of the community such as all nations in the world, all organizations in an industry, or all employees of an organization. The advent of more powerful computing has greatly expanded the size of networks that can be studied using a census approach. Due to computing limitations, prior to the 1990s, most census studies were limited to networks of no more than a few hundred (and often a few dozen). Currently, researchers are analyzing networks with thousands of nodes and tens of thousands of links.

General census data collection consists of survey questions that ask for the names of those people with whom the respondent talks to in his/her community. These names are then recorded either by their study ID numbers or names since they represent other individuals included in the census sample. A classic study using census data was Rogers and Kincaid's (1981) investigation of the communication networks of Korean women from 25 rural villages in the 1970s. All the married women in each village were asked to indicate to whom they went for advice about family planning. Rogers and Kincaid (1981) mapped these networks and showed how the network of communication influenced the spread of contraceptives in these villages.

Specific census data collection entails obtaining a roster of all the members of the community and asking the respondent to check those he or she knows (and/or how frequently the respondent communicates with each).

There is little difference in the specificity level between census nominations and that collected with a roster. Roster census data usually result in many more nominations (limited only by the number of people on the roster), whereas nominations are usually limited to five or seven close ties. The main challenge to census sample studies is defining the boundary of the community (Laumann et al., 1983). The roster method is quite commonly used in organizations in which the size is less than 100 or so. Quite often rosters are distributed as an aid for the nomination question. For example, in one study class rosters were distributed to six-graders in 16 southern California schools (84 classes), and students were asked to write down the ID numbers of their five closest friends. In school research, however, the network boundary can be the classroom, grade, or entire school depending on the research setting and school size.

Census data provide a complete map of the communication network so that researchers can study how information or behavior spreads through the network. This can be critical for organizational behavior studies in which knowing who communicates with whom is fundamental to organizational performance. Network data also provide a mechanism to change organizations either by realigning the communication network or by identifying change agents within the organization (see Chapter 11).

In some cases, the researcher may have the choice between using a nomination method or a roster one (Doriean, 1992). For example, in an organization, the researcher can give respondents a list of all the employees and have them check the frequency with which they work with each one or have them write the names of those they work with. The advantages of the nomination method are (1) it is an unaided recall; (2) may be less demanding for the respondent because he or she does not have to read every name on the roster; (3) the rank order of the nomination can be preserved and used as a proxy for tie strength; (4) the number of alters allowed for each respondent can be varied (i.e., selecting only the first five or four nominations); (5) the data entry and management are easier (i.e., the five ID numbers of those named can be stored easily with the attribute data); and (6) it is more likely to identify individuals outside the imposed boundary of the network.

The advantages to the roster method are (1) weak ties are measured as well as strong ones and (2) there is no ambiguity regarding the boundary of the network, everyone on the list is in the network. The roster method will usually record more links since respondents scan the list and indicate all of those network contacts, not just the top five or seven that occur to them. The strength or frequency of communication and contact can be measured with a roster, and this information used to reduce the number of links. For example, next to each name the researcher can ask the respondent to circle the number that represents frequency of contact and in the analysis decide to retain only those links in which the frequency is greater than some value. Often the best approach is to use the nomination format but provide a roster for the respondents to refer to. The roster can include names and ID numbers with the respondents instructed to simply write the ID numbers of his or her network nominations.

Two-Mode or Jointness Data

Two-mode data (also referred to as jointness or duality data) consist of recording instances in which individuals participate in or attend the same events. One well-known example of two-mode network data is that collected on intercorporate interlocks by recording the names of individuals who are on the board of directors for each organization in an industry. Since many individuals sit on numerous boards, they function as a network connecting these various organizations (Pennings, 1980). The two-mode methodology has been used to construct a large interlocking directorates database of the Fortune 500 companies (Mizruchi, 1982, 1992).

Two-mode data are often collected from archival sources, such as annual reports, and then converted to a network using matrix algebra. The original data consist of a table in which the rows are individuals and the columns are the organizations or events. This table is a matrix, which can then be transposed (rows and columns are switched) and postmultiplied to yield an individuals-by-individuals matrix representing the number of joint member-ships (see Chapter 8). The transposed matrix can be premultiplied (placed first) to yield an organizations-by-organizations matrix. Thus, one dataset provides two different networks an individual-by-individual network indi-cating joint participation in activities or organizational membership and an organization-by-organization network indicating the number of members in common (Breiger, 1974).

Figure 3–2 shows a small hypothetical example of two-mode data. Here, the rows in the table (or matrix) are people and each column represents an event the people attended. If person 1 attended event A, there is a 1 in the cell; otherwise it is 0. The data in Figure 3–2 show that person 1 attended events A and C; person 2 attended events A and B; and so on. We can trans-pose matrix A and flip the rows and columns, so that the rows are the events and the columns are people. By multiplying A by A' (A transpose), we get a matrix in which both rows and columns are people and cell entries indicate the number of events in common. We can also multiply A' by A and get a matrix in which both rows and columns are events and the cell entries indi-cate the number of people attending each event.

The classic two-mode study was the Southern Women study originally conducted by Davis, Gardner, and Gardner (1941), who extracted newspaper

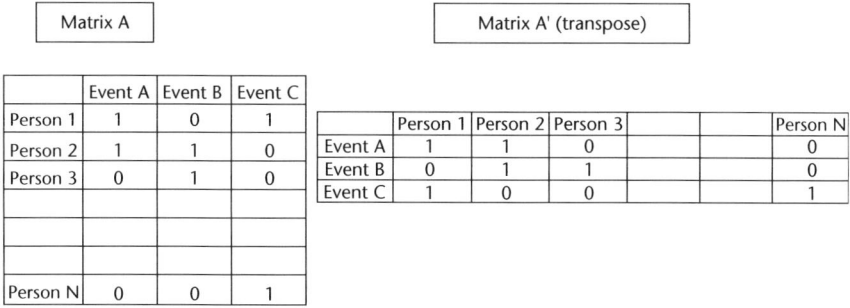

Figure 3–2. A small hypothetical example of two-mode data. Matrix A is the affiliation matrix indicating which events or organizations each person attended. On the right, matrix A' is matrix A transposed (flipped so the columns are rows and rows become columns). These matrices are now conformable, the number of columns in A equals the number of rows in A', and can be multiplied, yielding a person-by-person matrix indicating the number of shared events.

reports of social event attendance of 16 women at 12 events. These data constituted a 16 row–by–12 column table. Breiger showed how this table, treated as a matrix, could be pre- and post-multiplied with its transpose to return the women-by-women and event-by-event networks. Breiger's analysis showed that there were two cliques of women based on who attended which events together.

These five network data collection techniques are shown in Table 3–1 in order of increasing levels of relational information and decreasing levels of generalizability. That is, egocentric data provide more relational information than simple survey questions and sequenced data more relational information than egocentric, census data still more, and two-mode data provide the most relational information, since they provide an individual-by-individual matrix of connections, and also an organization-by-organization matrix.

While more relational information is provided at each level, there is usually some loss of generalizability when one uses the census and two-mode techniques. The first three techniques are often used with random sample selection procedures and thus can provide population parameter estimates. Snowball sampling, however, provides parameter estimates dependent on the starting nodes and dependent on the ability of follow-up with those named. Census and two-mode approaches retain some generalizability when communities (and organizations/events) are selected randomly. In addition, the characteristics of the communities sampled can be compared with known population estimates to determine the representativeness of studied communities. Increasingly, scholars are using the Internet and electronic forms of communication to gather communication network data. These data may come from tracking e-mail communications and provide a large repository of interpersonal communication. In addition to these five survey data collection strategies, network analysts often rely on data collected from archival sources.

Archival Sources

While the data collection techniques mentioned so far rely primarily on asking respondents to report their network, network data are often collected from archival sources such as computer logs, diaries, and telephone logs. For the Southern Women data, Davis et al. (1941) examined newspaper reports of women's attendance at social events over a 9-month period. These data were used to illustrate the two-mode network data methodology (Breiger, 1974). Diaries have been used to report size and composition of networks (Bernard et al., 1984). E-mail networks have also provided a direct tally of interpersonal communication behavior (Dutton, et al., 1987; Rice, 1982). Bibliometric network analysis consists of examining reference lists from publications to see who references whom. A network is then constructed to determine the structure of a scientific specialty (Harris et al., 2009; Hummon & Carley, 1993; Rice, Borgman, & Reeves, 1988). In short, aside from asking people directly about their networks, researchers have found many creative ways of uncovering this relational information.

The advent of social networking sites such as Facebook, Myspace, and LinkedIn has created a vast archive of social connectedness of large populations. Although much of these data remain in the private domain, researchers have begun creating large-scale networks of communications and connectedness in bounded populations such as universities (Kossinets & Watts, 2006; Lewis et al., 2008). Although few behavioral studies have emerged, there is considerable promise these investigations will yield considerable insights into the behavior change (see Christakis & Fowler, 2008, for an excellent example).

Data Management

Network analysis is often conducted by asking respondents to name other individuals with whom they discuss important matters. This name-generating technique elicits the names or ID numbers of the respondent's personal network. Data collected with survey and egocentric methods are analyzed using standard statistical packages such as SPSS, SAS, and STATA. Statistical analysis of egocentric data usually consists of the creation of various network measures such as the average, heterogeneity, and range of the personal network characteristics. For example, the General Social Survey (GSS) is a random sample questionnaire administered annually to track certain sociological variables. In 1985, this survey included a battery of egocentric questions designed to have respondents name up to five people with whom the respondent discussed personal matters. The respondent was then asked, among other things, to give the sex, religion, and age of these people. These data were then used to describe American discussion networks in the sense that the average age and the variation in religion could be calculated (as well as many other characteristics) (Marsden, 1987).

Egocentric data are often reshaped such that each tie or relation is treated as a case in the dataset. Such a permutation means that an individual who nominated two others contributes two cases to the new dataset and an individual who nominated four people contributes four. Once reshaped, the data are referred to as *dyadic,* and analysis proceeds by studying the dyads. Caution, of course, must be exercised when interpreting statistical tests since the usual assumption of independence is violated. Analysis of dyadic data is much easier, however, and standard statistical techniques such as multilevel (hierarchal) modeling exist to adjust for the nonindependence created by reshaping the data. For example, dyadic analysis permitted a test of the hypothesis that showed that participants in a needle exchange program were more likely to engage in risky behavior (sharing syringes) with friends they named first or second rather than those named third, fourth, or fifth (Valente & Vlahov, 2001).

In sequenced and census studies, the ID numbers of the nominees (also referred to as *alters*) are entered in the database. The respondents' ID and the ID numbers of the alters they nominated are then output separately into a "node-list" format file consisting of respondent and nominee's ID numbers. The node-list format is consistent with standard survey data storage formats in which each row represents a respondent. The network data may also be stored as "link-list" in which each row is the ID of the respondent and the ID of the alter. Other relationship information can also be included such as the strength or duration of the relationship. The link-list format is a dyadic format in which the number of cases is equal to the number of links. These data, either node list or link list, are then read into specialty network computer programs such as UCINET, Pajek, ORA, Visualizer, Inflow, or NEGOPY for analysis (see Appendix A).

These network computer programs convert the node-list or link-list data into a matrix in which the rows and columns represent the respondents in the study (see Huisman & van Duijn, 2005, for a comparison of network software). These programs also provide graphic displays of the network as well as calculation of common network indicators (Chapters 5 through 8). The network computer programs also convert the input data to program-specific format.

Some researchers study only one or few networks, either one community with multiple networks (e.g., advice, leadership, and friendship) or the same network in a few communities (friendship in three schools). For these researchers, the specialty programs mentioned earlier are excellent tools for analysis. And the output from these programs can be merged with other data the researcher might have available. Some researchers, however, study multiple networks—for example, friendships within multiple schools or interorganizational collaboration in multiple communities. For these researchers, computer programs that permit creating loops to cycle through each network are needed to do the analysis. Researchers can use SAS-IML or other matrix language programming modules available in statistical packages or programs designed to manipulate matrices such as R, GAUSS/SNAPS, or STATNET or write batch programs for UCINET or Pajek.

The choice of software is dictated in large part by the data. If the data are egocentric, then a statistical package (SAS, SPSS, STATA) is sufficient. If the data are census, then the choice depends on the number of networks. If three or fewer networks, the standard social network programs (UCINET, Negopy, ORA, Pajek, Visualizer) are preferred as they offer a much wider set of network measures and visualization features. With many networks to analyze, however, a programming language allowing repetition of network calculations will be necessary. (UCINET, Negopy, and Pajek have batch processing capabilities and so multiple networks can be analyzed using these computer packages, but the interfaces are less intuitive.)

For example, Figure 3–3 shows a simple 5-by-5 matrix where row 1 represents the ties between respondent one and the other four individuals in the group (usually the rows and columns both represent individuals). The rows represent the individuals *sending* the nominations and columns represent the individuals *receiving* the nominations. The first row represents the nominations of person one in which a "1" is put in the column of the person nominated. Each matrix cell indicates whether there is a tie between the two network members. For example, the "1" in row 1 column 2 indicates that person one knows person two, and the "1" in element 2,1 indicates that person two knows person one.

Matrix representation of networks enables quick computation of network properties. For example, a common measure of opinion leadership is the number of nominations received. Summing the columns of a matrix provides a score of how many nominations each person received. Figure 3–3 shows that person one received the most nominations (three) and hence may be an opinion leader in this network. These network scores are often output from the network computer package and merged with the original attribute dataset to compare network scores with other variables.

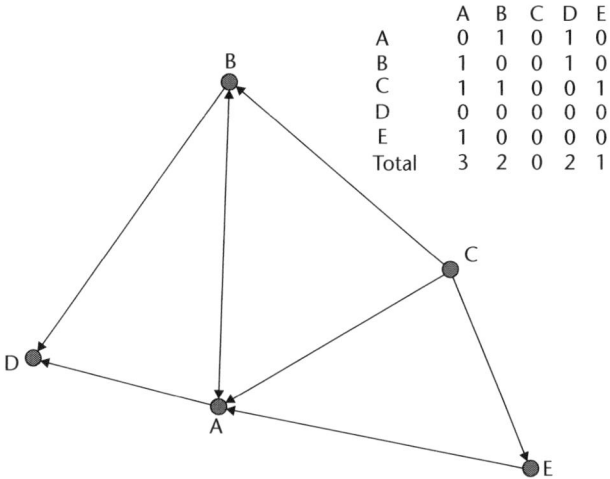

	A	B	C	D	E
A	0	1	0	1	0
B	1	0	0	1	0
C	1	1	0	0	1
D	0	0	0	0	0
E	1	0	0	0	0
Total	3	2	0	2	1

Figure 3–3. Small hypothetical example of a network of ties and its associated graph.

Sociograms

One of the unique features of network data compared with other types of data is that a diagram depicting relationships can be drawn. Earlier chapters have presented several examples of network graphs. Figure 3–4 shows a graph of the friendships between students within one classroom of a southern California middle school. Students were asked to name up to five of their closest friends in the class by writing their number from a roster. Each circle represents a student and the lines indicate who named whom as a friend. The arrowheads indicate direction of relationship since some people will name a friend who may or may not select them in return. For example, numbers 10 and 23 chose each other as friends, whereas number 3 named number 23 but number 23 did not name number 3. The lengths of the lines do not have meaning. People are placed on the graph based on how well connected they are; for example, those with many connections, such as number 9, are usually placed in the center and then other nodes arrayed around them. The graphic programs try to make the pictures readable by moving the nodes away from each other so there is space to see the nodes and the labels (the numbers) while at the same time trying to keep nodes that have similar links near one another. There is no one correct way to draw a sociogram since the position of the nodes is somewhat arbitrary.

Network diagrams are useful for showing the structure of a network and there are a variety of techniques and computer programs available for graphing networks (Blythe, McGrath, & Krackhardt, 1996). Drawing network diagrams is one of the most attractive features of social network analysis

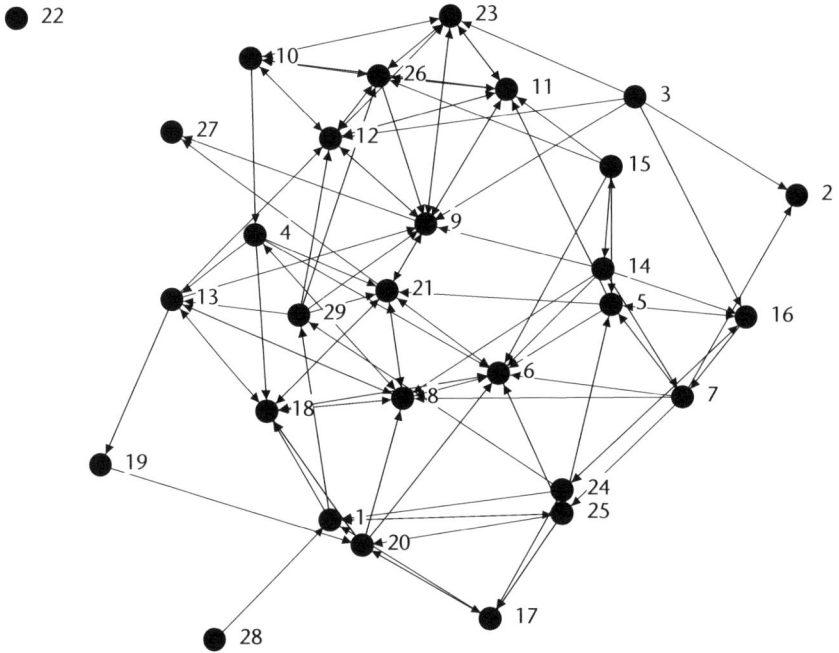

Figure 3–4. Sample social network in which students were asked to name their five closest friends in the classroom.

as it provides a visual depiction of the overall structure of communication (Freeman, 2000; McGrath et al., 2002). Once network data are collected, organizations, coalitions, and communities enjoy seeing their data reported back to them and viewing network diagrams, because most people know their own personal networks, but no one can see the overall network structure unless the data are aggregated.

In sum, there are three different types of studies one can conduct with network data. First, one can conduct an egocentric study with data on a person's personal network as reported by the survey respondent. These data can be analyzed on the respondents or the relationships by converting the data to dyadic. Second, one can conduct a sociometric study (either sequenced, census, or two-mode) with one or a few networks analyzed entirely in a network program (i.e., UCINET). Network variables derived from the analysis are often merged with a dataset containing other non-network information such as the age, gender, or education of the respondents. Third, one can conduct a sociometric study with many different networks analyzed in a program that permits the construction of "do" loops so the researcher can process multiple networks. Network variables derived from the analysis are often merged with a dataset as above, but now it is critical the researcher keep track of the unique identifiers for the networks (i.e., the ID numbers for the specific classes or schools).

Data Characteristics

Networks have been measured on kinship, marriage, advice, love, friendship, dislike, and countless other relations. The network question asked defines the type of network. A typical network would be created by asking a question such as, "Name five other people you talk to about important matters." Network data can be collected on a wide variety of substantive issues. For public health, it is advised to ask network questions such as, "Name five other people who you talk to about a health topic." General questions can be further *funneled* to ask the respondent to name those who he/she talks to about a particular health issue such as what contraceptive method to choose.

Network data are also directional so that ties may be *symmetric* (John talks to Mary and Mary talks to John) or *asymmetric* (John talks to Mary but Mary does *not* talk to John). Symmetric ties are reciprocal, whereas asymmetric ties are unreciprocated directly but may be reciprocated indirectly through intermediaries. Indirect reciprocation occurs when John talks to Mary, and while Mary does not talk to John, she does talk to Maria, who talks to John. Some networks are inherently asymmetric while others are symmetric. For example, if people are asked to indicate who they had lunch with, that suggests a symmetric/reciprocated relationship. On the other hand, advice seeking is asymmetric: the people I seek advice from may not seek advice from me.

Network data may be *binary* or *valued*. That is, network nominations can be used to record the presence or absence of ties but also may record how frequently individuals communicate with one another. For example, a researcher might be interested in determining how often members of a community talk to one another by asking if the respondent talks to his or her friends (1) less than once per month, (2) monthly, (3) weekly, (4) a few times per week, or (5) daily. In this manner, values can be attached to the ties corresponding to the frequency of interaction. Thus, a network link is composed of three components: its meaning (friendship, advice, etc.), its direction (whether symmetric or asymmetric), and its weight (the value of the link).

Network Variables

The network variables created from network data consist of two types: relational and structural. Relational variables are those that are constructed from the respondent's set of direct ties. One example of a relational variable is personal network density, or the degree to which a respondent's ties know one another. Structural variables are those that are constructed from the entire network of connections. One example of a structural variable is positional equivalence, or the degree two individuals occupy the same position in the network (White, Boorman, & Breiger, 1976). Table 3–2 provides a description of the distinction between relational and positional measures (see Burt, 1980, for further discussion). In a sense, the division between relational and structural variables is not rigid since relational and structural measures are often highly correlated.

Examples of *relational* variables include connectedness, reach, number of nominations received or sent, personal network density, constraint, reciprocity, group membership, and system density. *Connectedness* and *reach* measure the degree any member of a network can reach other members of the network. *Number of nominations sent and received* measures how many others an individual nominates and the frequency an individual is nominated, respectively.

Personal network density measures the degree an individual's set of ties know and nominate one another. Constraint is the extent to which a person's personal network inhibits him/her from reaching others in the broader network. *Reciprocity* measures whether a person's nominations are reciprocated, and *group membership* refers to network analysis procedures that determine who belongs to which groups in a network. Network *density* measures the proportion of ties in a network relative to the total number possible. Group membership and network density variables use the entire network for their computations and hence are more structural measures and lead to a more complex analysis of the structure of a network.

Examples of *structural* variables include centrality and positions. *Centrality* can be measured a variety of ways (Freeman, 1979)—for example, number of nominations sent and received are measures of centrality out-degree and in-degree, respectively. Centrality betweenness measures the degree an individual lies between other individuals in the network. Centrality closeness measures the degree an individual is near all other individuals in the network (Freeman, 1979). Centrality power measures the degree an individual can exert control over the network (Bonacich, 1987), and centrality flow (Freeman, Borgatti, & White, 1991) and information (Stephenson & Zelen,

Table 3–2. Relational and Positional Concepts of Network Structure

	Relational	Positional
Individual	Personal network density	Central or peripheral individuals
Group	Clique formation based on direct ties	Hierarchical partition based on tie similarity
Network	Dense vs. sparse networks	Set of positions; centralization

Adapted from Burt, 1980.

1989) measure the capacity of individuals to carry information within the network. Chapter 5 will describe centrality measures.

Positional analyses report the hierarchical structure of a network by partitioning individuals based on the degree of similarity in their network ties. Positional analyses do not provide individual measures but rather provide indicators of equivalence (similarity) for all pairs of individuals in a network. The simplest positional measure computes the proportion of common ties for each pair of nodes in a network. This measure presents the percent of links each pair of nodes has in common. The similarity criterion can then be used to form groups within the network based on their similarity scores.

Individual and Network Level

Many of these relational and structural variables exist at both the individual and system level. For example, personal network density may be measured for each respondent and may also be measured for the whole network. The various centrality measures can be computed both for individuals and for the whole network. Network centrality, referred to as *centralization,* measures the degree a network is centralized (the nominations are concentrated on one individual or a group of individuals).

Sometimes there can be many steps involved in the processing and managing of network data to extract the types of measures needed to answer substantive questions. The diagram in Figure 3–5 provides some assistance.

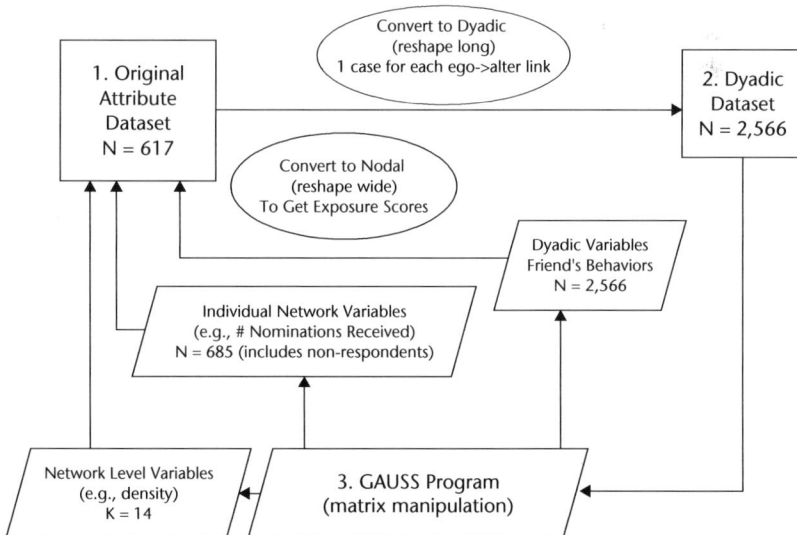

Figure 3–5. Illustration of the data management flow for a typical network study considering attribute and network data.

In a complete network analysis with sociometric data, there are a number of steps in the process. This example has an original set of survey data from 617 adolescents in 17 classrooms (in four schools). Respondents were asked to name friends in the class and to write the number from a roster they were provided. These data were then converted into a dyadic dataset that had one case for each relationship—the respondent and the identification number (roster number) of the person named as a friend. If a person named three people, then he or she contributed three cases to the dyadic dataset.

The dyadic dataset can then be read into a specialty computer program written in R, GAUSS, SAS-IML, STATA/MATA, or any other matrix level programming language. This program creates a data file that has the respondent's unique ID, the alter's ID, and any data needed for the alters. For example, the researcher may want to know the sex, ethnicity, age, and outcome variables for each person named. Specific relationship information may also be ouput for each tie such as whether the person was named first, second, third, fourth, or fifth; whether they reported doing any activities with that person; and so on. This dyadic data can then be used for analysis to determine if any relationship characteristics are associated with behavior. For example, it might be hypothesize that behaviors are similar between the respondent and friends named first or those of the same ethnicity.

The dyadic dataset can also be used to calculate the respondent's personal network composition and exposure variables. The dyadic dataset is "collapsed" on the respondent's ID. This converts the dyadic back to a regular attribute dataset but now it can have the average (or other statistic) scores for the network partners. For example, it is possible to calculate the percentage of the friends who are male and female, percentage of each ethnicity, and the number or percentage who engage in various behaviors. These variables can be used in analytic models to predict individual behavior based on average personal network attributes or behaviors. For example, adolescents with smoking friends might be more likely to smoke.

The GAUSS program (#3 in Figure 3–5) also creates individual network measures such as number of nominations sent and received as well as more complicated measures covered in later chapters (see Part III). These individual network measures can then be merged with the original attribute file and used as variables in analysis. For example, students who receive many nominations as a friend from other classmates (popularity) might be more likely to smoke (Valente et al., 2005). Currently, the GAUSS program is being translated for use in STATA/MATA to make them available to a wider audience.

The GAUSS program also creates network-level measures such as density or centralization (see Chapter 8). These network-level measures can then be merged with the original attribute file and used as variables in analysis. For example, peer influence on substance using behaviors may be stronger in densely connected school friendship networks than sparsely connected ones. Similarly, interorganizational diffusion of information might be faster in a densely connected network than in a sparsely connected one.

Efficient data management often requires knowing the right terms to use to get computer programs to perform the desired functions. In this case, the data were expanded to create a dyadic dataset and collapsed to create an attribute dataset. The average (or other statistic) of the alter data were calculated to compute average exposure. The dyadic data are in long form and the attribute data are in wide form. In STATA, the "reshape" command can be used to create long and wide forms of the dataset (Box 3–1).

Box 3–1. Reshaping Data from Wide to Long

Steps to Reshape Egocentric Data to Dyadic (Wide to Long)

1. Make a backup of the dataset.
2. Read the data and save it with a name specific to the network and alter. For example, for network 1, alter 1 save the data as net1_1.
3. Generate a variable called network and set it equal to 1.
4. Generate a new variable called "alter" and set it equal to 1.
5. Drop all network variables for alters 2 through 5.
6. Rename all network variables to be non-rank specific. For example, "sex1" should be "sex."
7. Save the dataset
8. Repeat steps 2 through 7 for each network and each alter. (A survey with 3 networks and up to 5 alters generates 15 new datasets.)
9. Append all the newly constructed datasets.
10. Tabulating the network and alter variables provides a count of how many dyads (relationships) were measured in the study.

Another, more elegant way to achieve the same result is to reshape the dataset from wide to long. In a wide dataset each observation is contained in a row with a unique ID number. A long dataset may have the same observation span many rows with an indicator for the unique contribution of each row. For example, to reshape the data in the STATA statistical package, one can use reshape command such as:

"reshape long reshape long net1_ID net1_age net1_educ net1_behavior, i(ego_name) j(alt 1-5)"

This last command reshapes the data from wide to long format creating five new cases for each unique value of "ego_name." The data will also consist of the values of the variables net1_ID, net1_age net1_educ and net1_behavior for each alter named.

Summary

This chapter provided an introduction to social network data collection and management methods. The chapter introduced the idea that network data provide measures at both the individual and the network level. Individual measures indicate a person's position in the network relative to others in the network. Individual measures also indicate network effects in terms of the properties of others a person is connected to, such as whether his or her friends are smokers. Network-level measures describe overall properties of the network such as its density or centralization.

The chapter then reviewed five types of network data collection techniques (survey, egocentric, sequenced, census, and two-mode), indicating their uses and advantages and disadvantages. The different types of computer software used to analyze these data were discussed as well as some general properties of graphs. The chapter closed with a discussion of relational versus structural network measures. The network paradigm is thus made up of these four components: (1) network data collection and management, (2) network data characteristics, (3) the distinct levels of analysis, and (4) network variables derived from the data.

4

Ego- and Personal-Network Effects

This chapter shows how researchers can collect network data from randomly drawn samples. The data only represent the respondent's personal network, usually from the respondent's perspective. The chapter then details the various measures derived from personal network data and the research questions and hypotheses that have been tested. A comparison between egocentric and sociometric data is presented. Although egocentric data are somewhat limited, they still provide powerful measures of interpersonal influence that are strongly predictive of behavior.

The network perspective emphasizes that individual attitudes, beliefs, and behaviors are often a function of the attitudes, beliefs, and behaviors of their friends, family, colleagues, and associates. Personal network exposure is the number or proportion of ties holding a particular belief or engaging in a particular behavior. Generally, network exposure is associated with adoption, and the degree of exposure required for adoption is a personal network threshold. Most of the evidence for network exposure and threshold effects comes from egocentric data, in which data on a person's social network are gathered by asking the focal individual and not necessarily interviewing his or her network contacts. Analysis of egocentric data is usually done with standard attribute-based statistical programs such as SAS, SPSS, and STATA.

Social networks are important influences on behavior for many reasons. First, social contacts provide information about opportunities, resources, products, and about everything people want or need. Word-of-mouth communication is frequently cited as one of the most frequent channels people report on how they first heard about something or what they know about it (Van den Bulte & Wuyts, 2007). Information about a job or service travels readily through interpersonal channels. Second, social networks also provide resources typically referred to as *social capital*. The resources available in networks often consist of how-to information such as how to perform a work-related task or get something done.

Social networks also provide role models for behaviors. It is easier for people to adopt a new behavior once someone they know has done so because they see how it is done. Role modeling is an important component of vicarious learning and building the self-efficacy needed to engage in new behaviors (Bandura, 1986). Finally, social networks can provide the support needed to continue adopting a new behavior even when it becomes difficult or challenging to do so. Thus, measuring social networks provides an important tool needed to understand human behavior. Personal networks can be measured using egocentric techniques and sociometric ones. This chapter explains the egocentric techniques.

Burt (1984) proposed a set of egocentric questions that were included in the General Social Survey (GSS), fielded in 1985 by the National Opinion Research Corporation. The survey consisted of a random digit dial sample of U.S. households and included for the first time a measure of social networks. After extensive pilot testing, Burt proposed the survey items reproduced in Appendix C. These questions were designed to measure Americans' close personal networks derived from responses to the name generator "Who do you talk to about important matters?" There are other questions one might use to generate egocentric names such as "Who do you talk with most frequently?" or "Who are your closest friends?" depending on the specific research questions and settings. The respondent only need provide the first names, nicknames, or initials since the researcher will not attempt to contact the persons named. The named persons are often referred to as *alters*.

Once the names are generated, the researcher asks a series of questions about each person named. For example, researchers generally measure sociodemographic characteristics of each alter, such as their gender, ethnicity, age, marital status, and how the respondent, ego, is related to each alter (e.g., family, friend, or colleague). The researcher can then assess substantive issues specific to the research, such as whether the person supports a political candidate, is a smoker, uses substances, practices safe sex, supports gun control legislation, or other research issue. Once the personal networks have been measured, the researcher can characterize people's immediate close social networks and determine whether the network characteristics are associated with substantive phenomenon.

For example, the GSS 1985 data were used to characterize Americans' core social networks (Marsden, 1987). Marsden (1987) showed that Americans generally had 3.0 (standard deviation [SD] = 1.7) close contacts and these contacts were quite homogeneous in the sense that people associated with others of their same ethnicity, age, and education levels. Marsden also showed that urban Americans had more heterogeneous networks than rural ones.

When constructing an egocentric survey, it is typical to measure the following characteristics:

1. Strength of relationship (e.g., closeness, acquaintance, stranger; how long known)
2. Frequency of interaction (e.g., how often talked to, how often consulted)
3. Type of relation (e.g., family, friend, coworker)
4. Socioeconomic characteristics (e.g., educational attainment, wealth, income)
5. Demographic characteristics (e.g., age, residential location)
6. Substantive characteristics (e.g., smoke, practice safe sex, practice family planning, support a candidate)
7. Content of communication (e.g., discuss politics, health, child rearing) or risk behavior (e.g., unprotected sex, share syringes)

Table 4–1 shows the kinds of measures derived from egocentric data. Typically, these measures are of one of two types: compositional measures and variance ones. Compositional measures are those derived by counting or taking the average of egocentric network variables. For example, the number or proportion of males in the personal network is a compositional variable.

Table 4–1. Egocentric Network Measures

Level of Measure	Example	Composition	Variance (Heterogeneity)	Population-Level Variance
Binary (0/1)	Smoking	Percent in positive category	IQV	
Nominal	Ethnicity	Percent in reference category	IQV	
Ordinal	Education	Average	SD	Mean of SD
Interval	Age	Average	SD	Mean of SD

SD, standard deviation.

For a behavioral example, the number of smokers in the personal network is a compositional variable. Variance measures are those derived by calculating the variance or SD of the egocentric network variables. For example, the SD of the age of the alters is a variance measure.

All of the measures taken on personal networks can be collapsed into compositional and variance measures. For example, the number or percentage of females and the IQV of the gender variable can be calculated. Each individual in the data can be characterized as the degree his or her personal network is female and the sample characterized as the extent to which the percent female varies. For relation type, the proportion or number of the personal networks who are family members and the diversity of that proportion can be calculated.

For binary variables, the proportion and variance will be highly correlated (although not linearly) since the variance is greatest when the networks are similarly distributed across the categories. For example, suppose a person has four friends—two male and two female. The personal network composition is 50% female with a maximum IQV. For other respondents with a larger percentage who are female, IQV decreases. For nominal, ordinal, and interval variables, the compositional and variance measures are independent. Ethnicity, for example, might be calculated as the percentage of the personal network who are Hispanic/Latino and the variance measure indicates whether the distribution of alters across other ethnicities is evenly distributed (high variance) or skewed to one or few other categories (low variance).

Likewise with interval-level variables such as the network alters' age, researchers calculate the average age of the network and its SD. These network variables can be used to explain individual behavior. For example, it might be hypothesized that adolescents with older and more varied (on age) personal networks are at greater risk for substance use or other risky behaviors. Adolescents with older friends, and some much older friends, are probably exposed to more risk behavior such as smoking friends or having friends who engage in unprotected sex.

Table 4–1 also has a column labeled population-level variance. This column indicates that the mean of the SD is a measure of the overall population variance. That is, the average of the personal networks' SD indicates how much the population network varies. A large average SD indicates that overall people are quite varied in the ages of their friends, whereas a small average SD indicates that people named others who all had similar ages.

In sum, the egocentric network nominations are used to characterize individual's personal networks. There are seven types of network questions asked to gauge these personal networks. Compositional and variance measures from these seven types are derived from these variables, and they can be used to describe personal networks of respondents and determine whether personal networks are associated with behaviors. In addition to the compositional variables, there are several standard measures calculated from the personal network data. Typical egocentric variables are size, personal network exposure, tie strength, concurrency, density, and constraint.

Measures

Size

A basic yet critical variable in network analysis is individual network size. Some people have small networks, while others have quite large ones. Although techniques exist for measuring a person's network size (Bernard et al., 1987), in egocentric research, size is simply a count of the number of names or nicknames provided in response to the name generator. Often size will vary from zero to 5 or 6 since name generators often limit the number of persons named, because each name will also require additional information to be recorded. Providing more names lengthens the survey and naming too many names can make a survey prohibitively long.

Some researchers have suggested allowing the respondent to name as many persons as he or she can or at least increasing the limit to 15 or 20 to measure size better. It may also be desirable to increase the size and only ask one substantive question for all alters named, and then administer the full battery of network questions to the first five named. This allows the researcher to characterize the close personal networks in detail and also understand the attitudes or behaviors of a larger number of the respondent's network, including the behavior of weak ties. It has also been suggested to allow the respondent to name many alters and then ask the network questions for a random sample subset of those persons named. This later technique enables the research to study network effects beyond the close (strong) ties.

Personal Network Exposure

Personal network exposure is the degree to which a focal individual's alters engage in a particular behavior. Egocentric data can also be used to show that people who engage in certain behaviors are more likely to have close personal network associates who also engage in those behaviors. For example, in a study of factors associated with the adoption of contraceptive methods in Bolivia, people who reported using a current contraceptive method had 63% of their personal networks who also used contraception, while those who did not use reported only 37% of their personal network used contraception ($p < .001$, $N = 5,691$). This difference persisted but diminished when the respondent's partner was removed from the calculation (54.4% versus

38.3%, respectively; $p < .001$, $N = 4,156$). The overall rate of contraceptive use (both traditional and modern methods) in these data was 55.7%. Thus, those who use contraception to limit their family size are more likely to have people in their network who also use contraception. This finding is not surprising given that people usually associate with others like themselves (the homophily principle) and that information about contraceptive availability and use would pass through social networks. Egocentric data can tell us something about how networks influence individual decisions. (Commands for calculating network exposure using egocentric data in STATA are available from the author.)

Personal network exposure is a fundamental and critical variable to be calculated in network research. It captures social influence by measuring the extent one's network engages in a behavior. There is often an assumption that the networks influence the respondent given that the respondent knows these alters engage in the behavior. This social influence and the assumption that people are influenced by their peers can be tested in at least two ways. First, social influence can be tested by asking the respondent to indicate whether he or she was influenced by each alter. For example, after eliciting network nominations to measure social influence on smoking the researcher can ask, "Did this person (name) offer you a cigarette?" Second, social influence can be tested by weighting exposure by tie strength or communication frequency. In this case, the behavior of the tie is multiplied by the frequency of communication or contact.

Tie Strength

A classic finding in the network field is the importance of weak ties and bridges for connecting different groups so that information and behavior can spread throughout a community or population (Granovetter, 1973). Strong ties, however, are important for disease transmission and behavioral adoption at the individual level. Strong ties are important because people are more likely to be influenced by those they are close to and have multiplex relations with than those to whom they are weakly connected. These weak ties are important at the global level but much less so as an individual makes a behavior change decision. It should also be noted that weak ties may be more important for information spread rather than behavior change since it is easy for individuals to accept or learn information, whereas behavior change is a more complex and cognitively challenging process. Weak ties are effective at transmitting information but less so for transmitting behavioral influence.

Valente and Vlahov (2001) conducted a study to test the importance of strong ties for social influence in the evaluation of the Baltimore Syringe

Exchange Program (SEP). In that study, participants were asked to provide the initials or nicknames of their five closest friends. For each friend named, participants indicated whether they engaged in any risk behaviors with each friend such as drinking alcohol, having sex, doing drugs, or sharing syringes. The last point was of particular concern because the needle exchange program is designed to reduce syringe sharing to reduce the spread of HIV. In another part of the survey, we also asked whether they had shared syringes with anyone in the past 3 months.

As Figure 4–1 shows, the amount of syringe sharing was about 30% at baseline and decreased as participants returned to the SEP and completed subsequent interviews. The decrease in syringe sharing is evidence of program effects for those who repeatedly return to the SEP and received behavior education. Figure 4–1 also shows the amount of syringe sharing with friends by the rank order of the friends named. The assumption is that friends nominated first are the closest friend, and the one named second, the next closest, and so on. The data show that syringe sharing—risk behavior—was more likely with friends named first or second rather than those named third, fourth, or fifth. This makes sense as the Baltimore injection drug users established bonds with these close friends and the trust relationship is solidified with syringe-sharing behavior. Further, these close relationships may also involve sexual relationships; thus, the syringe sharing is only one form of risk behavior for the dyad. Risk behavior among strong ties occurs in other studies as well. For example, studies have shown that adolescents are more likely to smoke if their best friend smokes (Alexander et al., 2001; Urberg et al., 1997).

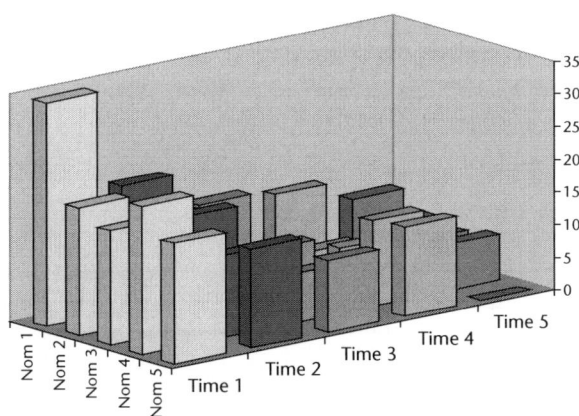

Figure 4–1. Reported syringe sharing among injection drug users by the order nominated (Nom 1 = first named) and survey wave (Time 1 = baseline). Injection drug users reported more syringe sharing with those first named, presumably their closest friends.

Serial monogamy or serial risk taking may seem a reasonable strategy to protect oneself from disease, particularly sexually transmitted diseases, but there is still some risk associated with the behavior. This is particularly true for injecting drug users, who may not have stable residences. In the Baltimore SEP, we found that only 29% of the close friends named at baseline were named 6 months later. This rapid turnover in networks means that the rational strategy of engaging in risk behavior only with closest friends loses its protective effect when those close friends change often. This keeps HIV spreading in the population.

Concurrency

Serial monogamy of course is not always the rule. Kretzschmar and Morris (1996; Morris & Kretzschmar, 1997) hypothesized that many people might engage in concurrent relationships (Figure 4–2). Concurrency occurs when a person is engaged in sexual or other risk behavior with multiple others within the same time frame. For example, node 1 in Figure 4–2, who has three serial sexual partners, offers less opportunity for disease spread in the community than node 2, who has three sexual partners but where the second partner overlaps with the first and third.

Concurrency is measured by asking respondents to provide information on the duration of the sexual relationships with all of their sexual partners. This is not overly burdensome, and many studies have shown this is possible (Morris, 2004). The researcher then calculates the relationship intervals and the degree of overlap between alters. Each person can then be characterized to the extent their sexual relationships overlap. Moreover, the extent of concurrency for the sample, and hence in the community, can be calculated.

There are other egocentric measures in addition to size, network exposure, tie strength, and concurrency. It is common, for example, to ask the respondent to indicate whether his or her friends know one another and how well they know one another.

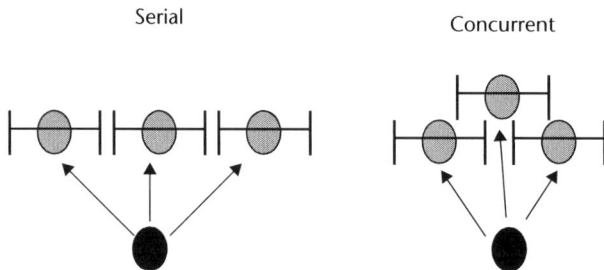

Figure 4–2. Sexual relations can be serial or concurrent. Serial relations occur in sequence with no overlap whereas concurrent ones contain overlap.

Density and Constraint

The survey example in Appendix C asks respondents to indicate which of their friends know one another. These data can then be used to construct a personal network density variable that reflects the extent a person's closest contacts are connected to one another. Figure 4–3 shows two personal networks, one that has some interconnectivity among alters (dense), and the other with alters that connect to others outside ego's immediate network (radial). Dense personal networks provide reinforcement for prevailing norms and practices and can provide protection from outside sources of influence or risk. Conversely, radial personal networks provide access to more information or influence that may be circulating in the network. Radial networks can be advantageous or disadvantageous depending on the topic or behavior being studied and its prevalence in the community or network.

Burt (1992) introduced a personal network measure called *constraint* that extends the personal network density measure by extracting more information from the pattern of relationships among the alters. Personal network density calculates the degree of connectivity among the alters nominated by ego. Constraint, on the other hand, measures the connections between alters from each alter's perspective. A constrained ego is one which the alters are connected

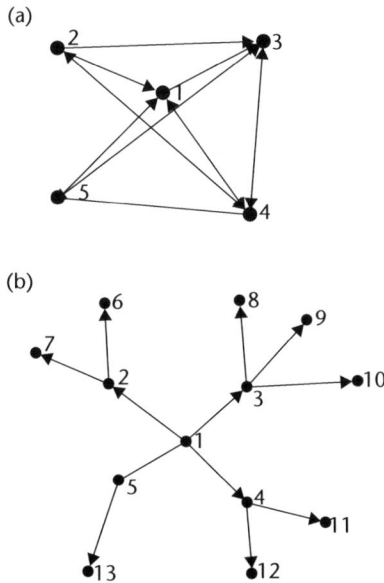

Figure 4–3. Personal networks can be dense in which the focal person's friends know one another (a) or radial in which they are not connected. (b) Burt (1992) defined radial networks as those with low constraint.

to each other and so ego's actions and perceptions are controlled by his or her personal network. In an un-constrained personal network, the alters are not connected to one another and so the personal network cannot collude to keep information from ego. Constraint is calculated as follows (Burt 1992, p. 55):

$$C_i = (p_{ij} + \sum_q p_{iq} p_{qi})^2, q \neq i, j \quad (4\text{-}1)$$

The calculation for constraint entails summing the degree to which each of the alters is connected to others in the personal network. Conceptually, the measures (density and constraint) are similar, but the key distinction is that constraint uses more of the information available in the personal network. Burt equates low constraint with occupying a position of structural holes. People with low constraint can access their networks better and span structural holes in the networks. Burt (2005) has shown that low constraint is associated with professional achievement and better performance.

Statistical Analysis

The measures and analyses mentioned thus far in this chapter are derived from data that could be collected randomly; that is, the respondents are not connected in a preexisting social network. Statistical analysis of associations between network variables and outcomes do not need to control for nonindependence of observations other than what would normally apply to the data. In a study of reproductive health practices in Bolivia, respondents were randomly selected households in the seven largest cities. Evaluation of communication campaign designed to promote reproductive health services was conducted using normal inferential statistical analysis.

In addition, egocentric network data were collected by asking respondents to name up to five people with whom they discuss personal issues. A series of questions were then asked about those named, including whether the alters knew one another, their gender, language spoken at home, frequency of communication, and whether the respondent thought each practiced family planning. For all of these questions, compositional and variance variables can be created from the data and treated as individual-level variables in statistical analysis.

Dyadic Data

As mentioned in Chapter 3, network data are often stored or converted to a dyadic format. *Dyadic data* refer to observations in which each case consists of the respondent and one network alter. In other words, in dyadic data, each case is a relationship pair. Dyads are the respondent (ego) alter pair, and dyadic data are the data associated with the respondents and alters. Sociometric data are often stored in dyadic format, and this is sometimes referred to as a *link-list format*. Egocentric data are often converted to dyadic format to facilitate statistical analysis. In addition, once in dyadic format, it is possible to calculate network exposure by merging on the alter ID and reshaping the data back to the original wide format (Box 4–1).

Box 4–1. Calculating Exposure

It is possible to calculate network exposure within statistical analysis programs such as SAS, SPSS, or STATA without relying on matrix manipulation or specialty network programs. To calculate exposure, the researcher converts a standard dataset to dyadic, or "long" in STATA terminology. The researcher then merges the dyadic data on the alter ID number (or name) with a dataset containing the behavior or attribute of interest. Now the researcher has a dyadic dataset containing the ego ID, the alter ID, and the alter's attribute. Converting the dyadic data back to a "wide" dataset and calculating the average of the alter behavior provides a network exposure score.

```
/* start with the original wide version of the dataset
and reduce to the unique subject ID the attribute of
interest and alter nominations */

use c:\data
keep net_id attrib nom1 - nom5
reshape long nom, i(net_id) j(alter 1-5)
sort net_id
drop if nom==.
save c:\dyadic, replace

use c:\data
keep net_id attrib
ren net_id nom
ren attrib alter_attrib
sort nom
save c:\ego_as_alter, replace

use c:\dyadic, replace
sort nom
merge nom using c:\ego_as_alter
sort net_id
drop if _merge!=3
drop _merge
save c:\dyadic_alter_beh, replace
reshape wide nom alter_attrib, i(net_id) j(alter)
save c:\ego_with_alter_behavs, replace
egen attrib_expos=rmean(alter_attrib1 alter_attrib2
alter_attrib3 alter_attrib4 alter_attrib5)
```

If the data are converted to dyadic format, the observations are no longer independent but are clustered on the respondent. Some respondents may have provided information on one alter while others provided information on four or five alters. Consequently, the analysis needs to control for clustering on the respondent ID. This is not difficult and usually entails specifying a multilevel or hierarchal model to explicitly account for the clustering. Sociometric studies, on the other hand, use data from a saturated sample such as a school or organization and so the statistical issues involved in estimating network effects are more complex (see Chapter 9).

Converting a regular attribute dataset to dyadic has certain advantages (Chapter 3 discussed how to do this). Because each case is the respondent and the data on the alter he or she named, analysis can be conducted to test how relationship characteristics are associated with behavior. For example, one might ask survey respondents to name their five closest friends and then ask for their gender, age, religious beliefs, and smoking behavior. The researcher can test whether people report smoking more with same-gender friends versus non–same-gender friendships.

It must be emphasized that dyadic data are not independent, that each case is not randomly selected from the population; rather, the cases are clustered on the respondent. In many cases, there may be multiple levels of clustering such that the cases are clustered by survey wave (e.g., baseline and follow-up) and the respondents. Researchers should use hierarchical linear models or random effects models or some other technique that controls for the nonindependence of the data.

Personal Network versus Sociometric Variables

Personal network exposure using egocentric data is usually easy to calculate in a statistical package, but this variable can be limiting when the researcher suspects that many respondents may not accurately know their alters' opinions or behaviors. These misperceptions can arise for many reasons. First, the respondent may not know his or her alters' attitudes and behaviors. Second, the respondent may purposively provide inaccurate information on his or her alters' attitudes and behaviors. Third, the respondent may misperceive the alters' opinions and behaviors because he or she wants them to be congruent with his own (reducing cognitive dissonance). Fourth, ego may misperceive the alters' opinions and behaviors because the alters tell ego things to pretend they hold a different opinion than they actually do. For example, people may say they support a political candidate in order to avoid an argument over political beliefs.

For example, personal network exposure was calculated on contraceptive use for women from voluntary associations in Yaoundé Cameron (Valente et al., 1997). Women were asked to indicate whether they had heard of family planning (FP) and any methods available to delay having children and to name their closest friends in their group. For each woman, knowledge of FP methods and use of a method (if any) was calculated. The methods her friends knew and used was also calculated (network exposure). Women were more likely to be aware of the same methods their friends knew and more likely to use the FP method their friends used.

Participants were also asked if they knew whether their friends used modern or traditional FP methods. Since the friends' reports of method use were also recorded, we could calculate whether the participant was correct or incorrect in her assessment. Finally, whether the respondent thought those friends encouraged them to use methods was also recorded. The study showed that perceiving friends to have encouraged use was the variable most strongly associated with method use, regardless of whether one's friends use, and regardless of whether one was correct or incorrect in her assessment of friends' use. This study highlighted the importance of perceived peer influence and that people may to some extent justify their actions by believing that others support and encourage those actions.

These analyses were possible because we recorded the participants' behaviors, asked who their friends were, and had those friends' self-reports. It is desirable to have alters' self-reports to calculate exposure to behaviors rather than relying solely on the participants' perceptions (Ianotti & Bush, 1992; Rice et al., 2003). And as will be illustrated, the basic diffusion model is one in which behaviors flow through networks such that network exposure is the fundamental building block for understanding networked diffusion and communicable disease spread. The egocentric results reported here, however, complicate analysis of personal network effects.

They indicate that tie strength may matter for some behaviors, meaning we possibly need to weight the exposure calculations by tie strength (Bauman et al., 2007). Weighting by tie strength is computationally easy, but substantively difficult because there are so many candidate weights to choose from. For example, one could weight ties by the frequency of contact or perceived emotional closeness. One could also weight on similarity of personal attributes such as stronger influence by those of the same gender, age, socioeconomic status, or any other attribute. There is a nearly infinite number of ways to include tie strength in exposure calculations.

Researchers have also proposed a threshold model in which people vary in the degree they are influenced by others in their network (Valente, 1996). Researchers may have incorrectly concluded there are threshold effects because there was an incorrect specification of the exposure that did not include correct weights for tie strength. Thus, there is tension between the proper exposure specification and threshold effects. If network exposure is not significantly associated with behavioral adoption, it may be due to threshold effects or inadequate modeling of exposure weights.

Snowball/Sequenced Data

Egocentric data provide a view of the respondent's network from the respondent's perspective. Once the names are generated, however, the researcher can create study designs in which the members of the personal network are also interviewed. This is referred to as snowball sampling and occurs when the researcher asks the respondent to indicate their friends (or other network members) and asks the respondent to recruit their friends. Snowball study designs are used in two types of studies: (1) when the researcher wishes to track behavior or communications among network members and (2) when using initial index cases to recruit their network members into an intervention or study.

There are two kinds of "snowballs"—one in which the interview attempts to contact and interview every one of the respondent's alters (all of their network) and the other in which some specified subsample of the personal network is contacted. When all members of the personal network are contacted, this is a "true snowball." The sample sizes in a snowball can grow quite rapidly. For example, 10 index cases can provide 10 names yielding a pool of 100 subjects who can also provide 10 names, resulting in 1,000 subjects in only two steps. Of course, the name generator or network definition might involve a concept that generates only few connections and this can slow the growth of the snowball. For example, the study might measure only current sexual contacts, so 10 indexes who have two sexual partners yields only a pool of 20 new subjects.

The second type of snowball entails interviewing some subset of each respondent's personal network; this sample can be randomly chosen in an effort to make estimates regarding a population parameter. The sample can also be defined as those who are closest to the respondents, thus capturing strong rather than weak ones. Most often, the researcher is interested in a specific type of tie and will follow up only with those. For example, the researcher might want to interview all the drug users in a community and so elects to have indexes provide the names of his or her friends who use drugs. This provides entrée into the drug-using community, and further interviews will yield the structure of the drug using network.

Klovdhahl (1989) suggested eliciting a high number of alters and then taking a random sample of them to see how the network grows. Because the alters are randomly chosen, study results provide valid estimates of network properties attributable to the network. After one or two generations, researchers will have a large pool of subjects in the study who will know one another and hence be linked into a network. If the researcher starts with a set of randomly chosen index cases, then the network results provide a potentially valid parameter estimate of network structure.

Snowball sampling can be used to verify respondent assessments of their network alters' behaviors. For example, a snowball study of adolescent smoking can be conducted in which the ego and alter are both asked about their smoking behavior and that of their peers. If these self-report measures are validated with a biomarker (say cotinine), the researcher can then determine whether respondents are accurate in their assessments of their network partners' behaviors. It may also be possible to use snowball sampling to follow the trail of a rumor or piece of gossip or information. For example, if respondents report that they first heard a news item from people in their network, these alters can be interviewed and a trace of the information followed. These applications, however, are somewhat limited, and consequently few examples of snowball studies exist. More frequently, however, snowball sampling has been used to recruit subjects into studies or interventions.

Networks for Recruitment

Snowball techniques can be particularly useful for recruiting people into studies or health promotion and disease prevention programs. Network recruitment occurs when individuals are identified via outreach, clinical, service, or other methods, and these index cases are instructed to identify network partners that can also participate in the study or receive some program. For example, many studies have been conducted among drug users in which people receiving treatment or participating in a study are invited to bring their friends or substance using partners to the study setting so they can also receive treatment.

The idea of using social networks to identify people at risk for disease is not new and dates back to the use of contact tracing by local health departments. When individuals were diagnosed with a sexually transmitted disease (STD), workers at the health department would ask that person to name those they had had sexual relations with over the past 3 or 6 months and to provide their addresses. The workers would then contact those sexual partners and inform them that they are at increased risk for an STD and should be tested. These sexual network contacts were then recruited for STD testing and treatment and also asked to indicate their sexual networks if they had an STD.

More recently, interventions have been conducted in which individuals are invited to bring their network partners, friends, or close associates into a clinical or outreach setting to be given health promotion materials/interventions. For example, Valente and others (2009) set out to determine if a clinic

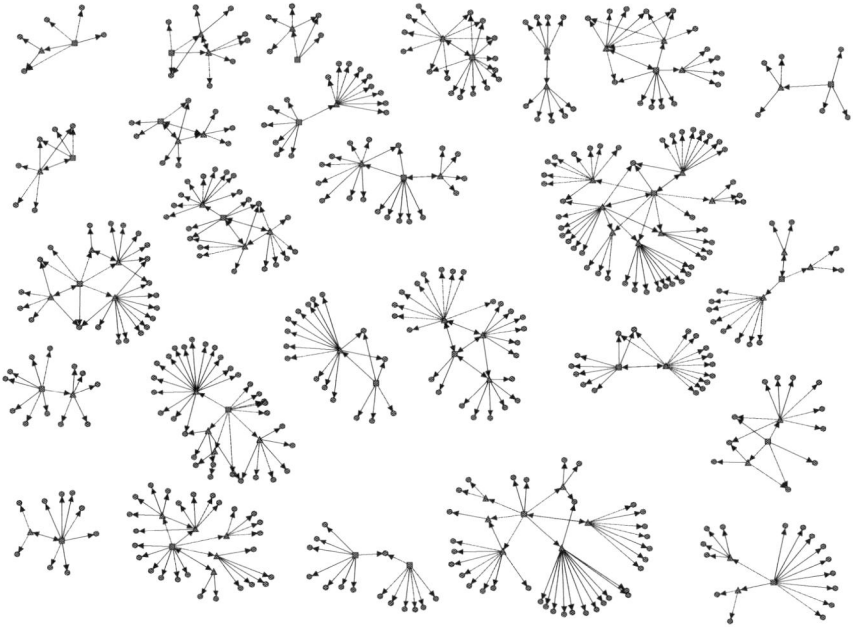

Figure 4–4. Networks of HIV-positive patients in which at least one alter was enrolled in an HIV vaccine preparedness study. Indexes are squares, enrolled alters are triangles, and nonenrolled alters are circles. Links are coded by willingness to invite the alter to participate in vaccine preparedness activities: solid arrows represent willingness, dashed arrows, not willing; dash-dotted arrows, absence of a response; and dash-dot-dot, enrolled but not named first-degree alters.

population of HIV-positive patients could be used to create a cohort of high-risk individuals who might be appropriate to receive an HIV vaccine. Figure 4–4 displays network linkages among indexes and alters in which at least one alter was enrolled in the study (794 links, 59.2%). Squares represent the 59 index patients; triangles, the 62 enrolled alters; and circles, named but not enrolled alters. Links are coded by willingness to invite alters to partici-pate in vaccine preparedness activities: solid arrows represent willingness; dashed arrows, not willing; dash-dotted arrows, absence of a response; and dash-dot-dot, enrolled but not named first-degree alter. The study showed that these indexes could enroll a cohort with the desired characteristics, but the networks were quite diverse.

The rest of this book will cover sociometric data and techniques used to analyze data from complete networks. It is wise to remember, however, that the complete network is composed of egocentric networks and that the sociometric data can be treated as egocentric. The building blocks of the sociometric data are the individual egocentric networks.

Summary

This chapter presented research on egocentric network data. Egocentric data are collected by asking people to name their closest friends or people they are connected to in some way. Egocentric data do not provide a connected network that can be mapped; rather they provide data that can be used to characterize each person's personal network environment. Egocentric data have been used to characterize the personal networks of populations. For example, data from the 1985 GSS were used to show that Americans have ties mostly to people like themselves (homogeneous) and that networks vary by geography (urban respondents had more heterogeneous networks than rural ones).

Many hypotheses regarding egocentric variables and behavior have been proposed and tested. Researchers have shown that behaviors are influenced by tie strength. For example, injection drug users were more likely to engage in risky behavior with close friends than with those less close and adolescents were more likely to smoke if their best friends smoke. Researchers have also shown that degree of concurrent sexual relationships in a community affects the prevalence of HIV. The chapter discussed how to convert egocentric data to a dyadic dataset, thus facilitating analysis and testing of certain hypotheses. The chapter closed with a discussion of the application of snowball sampling including network recruitment.

PART II

MEASURES

5

Centrality

This chapter provides background on the calculation, interpretation, and uses of various measures designed to determine which nodes occupy the center of a network. The chapter focuses on the three most common centrality measures developed by Freeman (1979): degree, closeness, and betweenness. Other centrality measures are also listed. The distinction between centrality and centralization is made, and extent of correlation among centrality measures reported. The chapter closes with a discussion of centrality and behavior change and how central individuals may affect the behavior of others.

When people are shown network diagrams, they frequently focus their attention on the nodes located in the center. Typically, people view being in the center of a network as a positive trait and see it as a good thing. Measuring the extent to which a node occupies a central position has been a critical focus of the network field. Central people often occupy important positions of prestige and visibility and, as noted in diffusion studies, may be influential in the spread of ideas and behaviors. Network analysts have developed numerous ways to measure centrality in a network (Borgatti & Everett, 2006).

Centrality measures for social networks were first developed in the 1950s by Bavelas, Sabidussi, and many other scholars from many disciplines (Borgatti & Everett, 2006; Freeman, 1979). The different measures and algorithms were summarized, expanded, and developed into an influential article by Freeman

(1979), in which Freeman introduced the modern typology of network measures by specifying that a centrality measure can have three properties:

1. It can be calculated on individuals referred to as point or node centrality.
2. This point centrality measure can and often should be normalized by the size of the network so calculations from different networks can be compared.
3. A network-level centralization score can be calculated indicating the degree of centralization derived from a specific measure.

Degree

The most frequently used centrality measure is degree, and it is an intuitive measure, easily calculated and easy to understand. *Degree* is the number of links to and from a person. In a directed (asymmetric) network, *in-degree* is the number of ties received and *out-degree* is the number of ties sent. Degree is characterized as a local centrality measure because it can be calculated without reference to the overall structure of the network. In other words, one can put a lens over a node's immediate ties and calculate centrality. Other centrality measures require information on the pattern of ties in the entire network to be calculated.

In-degree counts the number of times a person is nominated by others in the network. To make this measure comparable between networks of different sizes, this count is divided by the maximum number possible, which is $N - 1$. Theoretically, a person can be nominated by everyone else in the network. So the maximum possible in-degree is $N - 1$. The normalized degree centrality measure varies from 0 to 1. The formula for normalized degree is (Freeman, 1979):

$$C_D = \sum \frac{d_i}{N-1}$$

(5-1)

In-degree is a very useful measure, probably the most useful measure available to researchers. In-degree identifies opinion leaders in a network, and in friendship networks it indicates popularity. For example, popular adolescents are defined as those who received many choices as "friends" from their peers. In-degree can be used as a measure of social integration and used to identify opinion leaders to promote behavior change (see Chapter 11). In-degree is also a useful measure because a person can be nominated (and thus have an in-degree score) even if he or she does not complete a survey.

Out-degree is the number of names a person provides in response to a network question. Out-degree can be calculated as the total number of names provided or restricted to the number of names provided in the network (ignoring ties to people not predefined as being part of the network). In nomination studies (see Chapter 3), out-degree is often restricted to some maximum number. For example, a survey may ask people to name up to seven of your closest friends. In a roster study, out-degree can be as high as $N - 1$ (every other person but himself or herself). In a study assessing the number of sexual partners, out-degree is the number of sexual partners, which is a very important variable for understanding disease risk.

Out-degree is sometimes needed as a control variable in statistical analysis. For example, analysis showing that a network measure is associated with some outcome should include out-degree as a control variable because it may be that the measure of interest is related to the outcome because a person selected a large number of others in response to the network question. Out-degree is also used as a denominator when calculating network exposure or network composition terms to control for the size of one's network. Out-degree measures, to some extent, a person's socialness or sociality. Out-degree is often referred to as expansiveness.

Out-degree is also sometimes a useful indicator for personal attributes. For example, a network study can ask for the names of others to whom people go to for emotional support. Counting the number of others provides a measure of the size of one's emotional support network and this variable can be expected to correlate positively with health outcomes. Out-degree centrality provides a measure of network size, which can be very important. Out-degree, like in-degree, can be normalized by dividing scores by $N - 1$, the maximum possible. Degree scores can be calculated within standard statistical packages such as SAS, SPSS, and STATA when the data are dyadic (Box 5–1).

Closeness

Degree, as mentioned earlier, is considered a local centrality measure. Other measures of centrality require information on the pattern of links in the entire network. Freeman (1979) introduced two other centrality measures: closeness and betweenness. *Closeness* measures the average distance a node is from all other nodes in the network. It is calculated by summing these distances and then inverting the value to change the measure from a distance one to a closeness one. Point closeness then is the inverted sum of the distances, and normalized closeness is $N - 1$ divided by the sum of distances, making it an average closeness measure. Normalized closeness is calculated as (Freeman, 1979):

$$C_c = \frac{N-1}{\sum D_{ij}} \tag{5-2}$$

Box 5–1. Reshaping Data from Wide to Long and Calculating Degree

Using a simple dataset of nominations, the data are reshaped to dyadic format. If there are multiple networks in the data, the collapse command below is modified to include a variable indicating the separate networks. In this example, the data contain nominations of up to five alters.

```
/* Make Dyad */
use c:\data
reshape long nom, i(net_id) j(alt 1-5)
drop if nom==.
sort net_id
save c:\dyad, replace

/* Calculate indegree from dyad data */
use c:\dyad
gen one = 1
collapse (sum) one, by(nom)
ren one no_recvd
ren nom net_id
sort net_id
save c:\indegree, replace

/* Calculate outdegree from dyad data */
use c:\dyad, replace
gen one = 1
collapse (sum) one, by(net_id)
ren one no_sent
sort net_id
save c:\outdegree, replace

/* Merge In and Out Degree scores with data */
use c:\data
sort net_id
merge net_id using c:\outdegree
tab _merge
drop _merge
sort net_id
merge net_id using c:\indegree
tab _merge
drop _merge
save, replace
```

The maximum possible closeness score in any network is $N - 1$. When the distances to all nodes are summed and divided into $N - 1$, it provides a normalized version of closeness that varies from 0 to 1. Closeness has intuitive appeal as a centrality measure since someone who is closer to everyone else, on average, is in a central position. In geography, for example, St. Louis is in a central position in the United States because it is closer, on average, to all other U.S. cities. Los Angeles, on the other hand, may be near some cities, but it is far from many other cities, making it less central.

Unlike geography, however, social space is non-Euclidian; that is, the distance from A to B is not necessarily the same as the distance from B to A. Because networks are possibly asymmetric, the path from one person to another follows a direction along the lines. If one of those links is asymmetric, the path cannot be reversed. So the distance from one point to another may not be the same as the distance from that point to the original one (the distance from A to B is not necessarily the same as the distance from B to A).

Consequently, closeness centrality has a direction. One can calculate closeness based on the links directed to a person (in-closeness) or based on the links coming from a person (out-closeness). The calculations are the same (Equation 5-2) but are based on the direction of the person's direct links. The highest out-closeness is the person who can reach others in the fewest number of steps, while the highest in-closeness is the person others can reach in the fewest number of steps. Closeness has not been as useful a measure of centrality as in-degree and this may be in part due to its calculation.

Inverting the distance sums to calculate closeness is useful, but at the same time it can distort the measure in a nonlinear way. For example, a distance of 2 becomes ½ and a distance of 3 becomes ⅓ and so on. While inverting the distances and dividing into $N - 1$ (the maximum closeness possible) enables comparison between networks of different sizes, it also may not be the best way to convert distance into closeness. Valente and Foreman (1998) suggested *reversing* distances to make them closeness scores. Reversing distances entails subtracting the distances from the maximum possible in the network, $N - 1$. Valente and Foreman (1998) called this measure *integration* when calculated on in-distances and *radiality* when calculated on out-distances. The integration and radialiaty measures were found to correlate better with outcomes than closeness calculated by inverting distances.

Distances for Unconnected Nodes

One difficulty inherent in distance calculations for networks is the calculation of distances for disconnected nodes. Nodes that cannot reach one another in a network are an infinite distance from one another. Using infinity for the distance between disconnected nodes creates intractable mathematics for whole network calculations, however. Thus, some finite number is often used to represent the distance between disconnected nodes. The substitution of a constant for infinity is reasonable for several reasons. First, although the nodes are not reachable in this particular network, they might be reachable if the network was measured again or measured in a slightly different way. For example, two people might be connected in a friendship network but disconnected (unreachable) in an advice-seeking network. Given that they are reachable in another network, it seems logical to consider nodes as reachable in all networks.

A second reason to treat disconnected nodes as reachable rather than infinitely far apart is practical. Many network calculations require adding or inverting distances. Adding infinity to anything equals infinity and thus the calculations become meaningless. A third justification is that the lack of connectedness may be due to measurement error and the substitution minimizes the impact of this measurement error. Finally, on philosophical grounds, substituting a number for infinity may be justified because any person included in the study is thought to be somehow connected to the group and not disconnected from it entirely.

In sum, most network analysts treat unreachable nodes as being far away, but not infinitely far. Three obvious measures of distance for unreachable nodes are (1) $D + 1$ where D is the longest distance between connected nodes (the diameter) and (2) N or $N - 1$ (where N is network size). $D + 1$ assumes that two disconnected nodes are one step farther apart than the longest distance in the network. This works well for many applications because the disconnected nodes do not distort the distribution of distances too much. The disadvantage of $D + 1$ is that this distance is not a theoretical maximum. Another drawback is that since different networks within the same community or study may have different diameters, unreachable nodes in one network within the same community may have shorter distances than unreachable nodes in another. For example, a school friendship network may have a diameter of five and advice-seeking a diameter of seven and so students unreachable in the friend network may be calculated as closer than advice seekers reachable via six steps.

To address the limitations of $D + 1$, many researchers use $N - 1$ as the distance between disconnected nodes. $N - 1$ is the theoretical maximum distance for disconnected nodes because that is the maximum number of steps between any two nodes in a network. To understand how $N - 1$ can be the farthest distance, consider a set of nodes arranged in a line as a network that has the maximum distance between nodes. The distance from one end of the line to the other is $N - 1$. The drawback to using $N - 1$ is that average distances between nodes in a network of even moderate size can become quite large even with only a few unreachable nodes. These larger than expected averages hamper interpretation when reporting results and can distort analysis conducted with the metrics (for example, in a regression analysis).

In sum, researchers need to be conscious of the network structure and specifically aware if the network contains isolates or disconnected groups. Researchers needing to analyze the whole network including these isolates or dis-connections may prefer using a finite number rather than infinity for these distances. $D + 1$ has the advantage of providing average distances close to the existing average in the connected components but cannot be compared between networks. $N - 1$ as a value can be compared between networks of different sizes but inflates distance values considerably and so may perturb further analysis of the data (e.g., in regression equations).

Betweenness

The third measure Freeman (1979) proposed was centrality betweenness measured as the frequency a person lies on the shortest path connecting everyone else in the network. The concept of *betweenness* is very appealing as it measures the degree a node occupies a strategic position in a network, somewhat akin to bridging and centrality combined. Like the other measures, one can calculate a point measure and its normalized version. Point betweenness is calculated by counting the frequency a node lies on the shortest paths connecting all other nodes in the network. Normalized betweenness centrality is calculated as (Freeman, 1979):

$$C_b = \frac{\dfrac{g_{ij}\, p_k}{g_{ij}}}{n^2 - 3n + 2} \tag{5-3}$$

where $g_{ij}\, p_k$ counts the number of times point k lies on the geodesic (shortest path) connecting all other nodes (i and j) and g_{ij} is the number of geodesics in the network. Betweenness is the frequency a node lies on the shortest path connecting other nodes in the network. The maximum possible value that the numerator $[(g_{ij}\, p_k)/g_{ij}]$ can reach is $n^2 - 3n + 2$ and so this is the normalization factor (Freeman, 1979). Betweenness centrality is inherently directional since the geodesic (the shortest path) is directional. Consequently, separate calculations for in and out directions are not needed. Betweenness centrality captures the notion that a person with strategic contacts, say nominations received from leaders of two factions, inhabits a strategic position in the network even if his or her volume of contacts is not large.

One shortcoming of Freeman's (1979) betweenness measure is that it relies on the *geodesic,* the shortest path connecting nodes. It may be that some nodes occupy critical betweenness locations but not on the geodesic. Another criticism is that it takes a long time to calculate betweenness for networks larger than a few hundred members. Newman (2005) provided an alternative measure of betweenness calculated similarly but, rather than relaying shortest paths, samples all paths connecting two nodes. Brandes and Erlebach (2005) offered an algorithm that is more efficient for larger networks.

Although degree, closeness, and betweenness measure centrality, they each capture slightly different conceptions or functions of centrality. Degree, for example, measures local centrality, the extent to which a node is connected to many other nodes regardless of the location/position of those other nodes. In contrast, Freeman (1979) stated that betweenness centrality captured a gate-keeping function—if members high in betweenness opposed an idea, its diffusion to other segments of the group might be blocked. Closeness centrality captured a communication role such that people high in closeness can communicate an idea to many others rapidly.

The three measures, degree, closeness, and betweenness, often identify different nodes as being the most central and of course are not perfectly correlated. For example, the networks in Figure 1–1 displays friendship choices for sixth-graders in one middle school in southern California. Centrality (and other) scores were calculated for this network and the links and measures are reported in Appendix C. Students 21 and 7 have the highest degree scores each receiving 11 friendship nominations. These two students have the highest centrality in-degree. In this study, students were asked to name up to five of their closest friends and many of the students named five so they all have the same out-degree score. In sum, the three most prominent centrality measures identify different individuals as being most central and two of these measures, degree and closeness, are asymmetric, yielding different nodes as being most central depending on the direction of the links. Further, closeness and betweenness have several different ways they can be calculated. In addition to imperfect correlation, it is also the case that centrality measures vary in their robustness to missing data (Box 5–2).

The most central nodes on in-closeness were 29 and 10. These two nodes have the shortest average number of steps to be reached by everyone else in the network. Closeness centrality is an asymmetric measure; distances in one direction can be different than distances in the other direction. The in-closeness centrality measure determines the distances "to" each node and is based on the ties being directed to each node. Messages from other students can reach 29 and 10 more quickly, on average, than they can reach other students. Out-closeness centrality is highest for students 35 and 2. Notice that 35 makes five nominations and two of these nominations are

Box 5–2. Robustness of Centrality Measures with Missing Data

One nagging concern in the social network field has been missing data. Because sociometric studies use census sampling, it is desirable to interview all members of the community. Each person contributes $N - 1$ bits of information to the data, the ties or non-ties to everyone else. There has always been a feeling that response rates of 70% or 80%, although high by most scientific standards, are inadequate for network analysis and might make most network measures invalid.

To assess the effect of missing data on networks measures, a study was conducted using social network data from eight studies and 58 different networks (Costenbader & Valente, 2003). Centrality measures were calculated on all the networks; then 20% of the people were removed from the network, and the centrality measures were recalculated, and then correlated with the original measure. The process was repeated 25 times at each sampled level to get an average of the correlations. The average correlation indicates how well centrality measures assess centrality under conditions of missing data, that is, if the response rates were lower.

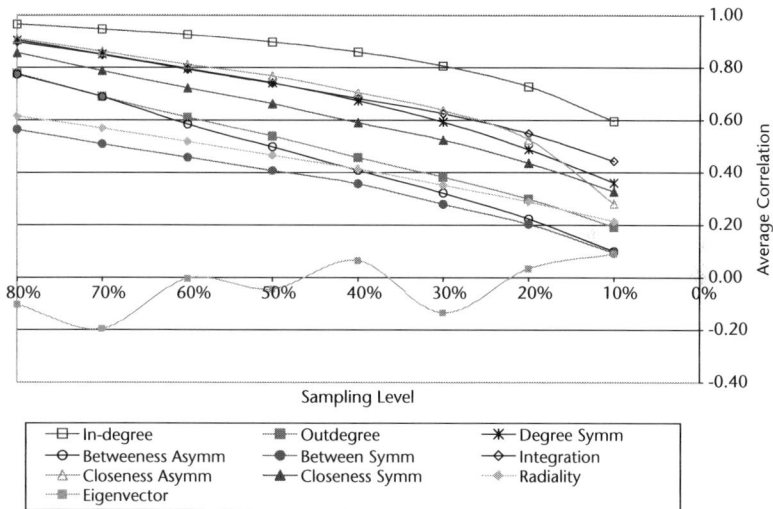

Figure 5–1. Correlations between centrality measures calculated on the complete network and that calculated on a sample decremented by 10% and repeated 25 times at each sampling level. Results show that in-degree is the most robust when sampled; it is 60% accurate when as little as 10% of the original network is used. In contrast, integration, radiality, and betweenness do less well, in part because these measures reflect more of the network structure. Eigenvector centrality seems to do the least well when the network is sampled.

(Continued)

Box 5–2. Continued

The exercise was repeated reducing the sample (i.e., increasing the missing data rate) to 70%, 60%, 50%, 40%, 30%, and 20%. Figure 5–1 shows the average correlations at decreased sample sizes averaged across all the datasets. The centrality measures were surprisingly robust. In-degree centrality was the most robust. The actual in-degree score and the one calculated on the 30% sample had a correlation of 0.80. Closeness and integration, the two distance-based measures, do the next best decreasing in the correlation linearly with the decrease in sample size. Betweenness does less well, correlating at less than 0.60 with the 80% sample and decreasing steadily to about 0.30 at 30%. The most disappointing measure was eigenvector centrality which correlated poorly with the measure from the full sample at even the highest sampling rate and correlated erratically throughout the experiment. The conclusion from this exercise is that those centrality measures which tap into the structure of the network the greatest are the most vulnerable to missing data and that simple measures like degree and closeness are the most robust under conditions of missing data.

The empirical analysis showed that no one factor was uniformly associated with measure instability. Response rate, density, centralization, and dummy variables for the various studies were all tested for their effect on measure instability. No one factor emerged that affected centrality measure robustness. Borgatti and others (2006) conducted similar analyses with similar results on simulated data.

students 2 and 23, who then link directly to the other group. Messages *from* student 35 can reach other students more quickly than messages originating from anyone else. In this case, in-closeness and out-closeness identify different nodes as the ones being most central. Substantively, this can be very important depending on whether one is concerned about sending messages or getting messages received or on transmitting infection or receiving it.

Betweenness centrality identifies node 27 as the most central. Student 27 lies on the shortest path connecting other students more frequently than any other node. If all the shortest paths connecting the people in this network were written out, student 27 would appear most often. In this case, 27 occupies a strategic position of importance by being the node that messages must pass through as they circulate through the network. If one wanted to disrupt communication flow, student 27 would be a critical person to inoculate with a specific message. If one wanted to disrupt the spread of infections, person 27 would be the most logical to immunize.

In sum, the three most prominent centrality measures identify different individuals as being most central, and two of these measures, degree and closeness, are asymmetric, yielding different nodes as being most central depending on the direction of the links. Further, closeness and betweenness have several different ways they can be calculated.

Which students are the most central? There are five: 21 and 7 (in-degree); 29 (in-closeness); 35 (out-closeness); and 27 (betweenness). Each one serves different functions in the overall structure of the network and each potentially can be used in different ways to mobilize action or accelerate change in the network. The different centrality measures might capture the different kinds of leaders one would expect to adopt an innovation or be used to promote it during different stages of diffusion. For example, since people high on betweenness act as bridges, perhaps they could be recruited to carry the innovation from the innovative stage to early adopters. Or these bridges should be inoculated so that diseases do not get transmitted from one group to another. People high on in-degree centrality can then be recruited during the early adoption stage to be champions since they are role models for many people. High in-degree people act as champions that move the innovation from the early adoption stage to the early majority stage. They can be proponents that can establish a critical mass in favor of the new behavior. As diffusion progresses, people high in closeness centrality can be recruited to ensure diffusion spreads to the maximum number of people. Although it is unlikely such data would be available to implement such a project, in an ideal world this is how diffusion might be managed.

One limitation to carrying out such a project is the intensity of the monitoring and data collection necessary to complete it. A second is that the three centrality measures (degree, closeness, and betweenness) are highly correlated (Valente et al., 2008), and so a person high on betweenness is often high on closeness or degree. Still if one wanted to maximize diffusion, such a project, or a variation on it, should be considered. (A variation might be using high in-degree champions but continuously reassessing the identification of leaders using the different centrality measures.)

Correlation among Centrality Measures

Although the three centrality measures discussed so far are correlated, the correlation is far from 1. To measure their correlation, the centrality measures degree, closeness and betweenness were calculated on 58 networks collected in eight studies (Costenbader & Valente, 2003). The correlations among these centrality measures within each network was then calculated

Table 5–1. Average Correlations between Centrality Measures (N = 58)

	1	2	3	4	5	6	7	8	9	Total
1. In-degree										
2. Out-degree	0.30									
3. Degree	0.78	0.71								
4. Betweenness	0.62	0.54	0.70							
5. Symmetric betweenness	0.69	0.50	0.85	0.67						
6. Closeness-in	0.55	0.16	0.45	0.37	0.30					
7. Closeness-out	0.18	0.81	0.56	0.39	0.38	0.01				
8. Symmetric closeness	0.40	0.64	0.66	0.37	0.44	0.42	0.65			
9. Eigenvector	0.71	0.69	0.92	0.64	0.72	0.44	0.55	0.63		
Average correlation	0.59	0.58	0.70	0.54	0.57	0.34	0.44	0.54	0.67	0.54
Standard deviation of correlations	0.21	0.21	0.15	0.14	0.18	0.18	0.26	0.13	0.15	0.14

and averaged across the 58 networks (Valente et al., 2008). The average cor-relations are presented in Table 5–1 and are generally pretty high, ranging from 0.18 to 0.92. The correlation between in- and out-degree was mod-est, 0.30, for example. Betweenness centrality was strongly correlated with degree and eigenvector (0.64) but not with closeness centrality. Closeness centrality was also associated with degree and with eigenvector centrality. The overall average correlation among all centrality measures was 0.54, indicating that these different centrality measures seem to represent a fairly consistent concept, centrality, but with some distinctiveness to the individual measures. Overall, degree had the highest average correlation (0.70) with the other measures (Valente et al., 2008).

Reciprocity was strongly associated with centrality measure correlations. If there were many reciprocated relationships in the network, the centrality measures were highly correlated. This strong correlation could be a func-tion of the symmetry status of the various measures—networks with higher levels of reciprocity will have higher correlations between asymmetric mea-sures than those with lower levels of reciprocity. For example, the corre-lation between in-degree and out-degree will be one when the network is perfectly symmetric because the in- and out-ties are identical. In addition, correlations between symmetrized measures were associated with the num-ber of components and network density, while asymmetric measures were not. Symmetrizing matrices before making centrality calculations should thus be done with caution and only if justifiable substantively. In addition, un-symmetrized centrality measures might be more distinct in densely connected networks with more components. The findings demonstrated that symmetrizing network data creates disparities between symmetric and asymmetric centrality measures (Valente et al., 2008).

Other Centrality Measures

Degree, closeness, and betweenness constitute the three main centrality measures, but at least seven other centrality measures have been developed, including eigenvector centrality (Bonacich, 1972; Seary & Richards, 2003), entropy (Tutzauer, 2007), information (Stephenson & Zellen, 1989), flow (Freeman et al., 1991), power (Bonacich, 1987), and complement (Cornwell, 2005). All of these centrality measures can be calculated in UCINET (Borgatti et al., 2004) and many other software programs (Huisman & van Duijn, 2005). Before using these measures, researchers should understand the advantages and properties of each measure. Eigenvector centrality is useful because it measures the centrality of a node based in part on the centrality of its neighboring nodes. Eigenvector centrality, however, uses symmetric data and is not robust to missing data. Power is very useful as a measure because it allows the researcher to vary the extent to which the centrality of one's neighbors is included in the calculation.

Link or Edge Centrality

Of interest in some applications is treating the links as nodes and the nodes as links. Link centrality analysis enables the researcher to determine which connections are most central in the network. Every link will have a degree of two (two nodes), but one can calculate closeness, betweenness, and other centrality measures based on the network of links. This might be useful if, for example, a researcher wants to identify which relationships are the most central. For example, a network of sexual contacts may be converted to links and the most central relationships might be the ones most effectively eliminated to stem the flow of STDs.

In the network of Figure 1–1, betweenness centrality was calculated on the links. (Degree centrality is not important as all links have degree one or two.) The link (edge) with highest betweenness centrality score was the link connecting students 27 and 29. Visual inspection confirms this is indeed an important link as it connects the girls on the left with the boys on the right. Removing this link would disrupt the flow of communication (or disease transmission) more so than the removal of any other link.

Centrality versus Centralization

Centrality measures can also be used to describe the extent to which a network is centralized. *Centralization* is the extent to which network links are focused on one or a few nodes in the network. A *centralized network,* sometimes referred to as a *hierarchical* one, concentrates links on one or a few people, while a *decentralized network* has links evenly distributed among the nodes.

A centralized network has most of its links connected to one or a few nodes. A star network (Figure 5–2) is a perfectly centralized network, whereas a wheel is decentralized. In the star, one node controls all of the activity, whereas in the wheel, every node is equally in control and has equal access to all others. Centralized networks are characterized by large variance in the individual centrality scores (some large and many small values), whereas decentralized ones have little variance in centrality measures (everyone has the same or similar scores). The star has one node with four links and four nodes with one link. In contrast, the wheel network has an equal number of links, two, for all five nodes.

One way to measure centralization is to calculate the standard deviation of the centrality scores (Wasserman & Faust, 1994). A centralized network will have a high standard deviation of centrality scores because some individuals have high centrality while many others have low centrality. A decentralized network, in contrast, has a low standard deviation of centrality scores because everyone has very similar scores. A network of five nodes in which everyone is connected to everyone else is perfectly decentralized and everyone has the same centrality degree score. In contrast, a network of five people in which four of them are all connected to one and the same person is perfectly centralized on that person and the standard deviation of the degree distribution is high.

A normalized centralization score is possible to calculate by taking the difference between the maximum score in the network and all other scores

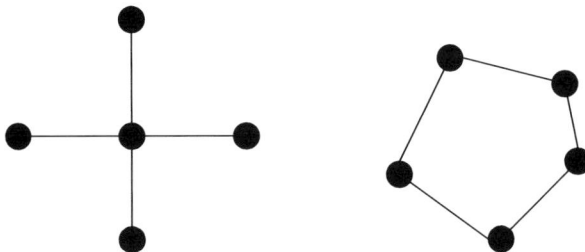

Figure 5–2. A perfectly centralized network on the left (a star) and a decentralized one on the right (a chain).

(see Chapter 8). This sum is then divided by the maximum value possible for a network. This centralization calculation logic is similar to using a standard deviation, which is a sum of differences, but instead divides by the maximum difference possible so the values range from zero to 1, with a perfectly centralized network having a centralization score of 1. The important concept to retain here is that centrality refers to the node or person-level measure and centralization to the network-level one. In other words, a person can have high centrality within a centralized or decentralized network.

Centrality and Behavior

Early studies showed that centrality was linked to task performance. Experimental studies showed that centralized groups completed tasks more efficiently than decentralized groups, although the centralized ones reported less satisfaction with the task (Shaw, 1971). Organizational behaviorists debate the merits of decentralized versus centralized decision-making with some industries favoring centralization while others favor decentralization. Trade flows and traffic research have an inherent interest in centrality as trade centers usually occupy central positions. At the same time, centralized traffic systems are subject to congestion and bottlenecks. Pitts (1979) showed that the city of Moscow emerged as an important and large city in part because of its position in the river trade network.

City planners need to calculate centrality on traffic grids to decide where to locate fire stations, police stations, and hospitals, as these should be in the center of their catchment areas. Central members can be drivers of diffusion, and those at the center of disease risk networks are at greater risk for the disease than those on the periphery. Ellen and others (2005) showed that adolescents in high STD prevalence communities who had larger social networks were more likely to contract an STD than those with smaller social networks. Rogers' (1962, 2003) studies of the diffusion of innovations concluded that opinion leaders, who are often at the center of networks, were more likely to be earlier adopters of innovations than were non–opinion leaders.

Rogers and Kincaid (1981) studied the adoption of contraceptive practices in 25 Korean villages from data collected in 1973. They found that there was usually a certain contraceptive method—IUD, condom, or withdrawal—that would become widespread in a village and this method would be the one also chosen by the women who received the most nominations as a family planning discussion partner. Again, in-degree centrality was associated with behavioral adoption, and in this case evidence that perhaps the behavior of the opinion leaders was imitated by many others.

Alexander and others (2001) found that popular students, measured as those who received many friendship nominations, were more likely to smoke than their less popular peers. Alexander and others (2001) also found that popular students were more likely to smoke in schools where the smoking prevalence in the school was high and less likely to smoke where the smoking prevalence in the schools was low. This cross-sectional study could only show a correlation between popularity and smoking but suggests that popular students embrace behaviors consistent with cultural norms and in turn may contribute to normative persistence.

Valente and others (2005) showed that adolescents popular in the sixth grade were more likely to become smokers in the seventh grade. Popular students were also more likely to become more susceptible to smoking (as measured by their refusal to state they would not smoke in the future) than their less popular peers. These effects held for change in smoking status as well as when restricted to nonsmokers in the sixth grade (smoking initiation). These analyses controlled for the many other factors associated with smoking including parental and sibling smoking, socioeconomic status, ethnicity, academic performance, age, and sex.

Why do popular students start smoking before their less popular peers? In part this perhaps is a function of the popular students' frame of reference. They anticipate that smoking will become widespread in their schools and so want to be earlier adopters of this behavior so they seem "hip" or "cool." They also want to retain their positions of popularity and so need to be trendsetters, and smoking will enable them to be seen as the trendsetters. In schools in which smoking will be seen as deviant behavior, popular students will not be more prone to smoke. It may also be that they possess some other characteristics that make them both popular and become smokers.

In-degree centrality is the most frequently used network measure of opinion leadership and has been used for decades. As early as the 1950s, researchers counted the number of choices each person received and used this count to indicate opinion leadership. Rogers and Cartano (1962) conducted an early study comparing the in-degree measure of opinion leadership with other measures such as self-assessment via survey. They found that the measures were somewhat correlated ($r = 0.35$) but not as strong as one might expect them to be. In more recent research, we conducted a survey of physicians using a validated leadership scale and found it correlated with in-degree centrality at 0.43 (Van den Bulte, et al., 2008).

The smoking studies showed that opinion leaders, defined as popular students, started smoking earlier than their less popular peers. These studies, and many others, describe a general model in which opinion leaders evaluate the relative compatibility and appeal of new behaviors as they are introduced into a community. If that new behavior seems to be one that will be embraced by the community, the opinion leader will adopt earlier than most everyone else in the community. In other words, if the behavior is culturally compatible, opinion leaders will adopt it early. Subsequently, many others will see the behavior of these opinion leaders, which will reinforce the acceptability of the new behavior, and its adoption by others will be accelerated.

Central people are in an advantaged position for access to information about what is happening in the community. They can scan the environment more effectively than others because of the many contacts they have and this scanning enables them to judge whether the new behavior will be acceptable to the community at large. Once central people sense or believe there will be widespread acceptance of the new behavior, they are likely to adopt it.

In turn, because of their central position, many others watch the central people to see how they will react to the new idea. The centrals are "on stage" more often than their peers and their behavior is monitored by more other people than nonleaders. As others monitor and emulate the behaviors of central people, their status as leaders becomes enhanced. Often then, widespread diffusion hangs in the balance while opinion leaders judge the acceptability of the new idea. Their endorsement means more than just another adoption, it signals community acceptance. This suggests that degree centrality would be an indicator more highly associated with accelerating diffusion than other centrality measures.

Not all opinion leaders are equal. Some leaders are local leaders while others are regional and still others national leaders. There are some leaders who command attention within their local community but not much beyond that. Still other leaders have regional influence so that they are well known and emulated by colleagues locally and regionally. National leaders have the most prominence. These leaders are recognized trendsetters and gatekeepers on a national level. National leaders may not be seen as local leaders within the community precisely because their contacts are outside the community. Since many people's adoption decisions are driven by their close personal networks, they may recognize national leaders as leaders, but perhaps will not emulate their behavior.

Behavioral diffusion is driven in large part by the behavior of local leaders. National leaders are usually perceived to be too different than those in the community and often do not provide the best role models as diffusion agents. National leaders function much like the mass media—their behavior may spread awareness about a new idea and legitimize it, but they often do not have direct influence on many others. The people they do influence are more likely to be regional and local leaders rather than nonleaders.

There is an element of network trust implied in these conjectures. People are influenced by those they trust. It is difficult to develop a trust relationship with a national leader whose sphere of influence is quite large. Local leaders can develop trust within the community and so their opinions are often more valued, and behaviors more often emulated than those of national leaders. Trust is often a prerequisite condition for interpersonal influence to occur.

Characteristics of Opinion Leaders

Leaders are just like followers, only more so. Leaders are often of slightly higher status than their followers but not much higher. National leaders are often perceived to be different than everyone else, but local leaders often have just a bit higher status than the people they lead in their community. Typically, leaders have slightly more education, have slightly higher incomes, and/or are somewhat better read on the topic. This happens because most people like to look up to others who are like themselves, only a little better in some way. It is difficult for people to relate to others who are very different from themselves. On the other hand, people can relate to others who are just one rung above them on the socioeconomic or status ladder.

Research also shows that leaders are more empathetic and good listeners; they learn from other people. Leaders are good communicators, enjoying interpersonal interaction. They are "people" people. Leaders also attend to media more, which provides them with the information they need to lead and to stay abreast of what is happening. The importance of opinion leaders for behavior change has led to the creation of opinion leader interventions designed to accelerate behavior change (see Chapter 11).

It should also be noted that leadership is sometimes distinguished between formal and informal leadership. Formal leaders are identified by their occupation (elected officials, company presidents, media personalities), whereas informal leaders are often harder to identify. At least 10 different techniques have been used to identify leaders (Valente & Pumpuang, 2007), and these different approaches often yield different types of people who may be differentially suited to different tasks.

Leader characteristics and abilities may also depend in part on the overall network structure within which the opinion leaders function. Being a central node in a centralized network has different implications than being a central node in a decentralized network. A central node in a centralized network can exercise considerable more power and influence than a central node in a decentralized network. Moreover, centralization may also influence how noncentral nodes relate to central nodes because noncentral members may feel vulnerable or dependent on the central members' attitudes. In essence, noncentral members may feel more empowered in decentralized networks than in centralized ones.

Summary

This chapter introduced the concept of centrality in social networks. The chapter provided the equations for the three most frequently used centrality measures—degree, closeness, and betweenness (Freeman, 1979). The extent correlation among centrality measures was presented as well as factors that influence correlations among measures. Overall, the correlation is quite high, 0.54, but far from unity and varies considerably between measures. There are also network properties such as reciprocity that affect the correlation among centrality measures. The greater the tendency toward reciprocity in the network, the higher is the correlation among measures. Thus, researchers should use caution when symmetrizing networks.

The chapter reviewed how each of these centrality measures might function in the diffusion of innovations and behavior change and discussed the roles of opinion leaders in the behavior change process. The distinction between centrality and centralization was emphasized. The interplay between centrality and centralization was discussed. Centrality measurement has been a key development in the network field. The central importance of central nodes and people in networks means that it is likely to continue this prominent role.

6

Groups

This chapter describes how network analysts define and measure groups. Components are the building blocks of group definitions and consist of all the nodes connected to each other through any number of steps in network. Nodes that cannot reach each other are in different components. More complex group definitions are then provided, namely, k-plexes and n-cliques, which permit variation in the degree of connectivity among group members needed to be a group member. The trouble with many group definitions, however, is that individuals can be members of many groups. While this reflects empirical reality, it can complicate statistical analysis. The Girvan-Newman (2002) algorithm is introduced, which provides mutually exclusive groups and a measure of how well the group definitions characterize the data. The chapter closes with a discussion of how groups influence behavior.

Most people enjoy being in groups. Groups help people define their identity and provide a sense of belonging. Belonging to a group signals to others our identity and how we relate to the rest of the world. Groups also provide protection. By belonging to a group a person does not have to defend his or her ideas, but rather can adopt those of the group and feel secure that others feel the same way he or she does.

Groups also provide the context for socializing, talking, and being with others. Humans are social animals; people like to talk and spend time with

others and groups can provide an organized, and sometimes not so organized, way to be with other people. But not just any other people: rather,
people who have similar ideas, attitudes, opinions, and behaviors. In sum,
people often join groups to be with others who are a lot like themselves or at
least share some particular trait.

Scholars have conducted a lot of research on groups, how they form, the
social pressure they induce, and the tendency for groups to reinforce existing
beliefs (Moscovici, 1976). Network analysts are concerned primarily with
providing network definitions for what it means to be in a group and how
to define and analyze groups from a network perspective. The starting point
is to take data collected on who is connected to whom, then define what it
means to be in a group in the network, and then create these network groups.
Whether the network groups match with other definitions of groups remains
a somewhat open research question. For example, to what extent do network-defined groups among high schools students correspond to commonly
labeled groups such as "jocks," "nerds," "geeks," "skaters," etc. (these are
often referred to as identities)?

Network analysts define groups as any subset of a network. For example,
the boys in a network of high school students (assuming it is coeducational)
can be defined as a group within the network. Generally, though, a subset of
a network is a group if it meets some network definition of being a group.
The simplest such definition is a component.

Components and *K*-Cores

A component consists of the connected nodes in the network, all nonisolates.
Everyone who can reach everyone else and be reached by everyone else is
in the same component. One can also define weak and strong components.
A weak component ignores the direction of the tie, while a strong component does not (Scott, 2000). In other words, strong components are nodes
connected to one another in both directions along every step in the path connecting them. A component is a simple concept but can be useful if one has
a large network that has several separate components. The components can
be extracted and analyzed as separate networks.

It is also possible to reduce a network by reducing it to only reciprocated
ties, and this reduction may create separate components. It is also useful
to describe a network by the number of components. A network with one
component is quite different than a network with many. Components then
simply determine whether nodes are connected and define groups based
whether the nodes can reach one another through any path of connections
in the network. Once a component analysis is completed, the researcher can

progress to determining the groups, clusters, and cliques within the overall network.

There are several different definitions of a group in a network, one of which creates group definitions based on the number of connections the nodes have in the network. A component consists of all nodes that have at least one connection. This concept of the number of links defining a group can be generalized by creating K-cores. A K-core is a subset of the network in which each node within the K-core is connected to at least K other people. Thus, a $2K$-core is the set of people connected to at least two other nodes. All the nodes with zero or one link are dropped from the network. Similarly, we can define a $3K$-core as all the nodes with three or more links. As K is increased, successive pictures of who is left in the network will look increasingly dense. Once nodes are dropped from the network, the links from and to it are also dropped so the K criterion is calculated on the remaining nodes and links.

The pattern of node removal as K is increased can be used to describe the network structure. For example, some networks have a core-periphery structure, which is a network with a set of dense connections among a subset of nodes and another set residing on the periphery with fewer connections (see Chapter 8). Most of the connections in the periphery are to the core and not to each other. Figure 6–1 shows a network of friendship links

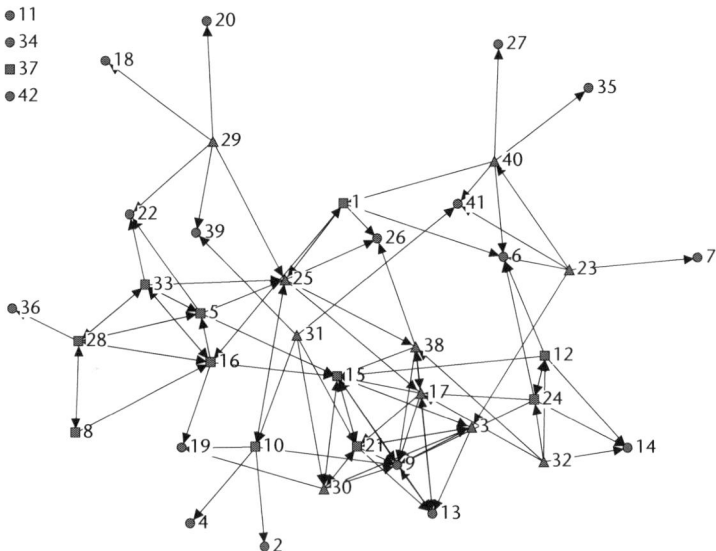

Figure 6–1. A network of friendship links between students in an alternate high school in southern California.

between students in an alternate high school in southern California. We ran the K-core routine in UCINET on this friendship network and it indicated that the cluster of friends in the lower middle of the graph constituted the K-core. Seven students, numbers 38, 15, 17, 21, 9, 3, 13, and 30, all remain connected to each other as K is increased from one to four.

The number of nodes dropped at each unit increase in K can be graphed as a histogram or bar graph at each increment of K. If the bars are all the same height, it indicates the same number of nodes were removed at each increase in K. If the bar graph is uneven or steeply increasing or decreasing, it indicates structural variations in which the number of nodes removed from the core changes abruptly. The pattern of this bar graph can provide an indication of whether the network has a core-periphery structure. If the bar graph is uniform across all bars, this indicates no core-periphery and little structure in the network. Conversely, if there is a sharp decrease in the bars, this indicates a core-periphery structure or at least considerable structure in the network. If there are a few nodes remaining after K is increased to a high number, then this indicates a K-core. If K is increased to seven and four nodes are left, these four nodes would be a $7K$-core, indicating these four nodes have at least seven connections in the network. If the number of nodes removed is dramatic, such that when K equals three all the nodes are dropped, then the network does not have a strong core-periphery structure. In general, the greater the percent decrease in nodes left in the core, the less a core-periphery structure exists. This is not a strict rule, though, because it may be that many nodes drop early but the core retains to high levels of K. Suffice it to say, it is instructive to look at the K-core collapse, the pattern of dropped nodes as k increases.

Although finding the core group is important, it is also important to understand how groups are distributed in the network and who belongs to which group. For this purpose, network analysis uses the concept of a clique. Strictly speaking, a *clique* is the set of points all directly connected to one another. A clique is a dense pocket of interconnectivity with every person directly connected to everyone else. Yet this definition of clique can be somewhat restrictive as it is common to have a group of people one might think of as a clique, yet every member is not directly connected to every other member.

The strict clique definition can be relaxed to define an n-clique, which is the path length at which members of the clique are connected. For example, a $2n$-clique is the set of people connected to each other within two steps. Two people are in the same clique if they are friends of the same friend. The n-clique definition allows people to be in the same group even if they are not directly connected to one another. One can also increase "n" to higher numbers such as $3n$-cliques and $4n$-cliques. Typically, though, values greater than two are rarely used because it seems counterintuitive for people to be in

Table 6–1. List of N-Cliques for the Network Given in Figure 6–1

Clique Members
1: 13 15 17 21 9
2: 13 15 17 38 9
3: 13 15 21 3 9
4: 15 21 3 30 9
5: 15 16 5
6: 12 14 24 32
7: 1 25 26
8: 1 40 6
9: 22 33 5
10: 23 40 41
11: 23 40 6
12: 17 24 32
13: 17 24 9
14: 12 24 6
15: 25 26 38
16: 17 25 38
17: 25 33 5
18: 16 28 33 5
19: 16 28 8
20: 21 30 31
21: 17 32 38

the same clique if they are three steps from one another. Table 6–1 reports the 2n-cliques for the network in Figure 6–1.

A second clique definition is a k-plex, which is defined as the set of points connected to all but k other nodes in the group. To find k-plexes, the researcher sets both "k" and "n" to the size of the groups. The minimum size for n, the size of the groups, is set to $k - 2$ (because values of n close to k return trivial groups) For example, $2k$-plexes with $n = 7$ will find all groups of size seven in which each person is connected to at least five others in the group. If k is increased to three, $3k$-plexes, all groups of size seven in which each person is connected to at least four other members would be reported. So as k increases, the number of groups identified in the network increases. In practice, one sets k and finds all of the groups as n increases from $k + 2$ to $n - 1$. For example, with $k = 2$ and $n = 4$, the $2k$-plexes are all of the groups size four and larger in which the members are connected to at least two others. Table 6–2 reports the k-plexes for our sample network.

The K-cores, n-cliques, and k-plexes provide good measures of network structure, and as the researcher studies a network, these group identification methods provide insight into the pattern of affiliations such that one can characterize the network according to who is in which groups with whom. UCINET returns a group co-membership matrix in which the numbers in the matrix indicate how many groups each person shares with everyone else.

Table 6–2. List of *k*-Plexes for the Network Given in Figure 6–1

Group Members

k-plex
Value of K: 2 (each member of a *k*-plex of size *N* has *N-k* ties to other members)
Minimum Set Size = 5
Input dataset: C:\MISC\DIFFNET\snbh\tprc_4
WARNING: Directed graph. Direction of arcs ignored.
Six *k*-plexes found.
1: 13 15 17 21 3 9
2: 13 15 17 21 38 9
3: 13 15 21 3 30 9
4: 13 15 3 38 9
5: 15 17 21 30 9
6: 17 24 32 38 9

The diagonal of this matrix indicates how many groups (cliques or *k*-plexes) each person belongs to. The group co-membership matrix can be used in subsequent analysis, for example, to investigate whether people who share many groups have similar attitudes and behaviors. (This would be done, for example, by correlating the matrix of shared groups with the matrix of attitude similarity; see Chapter 8.)

One problem with these group identification methods, *n*-cliques and *k*-plexes, is that they return lists of groups in which many people are members of multiple groups. This may reflect reality and be advantageous in some research analysis. On the other hand, for researchers studying behavior it can be difficult to conduct analysis comparing group membership to behavior because people are not classified in mutually exclusive groups. One solution is the hierarchical clustering analysis provided as part of the group analysis in UCINET. The hierarchical clustering output indicates group assignments at various cutoff levels. There is no rule to indicate where that level should be set. Further, when studying multiple networks in the same study, one might use different thresholds for different networks, thus creating potentially biased analysis. Fortunately, researchers have developed a grouping technique that partitions a network into mutually exclusive groups. This way each person belongs to one and only one group. The method also provides a measure of how well the data partition into these groups.

Girvan-Newman Technique

Girvan and Newman (2002; Newman and Girvan, 2004) used a technique of deleting selected links from a network to identify components. If one link connects two components in a network, then deleting that link would yield the two components, and the group structure of the network is nicely described by these two components. In this hypothetical example, the network structure is clear—one deleted link created two groups in which all the ties are contained within each group and there are no links between groups. Measuring how many links are within the groups and how many between the groups provides an indication of how well the group definitions characterize the network.

The problem now becomes which links to remove that are most likely to return separate components. Girvan and Newman (2002) suggested deleting those links that are most central in the network, the links with the highest centrality. Recall in Chapter 5 that it was mentioned briefly that centrality can be calculated on the network of links. Girvan and Newman suggested calculating centrality on the network of links (not the nodes). Every link has two nodes, but the location of those nodes affects the centrality calculations of the links. By calculating centrality on the links, researchers can identify those links that are the best candidates to remove to partition the network into mutually exclusive groups.

Grivan-Newman (GN) subgroups are derived by calculating betweenness centrality on the links, deleting the link with the greatest betweenness centrality, and then determining if there are any components. Each remaining component constitutes a group. After the link with the greatest betweenness centrality is located and deleted and any groups are detected, the process is repeated until the desired number of groups is reached. One can predetermine the number of groups desired, or the analyses can run until no groups greater than a specified size are detected. For example, if a researcher wanted to partition a large number of networks into six groups, then the number of groups can be fixed to six. On the other hand, the researcher can set the minimum group size, say three, and allow the algorithm to find multiple group structures and various group sizes.

The GN technique provides a partition of the network into mutually exclusive groups and it also measures how well the group partition characterizes the network. The measure for how well the groups characterize the network is called modularity (Newman and Girvan, 2004). Modularity is calculated by creating a matrix in which each row and column is one of the newly created groups. Each element in this new reduced matrix is the number of links from the original network between these created groups. The diagonal elements of the network are the number of links within each group. To calculate how well the group partition fits the data, the percentage of within group ties to between group ties is calculated. Newman and Girvan (2004) provides the equation:

$$Q = \sum_i (e_{ii} - a^2) = Tre - \| e^2 \|$$

(6-1)

where *Tre* is the trace of the matrix (the sum of the diagonal elements) and $\|e^2\|$ is the sum of all the elements in the matrix. Thus, this quantity, Q, indicates the percentage of ties in the network that occur within the groupings found by the algorithm. A Q of, say, 90% indicates almost all links are to members within the groups identified by NG, whereas one of 10% indicates that few are. The NG algorithm provides a way to partition a network into mutually exclusive groups and an index of how well that partition reflects the overall pattern of ties in the network. Thus, the researcher can choose among many competing partitions, selecting the one that best fits the data or selecting one with a less good fit but that is preferable for substantive reasons. A similar index, E-I, was suggested by Krackhardt and Stern, which takes the difference between the within-group and between-group links (Krackhardt & Stern, 1988). Figure 6–2 redraws the network in Figure 6–1 circling the groups identified by the GN algorithm in Netdraw. For example, 18, 20, 29 and 39 are in a group. From the picture the groups seem to make sense. The calculation of Q was 48.4%, indicating the 48.4% of the links are contained with the defined groups.

In some applications, the GN approach has clear advantages over *n*-clique and *k*-plex analysis because it provides a unique partition to the network and a measure, Q, that indicates how well the partition describes the network. One difficulty, of course is that networks with a high Q score will also

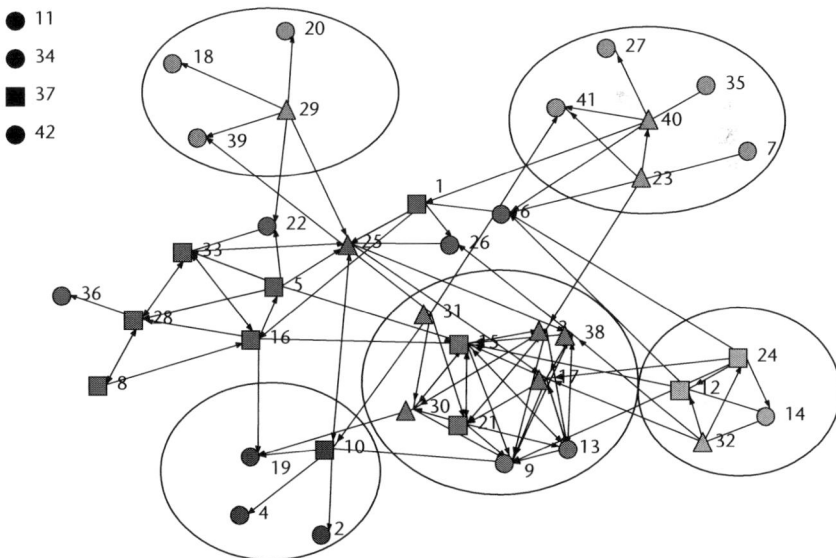

Figure 6–2. The network in Figure 6–1 with groups identified by the Newman-Girvan algorithm circled. Rates of smoking between groups varied, suggesting that group membership may affect individual smoking status.

have very distinct clustering results and networks with a low Q score are not modular and so are not well described by network partitions or clique/cluster analysis. The network in Figure 6–2 has a Q of 48%, which is pretty high, and so clique/cluster analysis and NG are somewhat descriptive of this network. In this example, there is considerable modularity in the network but there is no rule currently for what constitutes an acceptable Q value and this may vary by applications and research questions.

Groups and Behavior

Logic and empirical evidence indicate that people who belong to the same group will engage in the same behaviors. Groups have norms and members of the group are expected to uphold those norms. For example, if a person joins a chess club it is expected that he or she will play chess, enjoy chess, and value it as a game. Chess club members also probably value other games of mental acuity such as "Go" or bridge. Conversely, joining a sports team, such as football, signals athleticism and competition, which values physical strength.

In addition to these norms, though, groups also exert social pressure, sometimes subtly and sometimes overtly. To be a member of a group could mean that some members will have to display commitment to the group's values and group members may sometimes communicate to other members that they expect everyone to uphold these values. There is pressure to conform to group norms for behavior, sometimes overtly. The influence of group membership occurs both through selection and influence. A person selects a group to belong to because he or she is interested in the things that the group stands for. Once becoming a member, group members may pressure or persuade him or her to adopt the groups' norms.

Disentangling which comes first, selection or influence, is not always easy. Chance events may incline a person to join a particular group and then over time a person may feel pressured or compelled to adopt the group's norms. Moreover, once belonging to a group, the person may not want to risk the loss of camaraderie, companionship, solidarity, or belonging that would come from nonadoption of group behaviors. Both selection into a group and the influence of that group on individual attitudes and behaviors are processes that result in group members having similar attitudes and behaviors.

Groups also provide opportunities for information, resources, and support. Belonging to a group means that information available to the group will also be available to the individual and generally people will communicate more with group members than those outside the group. This increased communication means that members will be aware of and have access to whatever communication occurs within the group. It also means members may have access to resources that nongroup members do not have access to. For example, many people join a country club so they can network with other members.

In this sense, group membership provides one form of social capital. People usually trust others who are members of their group. *Social capital is the resources available from one's social networks.* Members of the same group tend to trust one another more than nonmembers, and because they are connected, there is more opportunity for a person to access the resources from others within the group. Thus, groups can increase connectivity among members and increase social capital.

Groups provide pressure for behavior change in another way. Interdependent innovations such as fax machines, email, text messaging, Facebook, and so on are innovations in which both parties have to adopt them for them to be used. Most (perhaps all) communication technologies are interdependent since their value is in the ability to provide communication and connection to others. If most members of a group adopt an interdependent behavior, then the nonadopters feel pressure to adopt. For example, if a person's friends begin to text message each other, he or she may feel pressure to begin text messaging to stay connected to the group.

The graph in Figure 6–2 also indicates whether each student reported being a current smoker. The symbols for the nodes correspond to the following: circle, no data; square, nonsmoker; triangle, smoker. Inspection of Figure 6–2 shows some clustering. Specifically, in the largest group, only two of the seven students for whom we have data reported being a smoker, whereas five of the seven students in the second largest group reported being a smoker. The other four groups report rates in between. We collapsed the grouping into three mutually exclusive groups, retaining the largest two and combining the other four, and compared the mean rates of smoking statistically. The smoking rates differed statistically significantly between groups (mean = 14.3% [SD = 37.8%], 71.1% [SD = 48.8%], and 57.1% [SD = 53.4%], respectively; $F = 2.79$; $p = .09$).

There is some evidence that belonging to a group is associated with behavior. At the most basic level, isolates have often been the last to adopt new ideas and practices across numerous behaviors (Valente, 1995). Isolates have few or no interpersonal sources of information or influence. Isolates often lack emotional and social supports necessary to adapt to changing circumstances. Joining groups provides a means to avoid being isolated.

Group Membership and Disease

Although belonging to a group can be advantageous in terms of access to information and resources, for disease spread, belonging to a group can increase risk. For example, belonging to a group of people who engage in risky sexual behavior may put one at increased risk of contracting a sexually transmitted disease. In general, group membership can protect one from disease as long as the incidence and prevalence of that disease in the group are low. Once prevalence reaches a critical threshold, however, being in the group puts one at increased risk since the disease will circulate rapidly in the closed group.

As long as the group is completely self-contained and has no outside contact, the group will remain immune and risk free. For example, communities that live in remote regions or on islands that are infrequently visited report being cold and flu free for some time. Eventually, however, a ship or airplane arrives bringing supplies, friends, families, and, of course, colds, the flu, and other illnesses (Gilmore, 1998). Group membership, therefore, can confer benefits, access to information, access to resources, and protection from disease if within-group prevalence is low. Conversely, group membership can be a liability if that group lacks resources or if disease prevalence is high.

Groups, Density, and Bridges

There is a tradeoff between the desire to form groups that are exclusive and consist of dense communications and commitments among its members versus having a group that maintains substantial ties outside the community. Earlier research has shown that community density was associated with more rapid diffusion of innovations (Valente, 1995). Dense networks provide more pathways than sparse ones, along which communication about new ideas and behaviors can flow. Sparse networks may not provide sufficient pathways for information to be circulated or for resources to be accessed, thus not conferring the benefits of the group. Density may also facilitate diffusion because dense networks may reflect a cohesive normative environment. A network with many links is more likely to have members who share common values or beliefs. Thus, a dense network may reflect a homogeneous community, and this homogeneity will facilitate information exchange and decision making.

Conversely, dense networks may not be efficient for several reasons. First, higher density may reflect more formal associations and these formal ties may not be as persuasive or trust-enhancing as informal ties (Krackhardt, 1992). Second, although there is a minimum density level needed for an organization or community to adopt innovations, once this level is reached, too much density may be a liability because it can limit connections to external information and resources. The lack of external ties then becomes a liability.

Organizational studies have shown that too much density can hurt performance (Oh et al., 2004; Uzzi, 1998). Finally, researchers have documented the tendency for groups to reinforce the opinions of members so that people fail to consider the perspectives of nonmembers. The relationship between density and performance, adoption behavior, or other outcomes is likely to be curvilinear as in Figure 6–3.

Figure 6–3 proposes that some basic level of density is necessary for organization, coalitions, and groups to function. The relationship between density and performance is likely to be nonlinear, the greater the density, the better the performance, or the more rapid the adoption of innovations. At some critical point, however, this relationship levels off and too much density begins to detract from performance. Exactly at which level density transitions from being an asset to a liability depends on the kind of performance or diffusion being studied and may depend on characteristics of the group members.

Support for this hypothesis was provided in a study of the effectiveness of satellite TV training of community coalitions to prevent substance use. Twenty-four community coalitions were randomly assigned to three conditions: control, satellite TV training, and satellite TV plus technical assistance. The coalitions were expected to adopt evidence-based programs for the prevention of substance use in their communities. Adoption was expected to be greater in dense coalitions and lesser in sparse ones. Surprisingly, however, coalitions that increased their density reported lower levels of program adoption (Valente et al., 2007). Figure 6–4 illustrates the

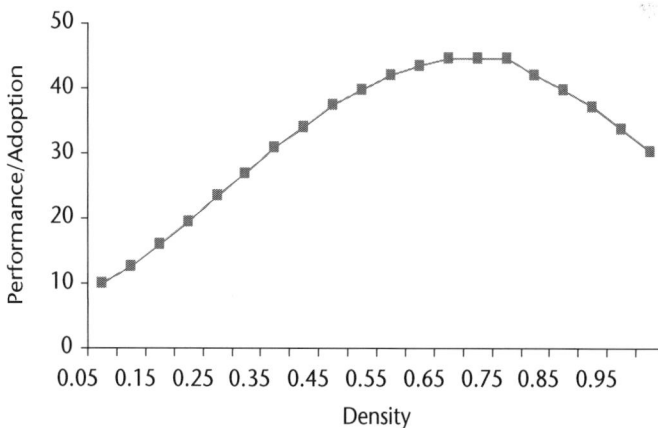

Figure 6–3. Proposed curvilinear association between performance or adoption and network density.

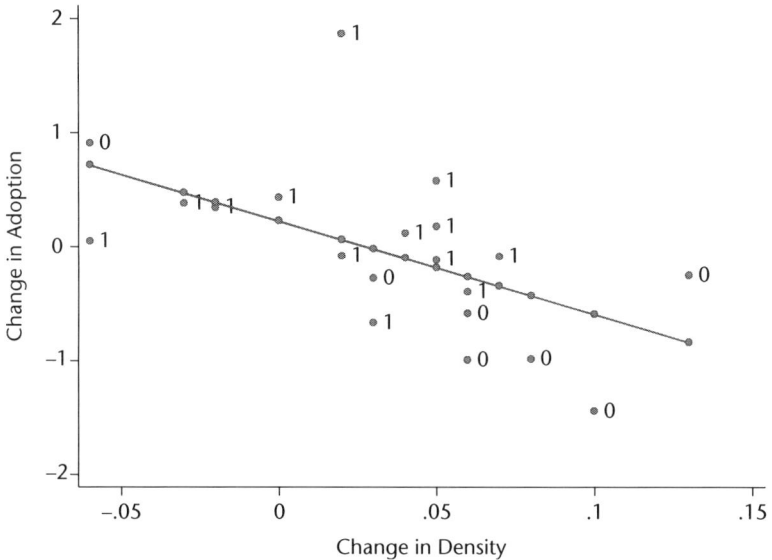

Figure 6–4. Decreased density was associated with increased adoption of evidenced based programs (or increased density was associated with less adoption). It is noteworthy that the communities labeled with "0" are the control ones and these control communities seem to pull down the association between density and adoption, indicating that they are responsible for this negative relationship.

main finding showing that an increase in density was associated with lower uptake of practices between year 1 and year 2.

The critical observation here is that too much density may restrict the formation of bridges between groups or from a group to outside information and resources. Most groups (organizations, coalitions, associations, etc.) need to balance the desire to create cohesion against the need to access new information and resources. Simply increasing the size of a coalition or hosting meetings designed to get everyone on the same page may not be the most effective means to create more effective organizations.

In follow-up analysis, we also showed that adoption of effective programs was also influenced by the centralization of the advice networks, after controlling for density (Fujimoto et al., in press). Decrease in centralization for the advice network and increased centralization in the discussion networks were associated with adoption. Networks based on friendships showed no consistent relationships to adoption. These analysis provide insight into the potential for optimizing networks for organizational and system performance. We return to this issue in Chapters 8 and 11 when discussing network-level indicators (Chapter 8) and network interventions (Chapter 11).

Summary

This chapter reviewed procedures and approaches to understanding how to define a group in network analysis. There are many different definitions of a group, but most agree that a group is a set of at least three people who are more closely connected to each other than to other people in the larger network. The definition of a clique was defined as a group in which each member is no more than n steps from every other member, a so-called n-clique. N can be varied to calculate different types of groups. k-plexes were defined as groups based on the number of other people in the group each person is connected to.

One challenge noted in this chapter is that many group definitions do not necessarily provide a mutually exclusive partition of the network into separate groups. That is, n-clique and k-plex analysis return a listing of many overlapping groups. This group analysis reflects the data and real world experience that many groups are not mutually exclusive, yet it can hamper statistical analysis of the relationship between group membership and behavior. The GN algorithm provides a means to identify groups in a network that are mutually exclusive and simultaneously provides an index of how well the network conforms to a mutually exclusive grouping pattern. We closed the chapter with a discussion of how groups may affect the diffusion of behaviors.

7

Positions

This chapter introduces positional analysis, which is conducted by defining positions in a network and reducing a network to these positions and mapping the relations between positions. The chapter also covers individual measures of positions in which nodes are defined as occupying the same position based on their connections to others or the similarity in their distances to others in the network. These individual equivalence positions can be used to group people into positions and to model the ways in which networks influence behavior.

Groups are aggregates of nodes/people who communicate or are connected to one another at a higher rate than others in the network. A network position, in contrast, is a set of nodes that occupy the same place or have similar relations with others in the network. Positions are composed of people who seem to be in the same space in the network, regardless of whether they are directly connected to one another, though they might be. Generally, a *position* is a set of nodes that has the same links to the same others or the same types of others.

The theoretical basis for defining positions comes from the sociological insight that people who occupy the same roles often act similarly. For example, fathers are alike even though they are fathers to different children. Network-defined positions constitute roles in the network and, consequently, people in the same position may behave similarly. Positional network analysis consists of (1) using mathematical algorithms to define distinct positions in the network, (2) studying how those positions relate to one another, and (3) determining how membership in a position might influence behavior.

Hummon and Carley (1993) studied publications in the *Social Networks* journal and concluded that the study of positions was the central theme in research on social networks up to the early 1990s. Position analysis has been popular in social network analysis because it uncovers macro-level structure of the network from micro-level analysis of network relations. Structural analysis is, to some extent, identifying positions in the network and then discovering how those positions relate to one another. Finding groups and measuring centrality and other network analysis activities are often considered less-structural analysis because they do not explicitly examine the interaction between micro- and macro-level network properties.

Position analysis is conducted at both the individual and network level. Individual position analysis is conducted by creating a measure of how equivalent two people are and then assigning a score for each pair of individuals based on that equivalence. Network-level position analysis is conducted by using mathematical algorithms to find positions in the network and then studying the relationships between these positions. Network-level position analysis consists of a set of positions and their interrelationships, whereas individual position analysis consists of a matrix of positional equivalence scores.

Network-Level Positions

Lorain and White (1971) wrote an influential paper in which they proposed that the relations between people in a network can be reduced to a set of positions and the relations between these positions also treated as a network (a meta-level network). In some research, the network representing the relations between positions is referred to as the *reduced-form network.* Lorain and White (1971) proposed that the network could be reduced to a set of blocks and the relations between blocks studied. This was called blockmodeling. Network researchers have developed different methods to identify the blocks (positions) and determine relations between positions (Doreian et al., 2005). The matrix or network that reports how the positions interact is referred to as the *image matrix,* the reduced-form network or matrix.

As in group definitions (Chapter 6), a strict criterion can be set for people to be members of a position and then the criterion gradually relaxed. As the definition is relaxed, it is possible to examine the pattern of positions created. The pattern of how members join positions can reveal facets of

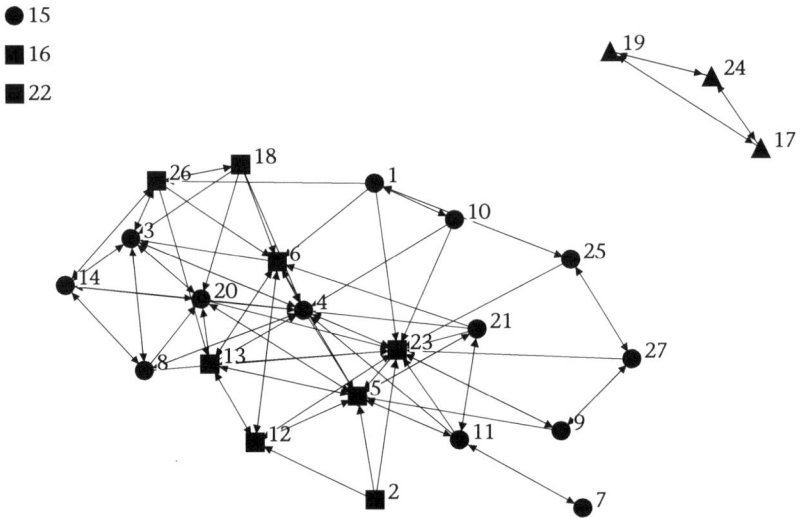

Figure 7–1. Network of class participants who knew one another at the start of the course. Shapes represent departments: square = A, circle = B, and triangle = C; number 23 is the Professor.

network structure and, of course, many different algorithms can be proposed for defining positions. In short, positional analysis and blockmodeling can get quite complex.

To illustrate how positions are defined, we use UCINET 6.0 (Borgatti et al., 2006) and the network shown in Figure 7–1, which shows who knew whom at the start of a course on network analysis. This course had 24 people initially, 3 of whom were faculty members, 1 who was the primary instructor, and 2 who sat in on many of the lectures to learn about social network analysis.

The class members were spread across three departments: A, B, and C. There were three faculty members in the course with one being the Professor, number 23. Casual inspection of the network shows some obvious structural patterns: (1) there were three isolates who were people registered for the wrong class and never attended; (2) there were three students from Department C who enrolled in the course and knew one another but no one in other departments; and (3) there might be some clustering based on other department affiliations but that is not clear from the graph.

A positional algorithm was applied to the data to determine if the different departments or statuses (faculty versus student) constituted distinct positions. The algorithm used was an optimization algorithm, which attempts to find the positions so that the blocks (the set of links within and between positions) have the least number of changes required to make the blocks all zeros or ones. A network divided into positions such that the blocks are all zeros or all ones is a perfectly partitioned network. This would indicate that all of the ties are within positions and there are no ties between positions. Notice the similarity between the positional approach and the Girvan-Newman method described in Chapter 6. The difference here is that the researcher specifies beforehand (a priori) which nodes belong to which positions.

Figure 7–2 reports the results of a blockmodel analysis of the network in Figure 7–1 using UCINET VI (Borgatti et al., 2006). Six positions were specified to test whether the four departments and two statuses (student and faculty) would yield different positions. Deciding on how many positions expected from a positional analysis should be driven by theory so that positional analysis confirms hypotheses rather than being treated as an exploratory approach in which one specifies various numbers in hopes of finding an interesting partition.

The results were interesting in that they partially confirmed intuition: department membership accounted for much of the variation in the network ties. Number 23 (B_F3), the instructor, was assigned a position by himself, which is not surprising because most of the students knew the instructor before the class. Positions 1 and 5 consisted of all Department B students (except number 2, A_F1), position 4 consisted of Department C students, and position 6 consisted of Department A students, one faculty member, and the "other" faculty member. Position 3 was mixed half Department A and half Department B.

UCINET also reports the number of "errors," which is the number of links that would need to be added or deleted to have a perfect blockmodeling structure. A perfect blockmodeling structure occurs when each block is composed of all ones (links) or all zeros (no links). For example, position one has 10 links to other people in position one. Since this value is below 50% of the total possible [28 = (8*7)/2)], it is more efficient to delete links (rather than add 18) to achieve a zero or one block. There are no errors between position 1 and position 2 because everyone in position 1 knew the person who occupies position 2. For links between position 1 and 3 through 6, "errors" consist of deleting links in those blocks as well, for a total of 22 errors. The errors in position 2 consist of one link within position 1, one with position 5, and one with position 6. Positions 2 through 6 had errors of 3, 11, 0, 8, and 9 for a total of 53 errors.

UCINET provides a display of the blockmodel network, the set of ties in the original matrix but with the people (nodes) sorted according to their position. One can easily see if there are links within and between positions; blocks with lots of zeros represent no connection between positions, whereas blocks with lots of ones indicate connections between positions. To determine how much connection is a *lot* of connection, a general rule is to compare densities within and between blocks with the density of the

```
Number of errors: 53
Errors per block
         1  2  3  4  5  6
        -- -- -- -- -- --
   1    10  0  2  0  3  7
   2     1  0  0  0  1  1
   3     1  0  2  0  5  3
   4     0  0  0  0  0  0
   5     0  2  2  0  2  2
   6     2  1  0  0  5  1
```

Blocked Adjacency Matrix

```
                      1 1 2 2   2     1 2 1 2 1   1 1 2     2     1     1 1
                    1 2 9 0 1 5 1 7   3   7 6 2 5 6 8   9 7 4   3 0 8 4 4   6 2 3 5
                    B A B B B B B B   A   B A A B A A   C C C   B B B B B   A A A O
                    ---------------------------------------------------------------
    1   B_S1   |      1   1     | 1 |         1     |         |         | 1       |
    2   A_F1   |                | 1 |               |         |         |   1   1 |
    9   B_S7   |            1   | 1 |               |         |         |       1 |
   10   B_S8   | 1              | 1 |               |         |     1   |         |
   11   B_S9   |            1   | 1 | 1             |         |     1   |       1 |
   25   B_S11  | 1          1   | 1 |               |         |         |         |
   21   B_S10  |       1        | 1 |               |         |     1   | 1     1 |
   27   B_S12  |     1     1    | 1 |               |         |         |         |
                    ---------------------------------------------------------------
   23   A_F3   |     1          |   |               |         |         | 1   1 1 1 |
                    ---------------------------------------------------------------
    7   B_S5   |       1        |   |               |         |         |         |
   16   A_S4   |                |   |               |         |         |         |
   22   A_S6   |                |   |               |         |         |         |
   15   B_S8   |                |   |               |         |         |         |
   26   A_S7   |                |   |           1   |       1 |     1 | 1   1   |
   18   A_S5   |                |   |         1     |       1 1   1   | 1       |
                    ---------------------------------------------------------------
   19   C_S2   |                |   |               | 1 1 |             |         |
   17   C_S1   |                |   |               | 1   1 |           |         |
   24   C_S3   |                |   |               | 1 1 |             |         |
                    ---------------------------------------------------------------
    3   B_S2   |                |   |           1   |       1 1 1 1 |           |
   20   B_S9   |                | 1 |               |       1     1 1 |         1 |
    8   B_S6   |                | 1 |               |       1 1   1 1 |         1 |
    4   B_S3   |                | 1 |               |       1   1   1 |         1 |
   14   B_S7   |                |   |         1     |       1 1 1 1 |           |
                    ---------------------------------------------------------------
    6   A_S4   |                |   |               |       1       1 |   1 1 1 |
   12   A_F2   |                | 1 |               |         |         | 1   1 1 |
   13   A_S5   |                |   |               |       1   1 | 1 1   1 |
    5   Oth_F2 |     1   1      |   |               |         | 1       | 1   1 |
                    ---------------------------------------------------------------
```

Density Table

	1	2	3	4	5	6
Dept B	0.18	1.00	0.04	0.00	0.08	0.22
Prof.	0.13		0.00	0.00	0.20	0.75
Mixed	0.02	0.00	0.07	0.00	0.17	0.13
Dept C	0.00	0.00	0.00	1.00	0.00	0.00
Dept B	0.00	0.60	0.07	0.00	0.90	0.10
Dept A	0.06	0.25	0.00	0.00	0.25	0.92

Image Matrix

	1	2	3	4	5	6
Dept B	1	1	0	0	0	1
Prof.	0	0	0	0	1	1
Mixed	0	0	0	0	1	0
Dept C	0	0	0	1	0	0
Dept B	0	1	0	0	1	0
Dept A	0	1	0	0	1	1

Figure 7–2. Blockmodel results for the network class data.

118

whole network. If block densities are larger than the overall network density, there is a connection or link between these blocks. In this case, the overall network density is 12.7%. This value (12.7%) can be compared to the densities of the subnetworks indicated by links between positions (the block of links indicating connections between positions). If the density between two blocks (positions) exceeds 12.7% (the overall average), then the blocks are connected. When densities are below the average, the blocks/positions are not connected.

It is worth reiterating the approach here. The overall network is partitioned into a set of positions. The links in the network are then reconfigured to show the links within a position and between positions. These are the "blocks." If the proportion of links (the density) connecting any two positions (within a block) is greater than that which occurs on average in the network (the overall density), then a link between positions can be inferred. The network has been reduced to a set of positions, and it has been determined at the macro-level how these positions relate to one another. This network of 27 people has been reduced to a network of six positions. The resulting reduced-form network is referred to as the image matrix. So the image network or matrix is the set of links between positions—in this case, a six-by-six matrix.

In this class example, position 1 is connected to positions 1, 2, and 6, because the densities (0.18, 1.00, and 0.22) all equal or exceed the overall density of 0.127. Similarly, position 2 is connected to positions 5 and 6, and so on. Note the image matrix does not have to be symmetric: relations from one position can be directed to another without those relations being reciprocated. For example, position 1 is connected to position 2, but 2 is not connected to 1.

A substantive aspect of blockmodeling and positional analysis is to label the positions and interpret the relations between positions. So rather than just say positions 1, 2, 3, and so on, the research can examine the attributes of the people in positions to determine if they can be logically grouped. For example, in an organizational study, the members of positions may conform mostly to organizational roles or task responsibilities (management versus sales, for example). Often, if a position is linked asymmetrically to another, researchers interpret this relationship as one of power or control. In this example, the positions are clearly indicated by department affiliations: Departments A, B, and C and the Professor. The positions conform almost exactly to the departments with the one exception being the mixed department.

Figure 7–3 graphs the image matrix providing a visual display of the positional relations. It reveals the structure of the network showing that Department C is isolated. It also shows the Mixed position reports knowing people in Department B, but those ties are not reciprocated. The Department A position has reciprocated ties with the Professor but not with the two

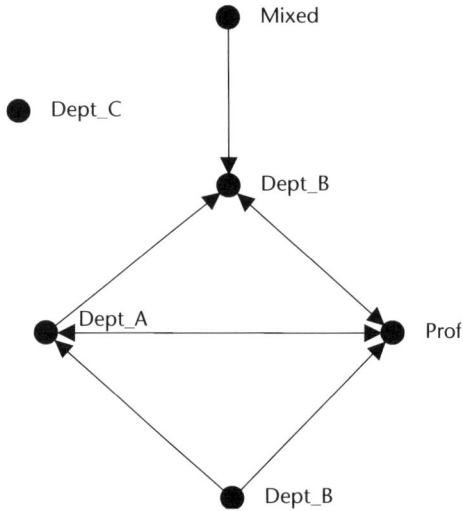

Figure 7–3. Graph of the image matrix providing a visual display of the positional relations. It reveals the structure of the network showing the Department C position is isolated while Department B at the top and the Professor occupy positions of power. Department B at the bottom reports ties to Department A and the Professor, but those links are not reciprocated at the positional (macro) level.

Department B positions. A naïve interpretation would lend one to believe the Professor is in the most comfortable position having two symmetric ties with Departments A and B and one incoming tie from Department B. Department B at the top, however, has a symmetric relation with the Professor and two incoming links from the Mixed and Department A positions. It is important to note that this type of position analysis can be conducted using attributes as the positional indicators. For example, the researcher could repeat this analysis by assigning four positions based on the department affiliations rather than letting the computer generate the positions.

It is perhaps instructive to compare this positional analysis to a group analysis (Chapter 6) of the same network. We ran the Newman-Girvan algorithm on these data and selected the best-fitting model. Some key differences emerged, including that the Professor was grouped with a new Mixed department group, which included students from Departments A and B and one other faculty member, and the other two faculty were grouped together. Thus, the resulting structure, using the Newman-Girvan group algorithm, was quite different from the positional analysis.

A network with several positions and an image network consisting of directional links pointing to one of those positions is an example of a hierarchical network. In this case, the network analysis has uncovered a situation in which one position holds a high status position and possibly members of this position enjoy a position of power. Although such a network is also likely to be centralized (see Chapter 5), the positional analysis and resulting image diagram provide a different, and possibly more informative, analysis of the overall network structure.

CONCOR

One of the most common structural equivalence position generators is CONCOR, which is an abbreviation of "converging correlations." CONCOR uses correlation analysis to find positions in a network and uses a square binary network as input. The first step is to compute correlations between the rows in the matrix. This produces a matrix of correlations with each cell indicating the degree of correlation between cases (the degree of similarity between two nodes). The rows in the correlation matrix are then correlated. This process is repeated successive times. Ultimately, the repeated correlations produce a matrix of all positive and negative ones, indicating cases perfectly similar and dissimilar. The network is then partitioned into two sets based on the positive and negative ones (the perfect correlations). CONCOR has thus produced a partition of the network into two positions. The process is repeated to divide the initial two groups into four groups (two for each initial position) and so on until each position has as few as two members. The researcher decides at which point to stop the CONCOR process and accept the positions identified.

CONCOR analysis is appealing because it provides an unbiased, mathematical partition of the network into positions, requiring little substantive or theoretical insight from the researcher. One limitation of the CONCOR approach is that the analysis is driven entirely by the performance of the mathematical process of correlating rows and columns. A second limitation is that using correlations to measure node equivalence may not necessarily be the best method for doing so (see later). Further, because successive iterations of the correlation matrix eventually produce ones and negative ones, correlations of quite different magnitude are eventually treated the same. That is, a correlation of 0.51 and one of 0.90 may both be eventually converted to 1s during the same partition. A third limitation is that CONCOR forces a bifurcation of the network into two positions, and then two more, and so on, whereas many networks and subnetworks may not conveniently be divided into two distinct positions.

These limitations aside, CONCOR does a good job of identifying positions based on node similarities. The process is automatic and correlations are a good measure of similarity. Further, the researcher can examine the successive partitions of the network into positions and choose to use a partition that conforms to some substantive knowledge of the data.

Individual Positional Measures

The preceding discussion provided a means of reducing a network to a set of positions and to map the relations between positions. It is often desirable to calculate the degree to which two people are similar, or occupy the same position in a network, without necessarily creating network positions. Individual positional measures provide measures of node similarity based on their connections in the network and in some cases based on all the links in the network. Individual position measures are dyadic measures as they are not measures for each person but, instead, are measures for every pair of people in the network.

The simplest positional measure would indicate the similarity of two people's contacts. For example, two people who are connected and not connected to exactly the same other people in the network are perfectly equivalent. Equivalent nodes occupy the same position. From a network perspective, two equivalent nodes are substitutable as they have the same exact relations with others in the network. Notice that two equivalent nodes do not have to be connected to one another to be equivalent. They can be perfectly equivalent and not connected. This measure of equivalence is referred to as *matches* in UCINET and is a simple comparison of two node's ties. Matches compare the links and nonlinks that each pair of nodes has with everyone else in the network, yet it may be more accurate to compare only the connections and ignore the nonconnections in the calculation. Because some network data are collected by asking for a person to list their five closest friends, the nonconnections that two people share are not as informative as the connections they have in common. Positive matches are the percentage of ties two people have in common and provide a good intuitive measure of structural similarity.

Figure 7–4 displays a structurally equivalent pair based on positive matches. Person A and Person B are connected to the same people and so they are perfectly substitutable and structurally equivalent from a network perspective. If Person A had one other connection, then it would slightly diminish the degree of structural equivalence or similarity between Persons A and B.

One useful measure of structural equivalence was developed by Burt (1987) based on distances. The distance measure of structural equivalence is derived from geographic measures in which two cities are similar if they are the same distances from other cities. For example, Chicago and St. Louis (two U.S. cities) are similarly distant from Los Angeles (LA), Denver, San Francisco, Seattle, New York (NY), Washington, DC, Atlanta, and so on.

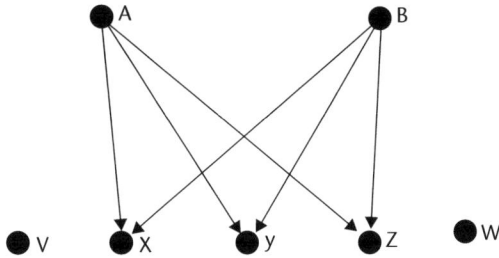

Figure 7–4. People are structurally equivalent when they are linked to the same other people. A and B have ties and non-ties to the same others in the network and so are structurally equivalent.

The difference in the distances between Chicago and every large city and between St. Louis and every large city is fairly small because Chicago and St. Louis are similarly distant from all U.S. cities. In contrast, the differences in distances between NY and LA to all the large US cities is quite large because the cities near NY are far from LA and vice versa.

The calculation of distance differences is referred to as *Euclidean distance*, and this provides a measure of structural equivalence. Two people are structurally equivalent to the extent they have the same distances to everyone else in the network. So a measure of Euclidean distances is given by Burt (1987) as:

$$D_{ij} = \sqrt{\sum_k (z_{ik} - z_{jk})^2 + \sum_k (z_{ki} - z_{kj})^2}$$

(7-1)

where z_{ik} is the distance from i to k measured as the number of steps in the network. This formula takes the difference of distances, squares each one (to get rid of negative values), and sums those differences. It is calculated in both directions (the distance from i to k and the distance from to k to i) because networks can be asymmetric. The distance from i to k and the distance from to k to i are not necessarily the same in network analysis. Using Euclidean distances to calculate structural equivalence is appealing because the measure considers the overall pattern of ties in the network, not just the direct ties for every pair of nodes.

Individual Measures as Positions

The individual measures of structural equivalence (SE), such as matches and Euclidean distance, can be used to find network-level positions. Once the matrix of SE scores are calculated, people can be grouped together based on their similarity of SE scores. For example, everyone with similarity scores of 1.0 can be considered a position; then that criterion can be relaxed to 0.95, 0.90, and so on, down to zero. The result is a series of position grouping based on a relaxation of the criterion of what it means to be in a position.

The pattern of position identifications can be graphically displayed so that the researcher can see which nodes belong to which positions at various cut-off levels. One can then examine the positional definitions and choose a cut-off value to use to define the positions based solely on the empirical pattern or based on some substantive criterion. Researchers can compare different individual (read dyadic) measures of equivalence to determine whether there are differences in the identified positions.

Positions and Behavior

Clearly, finding positions in a network and assessing the degree of equivalence between actors is interesting from a research standpoint and can have substantive meaning when trying to understand networks. Does positional equivalence influence behavior? From a disease perspective, it is not immediately obvious how position equivalence affects one's likelihood of contracting a disease because communicable diseases are spread by person-to-person contact. On the other hand, people in the same positions may be exposed to the same kinds of pathogens and so positional equivalence could be important to know.

For example, a positional analysis of sexual relations among a large network might reveal a set of positions such that one position is obviously a core group of sexually active individuals. Other positions that have contact with the core group may be at increased risk for sexually transmitted infections due to their contact with that group. All members of these positions may be at increased risk for disease. Although the risk factor is sexual contact, the positional analysis indicates why some people are at increased risk compared with others, even though their rate of sexual activity may be the same.

For behavioral influence, positional and structural equivalence measures may matter very much. In any given community, two people who occupy the same position in the network are likely to be very similar and they are likely to monitor each other's behavior. This is particularly true in business; firms that occupy the same position in a network of suppliers, clients, and regulatory agencies are likely to be quite aware of what their structurally equivalent firms are doing because these are cues to appropriate strategic action. In short, as Burt (1987) argued, social influence may in some cases flow via structurally equivalence rather than direct ties.

There are several reasons why influence may pass between SE people. First, competition often motivates action and SE people or organizations may feel in competition with one another and so monitor each other's behavior. Once one or a few people SE people engage in a behavior, others are likely to do so to remain competitive. Second, SE people, being connected to the same others, may be influenced by those to whom they are connected. For example, two SE professors are connected to the same students and so may get information and influence from those students. Finally, persons in the same position may have other attributes that put them in that position and these characteristics are associated with the adoption behavior. For example, managers in the same position may also be recipients of bonuses for adopting specific practices.

The influence of direct ties was labeled cohesive influence, and throughout the 1990s there were numerous comparisons between cohesion influence and that of structural equivalence. The central research question was: What influenced a person more in their adoption decisions—the behavior of people they are directly connected to, say as someone they turn for advice (cohesion), or the behavior of people who occupy the same position in the network structure (structural equivalence)?

In earlier analyses, Valente (1995) conducted position analysis (CONCOR) on 40 networks from three studies. Once the positions were established in each network, analysis (using ANOVA [analysis of variance]) was conducted to determine if behavioral adoption times were significantly different between positions. It was expected that people in the same position would have similar adoption times and people in different positions would have different adoption times. In 35 of 40 of the networks, the adoption times did not differ significantly between positions; thus, there was no support for the hypothesis that network position was associated with adoption.

The analysis was not necessarily comprehensive because there are multiple ways to determine positions in a network. Further, Valente (1995) did not examine each network to see if the CONCOR analysis produced similar positional structures. For example, did the networks have similar image matrix patterns or were they different between networks? Perhaps diffusion was a function of how the positions related to one another. It was also not clear how the network level positional analysis would compare to influences based on direct ties. One possible means to determine if network position affects behavioral adoption is to use individual positional analysis.

Network Weights

Valente (1995, 2005) compared network exposure based on cohesion with that based on structural equivalence in three diffusion network datasets. Exposure via direct contacts did not influence adoption, whereas in one dataset, Brazilian farmers' adoption of hybrid seed corn, exposure via structural equivalence did influence adoption. These models also included terms for infection (the degree one's number of nominations received affected adoption) and susceptibility (the degree one's number of nominations sent affected adoption). It was surprising that the network exposure terms were not more significantly associated with adoption, and in Chapter 10 more extensive treatment of these findings and analysis are provided.

It is important to note here, though, how we can use the construction of structural equivalence weights to create general social influence models based on many theoretical ideas of how social influence occurs. The cohesion social influence model states that a person is influenced by the behavior of those they are connected to. The exposure model is:

$$E_{Nt} = \frac{W_{ij}B_{it}}{A_{i+}} \tag{7-2}$$

where E is the exposure matrix, W is the network weight matrix, B is the behavior matrix, A is the original adjacency matrix, N is network size, and t is time. The behavior matrix indicates who has adopted the behavior at each time period. Exposure is calculated by multiplying the weight matrix by the adoption matrix and dividing by the number of network choices made. In the basic model, W indicates who is connected to whom (the adjacency matrix). This model can be expanded to include other Ws, types of connectivity or similarity.

W, for example, could be structural equivalence scores and exposure calculated on the degree structurally equivalent alters have adopted the behavior. W can be any permutation of A that indicates the degree of similarity (or difference) among the dyads. (Note W can also be constructed from attribute data by calculating the degree dyads are similar on some characteristics such as their education level, ethnicity, or attitude toward a behavior.) Different social influence processes can be modeled by changing W. For example, if the researcher thought that social influence would be stronger between people who shared some characteristics, say gender, then W could be created as a product of network connections and gender such that a tie in W existed only among people who nominated one another and were of the same gender.

Summary

This chapter provided an introduction to defining positions in networks. Positions are often defined as a grouping of nodes in a network based on the pattern of their connections to others in the network. Two people can be in the same position in the network if they have the same ties to the same others even though they might not be directly connected. There are many different algorithms used to identify structurally equivalent positions, notably the percentage of matches between two nodes or the degree of similarity in their distances to other nodes (structural equivalence).

Once these positions are identified, the researcher may reduce the network to these positions and create what is referred to as an image matrix. In an image matrix, each position is a node in the network and links are created between the nodes to indicate if there is a relationship between the positions. The image matrix provides a macro-structural view of the network. The chapter also discussed CONCOR, a popular algorithm used to find positions in a network.

The chapter closed with a discussion of positions and behavior and how diffusion and positional analysis may be used to understand how behaviors flow through networks. We then discussed how matrices of SE relations may be used to calculate SE-weighted network exposure. Persuasive influence may be a function of people directly connected (cohesion exposure) or may be driven by monitoring of structurally equivalent others, people who occupy the same position in the network.

8

Network-Level Measures

Network-level measures are measures calculated on the whole network. These measures provide indicators of network structure. Eight network indicators are reviewed: size, density, reciprocity/mutuality, triadic census/transitivity, average path length (APL), clustering, centralization, and core-periphery. The chapter then reviews two-mode data and closes with a discussion of network-level measures and behavior.

One of the more intuitive and interesting ways to study social networks is at the network level. The previous chapter discussed how a network could be reduced to a set of positions and the relations between positions were analyzed. Network-level measures examine the network globally, from a bird's eye view (if you will). Different networks within the same community can be compared. For example, how do friendship and advice-seeking compare in an organization? This chapter reviews various network-level measures and shows how network properties affect behaviors within those networks. Some might argue that because network measures ask about relations within the network, network-level analysis is the most appropriate level of analysis. The network-level measures will be presented, to some extent, in their order of complexity.

Size

Network size is an important structural property, and it affects many other network indicators. Network size may be dictated by the study setting or research requirements. For example, studying adolescents in schools means that network size will be the classroom, grade, or school size. In other settings, the researcher may specifically set the network size of interest, perhaps by studying organizations with 100 to 250 employees. Some researchers estimate that a practical size for a group is about 150 people and some evidence exists that 150 is an optimal size for a human group (Dunbar, 1993).

Size may also be a function of individual network size or of how many people a person knows or has a meaningful relationship with. There is a practical limit on the number of people one can know or can maintain relationships with. Some researchers estimate the average size of acquaintance networks in the United States is approximately 280 (Killworth et al., 2006). A team of researchers from the University of Florida has conducted several studies to estimate network size (Killworth, 1990). Although people may know as many as several thousand other people, the set of contacts they may be able to name on any given topic is likely much smaller.

Size also indicates something about the networks of study. If one studies middle schools in various U.S. states and there are over 1,000 students in the middle schools of some states yet less than 50 students in the schools in others, it indicates something about the schools. Larger schools may have a larger range of student characteristics and a more complex administrative structure than smaller schools. Also, in larger schools, the range of possible people a student can develop relationships with is greater than in a small school. Size may not be the most interesting network indicator and may only reflect the boundary of the network, but it is the primary network indicator. As mentioned in Chapter 6, networks are often composed of separate components, in which case it is important to report the size of the components. The next network measure is density, the number of links in the network.

Density

Density is the number of connections in the network reported as a fraction of the total links possible. Density is calculated as:

$$D = \frac{l}{N(N-1)}$$

(8-1)

where l is the number of links in the network and n is network size. Density is a key attribute of a network and should always be included as a covariate in analyses testing the effects of other structural properties. Equation 8-1 is applicable for asymmetric networks (in which the links are directed), but the numerator must be multiplied by 2 for undirected (symmetric) networks.

Density is also often calculated on subgroups within the network. For example, it might be hypothesized that network density differs by some attribute. Friendship networks among middle school students are often gender based so that boys are friends with boys and girls are friends with girls. Density can be calculated on ties among boys and between boys and girls. Density is a fundamental parameter for networks and subgroups within the networks. Density can also be used as a threshold value to determine interposition links as in blockmodeling (see Chapter 7).

There is an inverse relationship between size and density: as size increases, density decreases. Size is inversely related to density for at least two reasons. First, as mentioned earlier, there are practical limits to the number of other people a person knows or can establish relationships with. So as the boundary definition for the network increases, the limit on each individual's network size indicates that density will decrease. Second, in small groups, organizations, and communities, it is easier for people to know everyone in the network. For example, in a small organization of 10 employees, everyone will know everyone else and be pretty familiar with their day-to-day activities. Conversely, in a large organization of 250 or more employees, many employees will not know other employees. Consequently, all analysis of networks at the network level should include density as a covariate.

Although density is calculated as the proportion of links in the network, in nomination studies this formula may be modified to account for the limited number of network nominations solicited. In a nomination study in which the researcher asks respondents to name up to seven of their closest friends, the researcher may elect to report effective density, which is the number of links divided by size multiplied by seven. Thus, effective density is calculated as:

$$D_E = \frac{l}{N(\lambda)}$$

(8-2)

where l is the number of links, N is network size, and λ is the maximum number of nominations requested.

Mutuality/Reciprocity

Reciprocated or mutual ties are links in which the direction goes both ways: If A chooses B, then B chooses A. Reciprocity is often referred to as *mutuality* because reciprocated ties are mutual, and this term may be preferred because reciprocity can be a bit ambiguous. Reciprocity is ambiguous because there is both direct and indirect reciprocity (indirect reciprocity is when A chooses B but B does not choose A but chooses C who chooses A). Mutual, directly reciprocated, ties are symmetric while those that are not mutual are asymmetric.

Some relations (networks) are inherently mutual or symmetric, such as when asking, "With whom did you have lunch?" If a person had lunch with someone, it is expected that other person had lunch with the focal person. Conversely, other relations are inherently asymmetric such as, "Whom did you go to for advice?" It is quite likely a person goes to someone possessing greater expertise or authority for advice and that person is unlikely to reciprocate that nomination. Thus, measuring and understanding the degree of reciprocity in a network are important.

Reciprocity is measured (Borgatti et al., 2006):

$$R = \frac{\left(A_{ij} = 1\right) \text{ and } \left(A_{ji} = 1\right)}{\left(A_{ij} = 1\right) \text{ or } \left(A_{ji} = 1\right)} \tag{8-3}$$

where A_{ij} indicates a link from i to j. A high degree of reciprocity indicates that people choose one another. This also means that people are choosing one another and not others and this can create more clustering within the network, thus increasing the distances in the network. Reciprocity can be an individual-level measure and a network-level one. At the individual level, reciprocity is a count or the proportion of reciprocated ties. At the network level, it is reported as the proportion of reciprocated links in the network (Equation 8-3).

Reciprocated ties may also suggest stronger ties. For example, in friendship networks, best friend ties are more likely to be reciprocated, whereas those among less close friends are less likely to be reciprocated. Tie strength can be measured as the order in which one provides names in response to a survey question, assuming that people provide the names of their closest friends first and less close friends later. Reciprocity can be included in this calculation by defining *closeness* as reciprocated friends.

For some behaviors, reciprocity may be associated with a greater likelihood of engaging in the behavior together or for the pair to influence each other. For example, several studies have shown that people are more likely to engage in risky behavior with closer ties than with distant ones (Valente & Vlahov, 2001). Risky drug and sexual behaviors occur more frequently with close and strong contacts because there is a higher degree of trust and intimacy with these close contacts and it would be impolite to use protective measures with such close friends. For example, two people engaged in a romantic relationship often do not use condoms as protection because they want to communicate their trust and commitment to one another. In contrast, condom use may be more prevalent among casual sexual partners because there is no need to communicate trust and intimacy. In short, one might expect more behavioral influence between reciprocated relationships.

Triads/Transitivity

Reciprocity compared the links between two nodes, but what about the links between three nodes? The links between three nodes are referred to as *triads,* and in a directed network there are 16 possible combinations of links connecting three nodes (Holland & Leinhart, 1979). One measure of network structure is to describe the prevalence of these 16 types for the network (Figure 8–1). Of particular interest is transitivity in the network's triads. Transitivity in a network exists when there is the following combination of links among three nodes: if A → B, and B → C, then A → C (number 030T in Figure 8–1). This triad is considered transitive because A and B both have the same relationship to C.

Transitivity forms the basis of much sociological thinking about how people function in groups. Balance theory argued that people preferred a

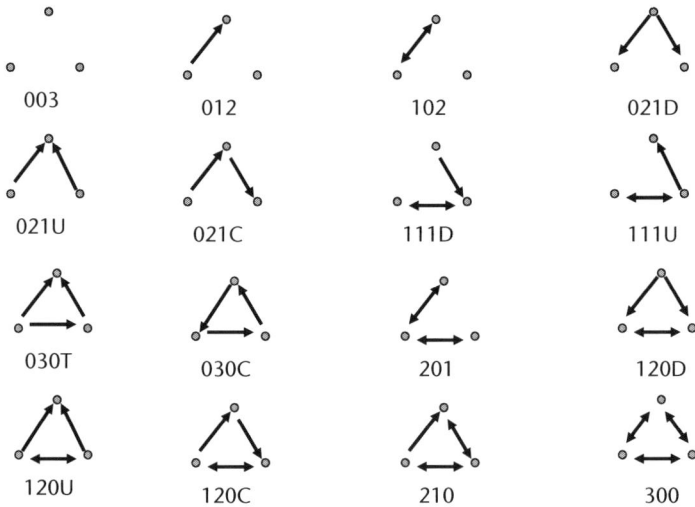

Figure 8-1. There are 16 possible configurations for the links between three nodes. These configurations are referred to as the MAN distribution for the number of mutual (M), asymmetric (A), and null (N) links among the nodes. Code 120 refers to 1 mutual, 2 asymmetric, and zero null links in the triad.

balanced environment with the people around them (Heider, 1958). If A and B are friends (from A's perspective) and A likes C, then A would want B to also like C. In balance theory, C could be a person or an attitude or object, such as a political opinion, a new product on the market, a behavior, and so on. People struggle to keep their world in balance, and Festinger (1954) introduced the idea of *cognitive dissonance,* which is the discomfort one feels when their environment is out of balance. Festinger (1954) argued that people will try to reduce their cognitive dissonance by trying to bring balance in their life—by trying to reduce intransitive triads.

The tendency toward transitivity is the basis for the strength of weak ties theory proposed by Granovetter (1973). As Granovetter (1973) stated, the tendency for transitivity means that triads like number 201 in Figure 8–1 were uncommon (referred to as the forbidden triad [Granovetter, 1973]). So intransitive triads are rare, and because they are rare, there are few weak ties in the network. Yet the scarcity of these weak ties makes them strong in terms of their information capacity.

Researchers conduct transitivity analysis by reporting the proportion of transitive triads in the network. Networks with high levels of transitivity are thought to be cohesive and, thus, in a broad sense may be thought of as effective. Researchers conduct triad analysis by calculating the proportion of triads in the network that can be classified in the 16 categories Holland and Linehardt (1979) defined. These categories are often referred to as the MAN categories since there was a three-digit code defined for each category corresponding to the number of mutual (M), asymmetric (A), and null (N) links in each triad. So a code of 111 indicates one mutual tie, one asymmetric tie, and one null tie as the links among the three nodes, and a code of 210 indicates two mutual ties, one asymmetric, and zero null ones as the links among the three nodes.

So any network can be described in terms of the proportion of triads in the network of each of the 16 types. This is called a triad census. Understanding triads and their distribution in the network is important because triads have provided the basis for many social network effects (Faust, 2008). The strength of weak ties, for example, is predicated on the notion that there are few 201 triads (two mutual links and one null) and therefore weak ties are rare. Burt (1992) used triad census to stress the importance of structural holes, and Fernandez and Gould (1994) used triads to develop measures of brokerage. Faust (2008) has shown that using limited choice sociometric surveys (fixed number of nominations) result in networks that have a limited distribution of the triad census.

The reader might expect the next network structural property consists of analysis of four nodes, because reciprocity involved two nodes and triads/ transitivity involved three. Analysis of the properties of four nodes, however, is considered group analysis, and group calculations were discussed in Chapter 6. One network property in connection with groups is the number of components. It is important to determine the number of components in a network. The next network-level property concerns the number of steps it takes to transverse the network.

Diameter/Average Path Length

Two fundamental properties of a network are its diameter, the length of the longest path in the network, and the average distance between nodes. Networks with the same number of nodes, and even the same density (number of links), can have different diameters because the diameter is the number of steps in the longest path in the network. The network in Figure 8–2 shows who went to whom for advice in one community coalition designed to promote community-based substance abuse prevention activities (Jasuja, 2005; Valente et al., 2007). The length of the longest path in this network

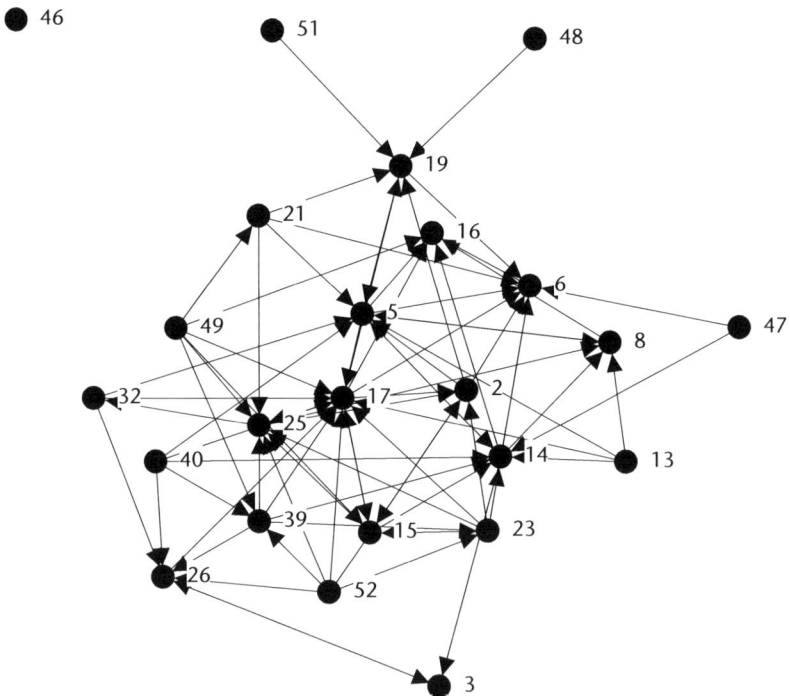

Figure 8–2. Network from one community coalition indicating to whom they turned for advice about prevention.

is five. For example, to go from person 3 to person 10 requires five steps: $3 \rightarrow 26 \rightarrow 17 \rightarrow 2 \rightarrow 5 \rightarrow 10$. There are numerous five-step paths in the network, and because this is the maximum in the network, it is the diameter. Network diameter then is the maximum distance between nodes in the network.

Average path length in a network is also an important structural property. The average path length (APL) is the average of the distances between all the nodes in a network. (APL is sometimes referred to as the characteristic path length.) A small APL indicates a cohesive network, while a large one indicates greater overall distances between nodes. For the network in Figure 8–3, the average distance between reachable people was 2.28. So, on average everyone in this network is 2.28 steps away from everyone else in the network provided they could reach one another. The APL is calculated by calculating the distances between all pairs of nodes in the network and then calculating the average (being sure to omit the diagonal).

Diameter and APL provide an overall indication of the structure of the network. Low diameter or low APL indicate a cohesive network with little clustering. The researcher need not know anything about specific group or positional distinctions but instead relies only on this one numeric indicator to draw conclusions about network topography. On the other hand, a network with large diameter and small APL may indicate that there are branches or spurs to the network that are mostly inaccessible to others in the network. One way to test the network structural tendencies would be to generate a sample, say 1,000, networks with the same size and density as the empirical (focal) network and calculate the diameter and APLs for these simulated networks (see Chapter 9). The researcher can then compare the empirical network indicators (diameter, APL) with the randomly generated distribution of networks with a test (a t-test) to determine if the network indicator is larger or smaller than would be expected by chance.

Density and Cohesion

All things being equal, as size increases, so does the APL, although not as much as one might think. On the other hand, the relationship between APL and density is nonlinear. As density increases, APL decreases, because high-density levels provide many paths along which to connect nodes. Research has shown, however, that the relationship between density and cohesion (APL) is not uniformly negative.

Figure 8–3 graphs changes in cohesion calculated for link deletions and additions for a large sample of randomly generated networks of size 10 for

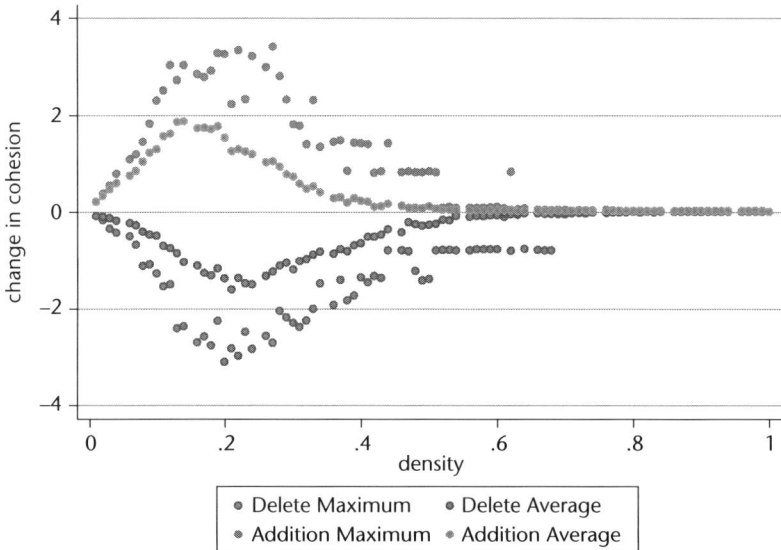

Figure 8–3. Maximum and average changes in cohesion scores as links are subtracted and added to the network by density. There is a sweet spot in social networks when density is between 15% and 25%, in which link changes have a profound affect on network cohesion. When density is very low and when it exceeds 50%, individual link changes have little effect on network cohesion because there is either no network (density is too low) or too much network (density is so high that individual links have little meaning).

levels of density from 1 to 100 percent. At each density level, 50 different networks were created (because there are many different network structures at each density level). Notice that changes in cohesion (maximum and APL for the network) peak between 15% and 25% densities, indicating that networks in this density range can have their cohesion changed the most by the deletion of links. At 50% density and above, link changes have little effect on cohesion, because there are many redundant paths between nodes.

These simulated data indicate an interesting characteristic about networks. Density values above 50% indicate networks that have many redundant paths between nodes. Deleting links, or even nodes, in such networks will have little effect on overall network properties. Networks with 50% or greater density do not contain much structural information and in many cases are not likely to be interesting substantively. In such cases, it will probably be desirable to "prune" the network so that the researcher can find the hidden structure within the tangle of links. The pruning can be conducted several ways, perhaps first by considering stronger ties if the links are weighted. Next, the researcher can consider only reciprocated ties.

Clustering

Network clustering is a measure of the degree of "clumpiness" in a network. A network with high clustering indicates that nodes are connected in dense pockets of interconnectivity, whereas one with low clustering has few pockets of interconnectivity. Clustering provides an index of the degree of structure in the network. So while the group and position analyses provided in Chapters 6 and 7 detail ways to find groups and positions, clustering provides a single measure of how much the groups and positions define or characterize the network.

Clustering is calculated by computing the average of each node's personal network density (Watts & Strogatz, 1998). Personal network density is the degree to which a person's ties are connected to one another. Figure 8–4 illustrates the calculation of personal network density—the person A on the left has three contacts (depicted as the thick solid lines, connecting A with x, y, and z). And x and z are connected to each other (as indicated by the heavier solid line connecting them). The five dashed lines indicate potential links among A's alters, but they are absent. So the personal network density for A is 1/6, one tie of six potential ones. In contrast, person B has three links connecting the people in his personal network, and so has a personal network density of 3/6, or 50%. The average personal network density for all the nodes in a network is the clustering coefficient.

A network with high average personal network densities indicates that people connected to a third person tend to be connected to each other. Notice this is similar to the triadic transitivity concept discussed in the previous section. Thus, transitivity indicates clustering. When personal network densities are low, transitivity is lacking and people are not more likely to know one another when connected to the same third party. Therefore, low

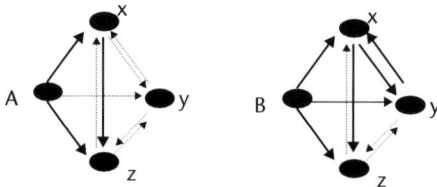

Figure 8–4. Calculating personal network density. The solid lines represent links, and the dashed ones potential links. Personal network density is 1/6 for Bob, whereas it is 3/6 for Paul.

personal network density indicates a lack of clustering. Another way to calculate clustering is to calculate the ratio of closed triads to all possible triads in the network (Luce & Perry, 1949; Wasserman & Faust, 1994).

Clustering can accelerate behavior and disease spread within groups but will inhibit spread between groups. The average personal density in the network indicates the degree of clustering, and high rates of clustering indicate a network with pockets of interconnectivity separated by bridges that link these cohesive subgroups. The cohesive groups can be protective from a public health perspective as long as disease or risk behavior does not penetrate them. Once a disease penetrates these cohesive subgroups, however, it is likely to spread quickly, infecting everyone in a short period of time.

In clustered networks, then, how the clusters are linked to one another becomes critical. Two different types of network structures exist that link clustered subgroups: (1) a bridge structure in which the clustered subgroups are linked by bridges, and (2) a centralized structure in which the subgroups are linked by central nodes who occupy powerful positions in the network. The best indicator to distinguish these two types of structures is centralization.

Centralization

Centralization is the degree a network's ties are focused on one person or a set of people. In centralized networks, one or a few people hold positions of power and control in the network, whereas decentralized networks have diffuse power and control structures. Figure 8–5 shows two pairs of networks with the same densities, yet different centralization scores. The networks on the left are decentralized (e.g., centralization = 9.1%), while the ones on the right are centralized (e.g., 50.9%). It is important to stress that density and centralization are not correlated and are independent structural measures of the network. A dense network can be decentralized or centralized, and a sparse network can be decentralized or centralized. The centralized networks on the right (one dense and one sparse) have a node at the center of the network that receives a disproportionate amount of ties.

Centralization was discussed in Chapter 5 in reviewing centrality measures. Recall that there were numerous individual centrality measures and each one has a network-level counterpart. For example, centrality degree measures the number of links a person sends and receives. Degree centralization degree (NB: centralization for the network level) indicates whether one or some nodes send or receive a disproportionate number of links and can be calculated on in-degree and out-degree. Centralization is calculated

Low Density Networks (18.2%)

Decentralized (0.0%)   Centralized (87.3%)

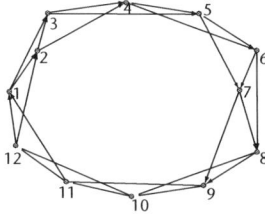

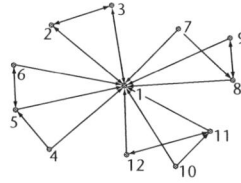

High Density Networks (36.4%)

Decentralized (9.1%)   Centralized (50.9%)

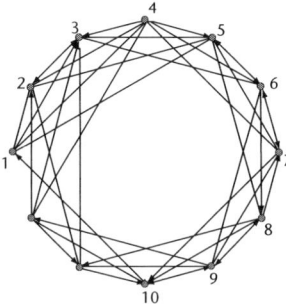

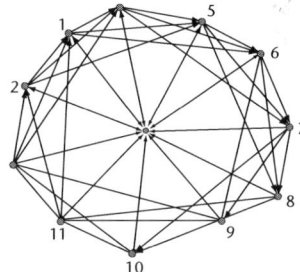

Figure 8–5. The top two networks have equal network density, 18.2%, yet the one on the left is decentralized (centralization = 0%) and the on the right is centralized (centralization = 87.3%). Similarly, the bottom two networks have equal densities, 36.4%, yet dramatically different centralizations (9.1% and 50.9%, respectively).

by determining the maximum individual centrality score in the network and subtracting it from all other individual scores in the network. These differences are summed and that total is divided by the maximum sum of differences theoretically possible in a network of that size (which happens to be given conveniently by a formula). For example, the formula for centralization degree (CD) is (Freeman, 1979):

$$CD = \frac{\sum (Max(C_{Di}) - C_{Di})}{n^2 - 3n + 2}$$

(8-4)

where $Max(C_{Di})$ is the maximum centrality score in the network, C_{Di} indicates the individual centrality scores, and n is network size. A similar formula exists for centralization based on centrality closeness, betweenness, and others. Another way to calculate centralization is by simply calculating the standard deviation of the centrality scores for the network. A large standard deviation indicates a lot of variation in the individual centrality scores, whereas a small one indicates little variation and hence a decentralized structure.

With nomination data, in-degree centralization will usually be greater than out-degree centralization. Typically, nomination data limit the nominations the respondent can provide. This limits the number of out-degree nominations, and so the variance in out-degree is smaller, making out-degree centralization smaller. In contrast, the nominations received distribution can be quite varied because one person or a few people will receive many nominations and so the out-degree distribution is greater. This, of course, depends on the data and the extent of actual centralization in the network.

Centralized networks have the potential for fast diffusion because people at the center of the network can act like broadcasters and reach many people quickly. Conversely, centralized networks may have slower diffusion because the central nodes are gatekeepers and have a disproportionate amount of influence in the network. If the central nodes delay adoption or if they do not support the new idea, then diffusion will be slowed in centralized networks. Thus, centralization has the net effect of placing more power and control on the central people, the opinion leaders. Opinion leaders are more critical to behavior spread in centralized networks rather than in decentralized ones.

The net effect, then, of centralization may be on the shape of the diffusion curve rather than on how long it takes for diffusion to reach saturation. Centralized networks will have steeper diffusion and the time until diffusion takes off rapidly will depend on the attitudes and behaviors of the central people. If the central people are resistant, then the diffusion will remain at a low level until leaders embrace the new idea and then it will increase rapidly. Conversely, if the central people embrace the idea early, then diffusion will accelerate rapidly. A more nuanced version of centralization is the idea of a core-periphery structure.

Core-Periphery

Many empirical networks exhibit a core-periphery structure. Core-periphery structures are networks in which there is a group of nodes who are densely connected to one another (the core) and a separate group of nodes loosely connected to this core and loosely (or not at all) connected to each other (the periphery). Core-periphery networks may have somewhat low centralization scores because the people in the core all have similar centrality scores. Yet, there is still considerable structure in the network but it is not a centralized structure, or a clustered structure, rather a core-periphery one.

The degree to which a network has a core-periphery structure is determined by fitting a core-periphery model to the data (Borgatti & Everett, 1999) by permuting the data matrix repeatedly such that nodes are alternatively in the core or periphery. The various empirically based core-periphery structures are correlated with an idealized core-periphery structure (connections among core nodes and with peripheral nodes and no connections between peripheral nodes). The best model is the one in which node assignments in the data have the maximum correlation with the idealized core-periphery structure. This correlation is the fit index indicating how well the data conform to a core-periphery structure (Borgatti & Everett, 1999).

Figure 8–6 displays a collaboration network that has a modest core-periphery structure typical of coalition networks (Valente et al., 2008b). The fit index for this core-periphery structure was 0.362, which is the correlation coefficient between the observed data matrix and a hypothetical ideal core-periphery matrix (Borgatti & Everett, 1999). The fit index can be interpreted as a correlation coefficient, indicating that these data only modestly conform to a core-periphery structure. Core organizations in Figure 8–6 ($n = 18$) are

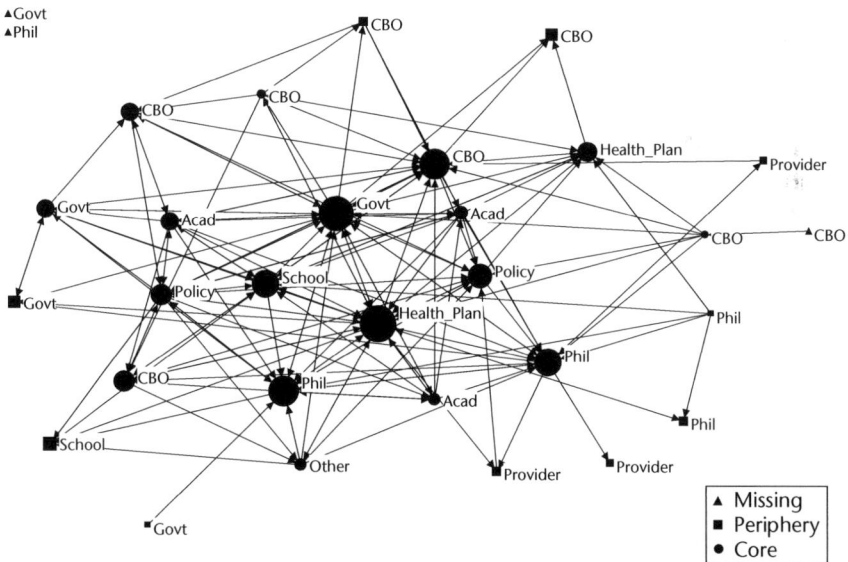

Figure 8–6. The network of collaboration among 31 organizations that participated in a coalition to expand children's health insurance. Circles are core organizations, and squares are peripheral ones. Nodes are sized based on in-degree in the collaboration network and positioned using spring embedding.

depicted as circles and peripheral ones (n = 13) as squares. In this study, there were many different types of organizations in the core of the network including government, health plans, school, philanthropic, academic, policy, and community-based organization/advocacy. Thus, the coalition was not dominated by one or a few organizations or organization types; rather collaboration was shared by many different types of organizations. It was also the case that being in the core was a function of organizational members' meeting attendance, involvement in coalition activities, and a higher percentage of the organization's goals being related to children (Valente et al., 2008b).

These are the primary indicators used to describe network structure: number of components, size, density, reciprocity, triad census (especially transitivity), APL (distance), clustering, centralization, and core-peripheriness. Table 8–1 reports the averages, standard deviations, and ranges for these network indicators for 24 communities from the STEP study. These are baseline network data derived from asking coalition members to name the other members they turned to for advice on prevention issues (Valente et al., 2007). The average size was 22.04 members, ranging from as few as 4 to as many as 41. There was an average of 12.7 components in the networks, and all of these consisted of one large component with each isolate being considered a separate component. The average density was 13%, with 20% of the ties being reciprocated. Some 37% of the triads were transitive, with one network having all triads transitive.

The APL in the largest connected component was 2.2, ranging from 1 to 3.1. This indicates that most coalition members could reach everyone else in the coalition (if they could reach them at all) in three or fewer steps. The maximum path length was 5.1, ranging from 1 to 8. The clustering coefficient

Table 8–1. Selected Metrics for 24 Coalition Advice Networks

	Mean	SD	Range (Min, Max)
Size	22.04	8.58	4, 41
Density	0.13	0.06	0.06, 0.33
Proportion of reciprocated ties	0.20	0.08	0.05, 0.40
Proportion of transitive triads	0.37	0.16	0.19, 1.00
Average geodesic distance*	2.16	0.45	1.00, 3.14
Maximum geodesic distance	5.08	1.64	1, 8
Number of component	12.67	5.56	3, 24
Clustering coefficient	0.31	0.13	.15, .67
Norm. In-degree centralization (%)	34.63	11.27	16.63, 54.50
Norm. Out-degree centralization (%)	18.06	7.89	8.41, 44.44
Number of isolates	2.92	8.58	0, 8

*Computed among reachable nodes.

average was 0.31, indicating moderately clustered networks. The networks were more centralized on in-degree (34.6%) and then on out-degree (18.1%), which is common in nomination studies because most respondents provide a similar number of nominations given the restriction on the number allowed and yet people/organizations can receive as many nominations as there are others in the network. There was an average of nearly three isolates per coalition.

As mentioned earlier, network indicators vary with one another and with outcomes. For example, size was negatively associated with density: the larger the network, the less dense it is ($r = -0.68$). Size was also negatively associated with the percentage of ties reciprocated ($r = -0.55$), the percentage transitive ($r = -0.63$), and clustering ($r = -0.59$). Size was positively associated with average path length ($r = 0.80$). Thus, in this study, the larger the network, the more likely that people do not reciprocate nominations and form tightly nested triads in which everyone knows one another. Density was also associated with other metrics. For example, density increased reciprocity ($r = 0.48$) and transitivity ($r = 0.80$) and decreased the APL ($r = -0.69$).

One thing to note is that the APL will vary significantly depending on how disconnected nodes are treated. For the 24 networks in this study, the mean APL was 2.16 (SD = 0.45) when measured only among connected nodes in the largest component. The APL would increase dramatically if $N - 1$ was used as the distance between disconnected nodes to 18.9 (SD = 8.22) and 5.60 (SD = 1.57) when $D + 1$ was used where D equals the maximum distance between connected nodes. The lay public has become quite familiar with the small world concept associated with the term "six degrees of separation" (see Chapter 1). The measure of "six degrees" is the APL, and to report APL in a way that is consistent with "six degrees" concept one would consider only connected nodes, although in some instances it may be preferred to calculate network properties with the inclusion of disconnected nodes.

It is also possible to determine if network-level characteristics are associated with network-level outcomes such as how successful the coalition has been at achieving its objectives. These network-level outcomes can be derived from external indicators (Did the coalition achieve extramural funding?) or from aggregates of individual responses (How effective do coalition members report the coalition as being"). In the STEP study, coalition density was negatively associated with adoption of evidence-based practices (Valente et al., 2007), whereas centralization was positively associated adoption of evidence-based practices (Fujimoto et al., in press).

One would expect networks with shorter overall path lengths to be more cohesive and conducive to the adoption of new behaviors. Because shorter APL indicates a shorter distance between everyone in the network, information has to travel less far to reach everyone and so diffusion should be facilitated. The tendency toward reciprocity and transitivity, however, will lengthen overall path lengths because it creates clustering in the network.

Two-Mode Data

In Chapter 3, five different types of network data collection were provided and the notion of two-mode data was introduced. Two-mode data are data derived from information on events, organizations, or situations in which people participate. For example, one might have data on the departments to which the employees in an organization belong. Two-mode data are arrayed in a table referred to as an *affiliation matrix*, in which people are the rows and the events or organizations are the columns. The events (columns) should be binary vectors in which a 0 means the person does not belong or did not attend the event and a 1 means the person attended or belonged. Table 8–2 provides an example from the class network shown in Figure 7–1. The students in this class were from different departments within the university. (The affiliation matrix in Table 8–2 is also sometimes referred to as an *incidence matrix*.)

The data show that every student belonged to one department, and one faculty member belonged to two departments (was jointly appointed). The two-mode data can be used to construct a person-by-person network based on shared departments by multiplying the Table in 8–1 by its transpose. The transpose of a matrix is the matrix turned on its side. So this affiliation matrix has 27 rows and 4 columns (ignoring the row and column labels) and its transpose has 4 rows by 27 columns. These two matrices can be multiplied because they are conformable (the number of columns in the first matrix equals the number of rows in the second one) and the resulting matrix has 27 rows and columns (is a 27-by-27 square matrix, which are the outside dimensions of the two matrices).

The product of these two matrices indicates which people are in the same department and the network can be graphed (Figure 8–7). The network shows connections between all of the people in the same department. There is one link connecting the two departments, the faculty with appointments in the two departments. The network has been constructed from information only about who belonged to which department. A matrix (network) of department-by-department affiliations can also be constructed from this same data. The cells of the department-by-department matrix indicate the number of students who share departments. The department-by-department matrix is created by multiplying the transposed matrix by the original one (reversing the order of the multiplication) so the first matrix is 4×27 and the second is

**Table 8–2. Departmental Affiliations of the
Students (27 × 4 Matrix)**

	Dept. A	Dept. B	Dept. C	Other
A_S1	1	0	0	0
PD_F1	0	1	0	0
A_S2	1	0	0	0
A_S3	1	0	0	0
Oth_F2	0	0	0	1
B_S4	0	1	0	0
A_S5	1	0	0	0
A_S6	1	0	0	0
A_S7	1	0	0	0
A_S8	1	0	0	0
A_S9	1	0	0	0
B_F2	0	1	0	0
B_S5	0	1	0	0
A_S7	1	0	0	0
A_S8	1	0	0	0
B_S4	0	1	0	0
C_S1	0	0	1	0
B_S5	0	1	0	0
C_S2	0	0	1	0
A_S9	1	0	0	0
A_S10	1	0	0	0
B_S6	0	1	0	0
A_F3	1	1	0	0
C_S3	0	0	1	0
A_S11	1	0	0	0
B_S7	0	1	0	0
A_S12	1	0	0	0

27 × 4. Thus, the affiliation data provide two networks that can be graphed and correlated with attributes or other networks.

For example, it might be hypothesized that department affiliation was associated with the network of who-knew-whom when the class started. The correlation between the department affiliation matrix and the choices of who knew whom is calculated using a technique known as the Quadratic Assignment Procedure (QAP) available in statistical programs (Krackhardt, 1987, 1988; Borgatti et al., 2006). QAP provides a means to correlate to two matrices that accounts for the dependencies in the matrix.

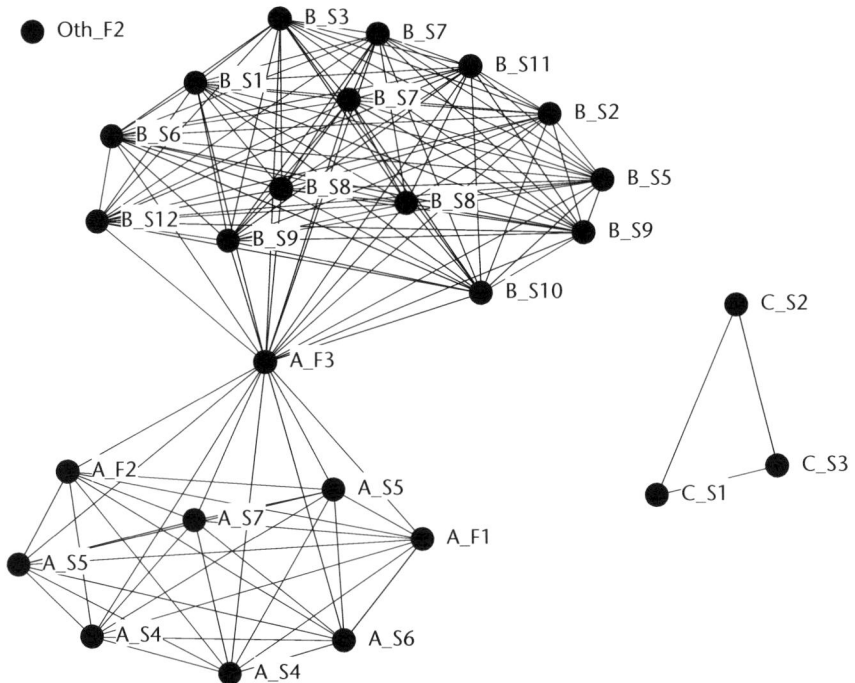

Figure 8–7. Graph of two-mode data, in which links indicates people who belonged to the same department derived by converting an affiliation matrix (department membership) into one mode adjacency matrix.

In this case, the "know" network shown in Figure 7–1 was regressed on the network derived from departmental affiliations using the two-mode technique (Figure 8–7). The standardized regression coefficient (β) was 0.23 ($p < .001$), indicating that department affiliation was weakly associated with who knew whom at the start of this class. The correlation was not as high as expected, although it is statistically significant.

Individual Network-Level Interactions

One theoretically interesting avenue of research is the interaction between individual-level and network-level measures. These interactions can be of two types. First, interactions between individual measures such as centrality can be studied in the context of a network metric such as centralization. For example, are central members of an organization more likely to be successful in a centralized organization than a decentralized one? In this case, the overall network structure is hypothesized to affect the interpretation of the effects of the individual metric.

The second type would be an interaction between a network-level metric and network influence. For example, it might be hypothesized that social influence is stronger in dense networks than in sparse ones. Dense networks have more connections and so more opportunities for information to flow, and they may be indicative of a norm in which communication occurs. Conversely, dense networks may be "noisy" and so social influence for each individual competes with others in the focal person's personal network. Therefore, the other hypothesis is that social influence is stronger in sparse networks. One way to test this proposition would be to compare network exposure based on the number of ties who engage in the behavior compared to the same measure divided by the number of ties (comparing network exposure as a count versus a proportion). Another way would be to use data from multiple networks with identical measures so that social influence can be compared across sparse and dense networks.

One might also think that social influence varies by network position. For example, are people on the periphery of the network more likely to be influenced by peers than those at the center? Because people in the center have more connections or occupy a privileged position in the network, they can be more selective about how others influence them. People on the periphery, in contrast, may only learn about behaviors from one person and so may be more susceptible to that person's influence. Given the plethora of network level and individual level measures, the number of hypotheses is enormous.

Summary

This chapter described the network level of analysis in network analysis. Network-level indicators are those measures which describe the entire network. Size is the most basic network measure, and network density is a fundamental property. Mutuality, or the extent to which ties are reciprocated, is also a network level property and indicates whether there is a tendency for ties in the network to be reciprocated. Network researchers also examine the way three nodes are connected. Triads, three nodes, can be connected in as many as 16 different ways and researchers have documented these ways in what is known as a triad census. Every network can be described by the frequency the triads in the network occur in the 16 different possible permutations. Of particular interest are transitive triads, those in which A $\rightarrow$ B and B $\rightarrow$ C implies A $\rightarrow$ C.

A useful network metric is the APL of the network. APL is often used as a measure of network cohesion in which networks with low APL are considered cohesive. Networks with an APL greater than expected by chance are considered fragmented. The chapter showed how APL and density correlate. Another network indicator is analysis of whether the network has a core-periphery structure. The chapter included a discussion of two-mode data and how it is used to create networks of people-by-people and group-by-group. The chapter also provided an example of two-mode data and how it can be correlated with other networks to answer substantive questions. The chapter closed with a discussion on network-level influences on behavior.

PART III

APPLICATIONS

9

Exponential Random Graph Models, P* and Actor Oriented Models

This chapter describes in nontechnical terms how researchers can determine whether empirical networks exhibit certain structural properties (centrality, triadic transitivity, etc.) using a statistical test. These models are referred to as exponential random graph models (ERGMs), named after the technique used to generate simulated networks, which can then be compared to the observed network to statistically assess network properties. Here we try to provide a simple introduction so researchers can seek out more advanced materials and tutorials to learn how the analysis is conducted (Burk et al., 2007; Harrigan, 2009; Snijders, 2001; Snijders et al., 2007).

ERGM is derived from the P* model, which provided the basis for early statistical analysis of networks. The critical innovation in the P* model was the use of logistic regression analysis to determine the factors (individual characteristics and network metrics) associated with a link between two nodes. This chapter first provides an introduction to the dyadic approach used for many years. The chapter then describes the exponential random graph model (ERGM) approach used primarily with cross-sectional data. The chapter then provides an exposition of the actor-oriented co-evolution model, which extends the cross-sectional ERGM framework to model longitudinal processes. These models can be used to determine what behaviors drive social network evolution and whether social relationships influence behavioral changes. This actor-oriented co-evolution model is very flexible, permitting many kinds of hypothesis tests. The chapter includes some public health examples.

In Part II of this book, many social network measures were presented that treated social networks as static configurations. The network did not change and behaviors were often described as something distributed on the network. Networks were described by creating indicators for their structure such as density or centralization and network members were characterized by their positions in the network, such as their centrality. Individual and network measures could then be correlated with individual or group behavior. For example, an individual's centrality (in-degree) was found to correlate with smoking behaviors and density scores were associated with the rate of behavioral change. The language used so far often conveyed the concept of a fixed network with an idea or a behavior spreading through it much like cars moving on roads.

In reality, however, networks change. Individuals make new friends and lose track of old ones. Behaviors also change, of course, with some people trying a new activity for the first time while others quit after some experience. Sometimes relationships change because of the behavior change, while in other cases people change behaviors because their peers have changed theirs. For example, if an adolescent thinks smoking is cool, he or she may want to form friendships with smokers. Alternatively, an adolescent may start smoking because his or her friends have started. Consequently, researchers have been interested in finding ways to analyze network and behavior changes simultaneously. To study the co-evolution of behavior and social networks, researchers have developed models that attempt to estimate the probability that individuals form ties in a network based on the existing relationships and behaviors. A second limitation of much prior research on network effects is that statistical associations between network exposure (i.e., behavior of one's friends), network indicators (e.g., centrality, density), and behaviors (attributes of the individual) have not completely accounted for dependencies between the actors. For example, suppose a statistical analysis shows that people who smoke are more likely than nonsmokers to have smoking friends. This association may be a product of both the focal person and the network alters being connected to a third person who is also a smoker.

Until the relatively recent ERGM and co-evolution models, many people were unsatisfied with network analysis research without any indication of whether the network measures were expected and normal or whether one network structure could be considered to be "better" than another. The quest to develop statistical models appropriate for network data spans many decades (Holland & Leinhardt, 1979) and several teams of researchers. Fortunately, much progress has been made and a set of tools emerged that enable researchers to determine whether a given network can be considered to have certain structural tendencies (e.g., Is the network transitive?), whether behaviors drive network structures (e.g., Are smokers more likely to be selected as friends?), and how network relations influence behaviors (e.g., Do popular individuals have a greater influence on their friends?) over time.

Estimating the Link

Conceptually, to test the probability of observing network as a function of the structural characteristics within the network (e.g., number of ties, reciprocal ties, transitive triads, etc.) was conducted by estimating the probability of a link. Early work used maximum pseudo-likelihood estimation (MPLE) to estimate the contribution of relevant structural properties to the observed network. Essentially, this approach uses logistic regression to estimate whether the property increases or decreases the likelihood of observing a tie between two nodes, while accounting for other structural tendencies in the network. For example, an analysis including two parameters for density and reciprocity where the estimate for reciprocity is negative would indicate that there is a tendency for ties not to be reciprocated after controlling for the total number of ties observed within the network.

A useful introduction to MPLE for estimating network parameters was provided by Crouch, Wasserman, and Contractor (1998; also see Anderson et al., 1999) in which they illustrate the technique using both hypothetical and empirical data. In their hypothetical example, a small network of six nodes with 12 links is proposed that has one binary attribute distributed within it. Crouch and others (1998) explain that this network consists of 12 ties and 18 non-ties and the matrix is reshaped to a vector (a column with 30 entries) of 1s and 0s. Additional vectors are stored next to the link vector that represent whether the two nodes share the attribute, whether the tie should exist under conditions of mutuality, whether it should exist if mutuality occurs within the attribute, and whether the tie should exist under conditions of transitivity. In other words, variables are constructed that represent each tie's contribution to the structural properties of interest and, using logistic regression, model parameters are estimated that allow one to test whether these properties contribute significantly to the presence or absence of a tie.

Vectorizing the Matrix

As mentioned on the estimating a link section, the process of estimating an network effects originally involved vectorizing the matrix. The matrix of i-to-j links can be converted to a vector; that is, the rows of the network are stacked under one another to make one big column in which each row indicates the value of a specific i and j linkage, whether 0 or 1. This now becomes a vector that can be treated like any other vector, and we can perform a (logistic) regression to determine the things associated with elements of the vector being 1s rather than 0s. The link vector is the sequence of 0s and 1s representing who is connected to whom reformatted as a column. This link vector, the links and nonlinks in the network, is the dependent variable to be predicted with the understanding that the row entries are not independent observations. They are not independent because the same person contributes multiple cases to the dataset. This dependence violates the assumption of independence in normal regression analysis. Multilevel models (also known as random effects models) have been developed to cope with this nonindependence in survey research, and the network effects were developed to specifically model dependence in the network.

Maximum pseudo-likelihood estimates (MPLE) work by analyzing the factors associated with an element in the link vector being a 1 rather than being a 0. Node characteristics and structural properties are merged with the link vectors and statistical analysis can be conducted to determine if any of these are associated with a link. In sum, the network is converted to a vector (column) in which each element indicates whether there is a link between two nodes. This dyadic relational data is the outcome to be predicted. Vectors for the node attributes and vectors for the dependencies (network structure) are merged with the dyadic relational data. Then a logistic regression is calculated with the dyadic relational data (link vector) as the dependent variable and the other vectors as independent.

Figure 9–1 provides an illustration of how data can be reshaped for statistical analyses using a hypothetical group of 10 people with two attributes, sex and age. For example, person 1 has 4 outgoing ties, is male and 24 years old. To analyze these data, the data are converted to dyadic so each observation is the relationship between two people. The first two columns index the rows and columns to keep track of the people so the first 10 cases are person one's outgoing relations. P is the column indicating whether there is a link between the two people. Out is a count of the outdegree (number of nominations) for that person. R indicates whether the relationship between the two people is reciprocated (mutual) and T indicates whether the pair is in a triadic relationship. H_s is a variable indicating whether the pair are the same (homophilous) on sex. D_a is a variable indicating the degree of difference between the pair on age.

The statistical analysis then estimates whether these constructed variables (D, R, T, H_s, and D_a) are associated with P, the link between the two people. (Reflexive, or relations with oneself, are removed.) Of course these are not the only, nor necessarily the best variables to be constructed from this type

	1	2	3	4	5	6	7	8	9	10	Sex	Age
1	0	1	0	0	1	0	0	1	0	1	Male	24
2	1	0	0	0	0	0	1	0	0	0	Male	25
3	0	1	0	0	0	0	0	0	0	0	Female	25
4	0	0	0	0	0	1	0	0	0	0	Female	27
5	1	1	0	0	0	0	1	0	0	1	Female	32
6	0	1	0	1	0	0	0	0	0	0	Female	32
7	0	1	1	0	1	0	0	0	0	1	Female	26
8	0	0	0	0	0	0	0	0	0	0	Male	23
9	0	0	1	0	0	1	0	0	0	1	Male	35
10	1	0	0	0	0	0	1	0	1	0	Male	37

Reshaped data

i	j	P	I	Out	R	T	H_s	D_a
1	1	0	1	4	1	0	1	0
1	2	1	1	4	1	1	1	1
1	3	0	1	4	1	0	0	1
1	4	0	1	4	1	0	0	3
1	5	1	1	4	1	1	0	8
1	6	0	1	4	1	0	0	8
1	7	0	1	4	1	0	0	2
1	8	1	1	4	0	0	0	1
1	9	0	1	4	1	0	1	11
1	10	1	1	4	1	1	1	13
2	1	1	1	5	1	1	1	1
2	2	0	1	5	1	0	1	0
2	3	0	1	5	0	1	0	0
2	4	0	1	5	1	0	0	2
2	5	0	1	5	0	1	0	7
2	6	0	1	5	0	0	0	7
2	7	1	1	5	1	1	0	1
2	8	0	1	5	1	0	1	2
2	9	0	1	5	1	0	1	10
2	10	0	1	5	1	0	1	12

i	Row i
j	Column j
P	Tie
D	Density
Out	Out-degree
R	Reciprocity
T	Transitivity
H_s	Homophily on Sex
D_a	Difference on age

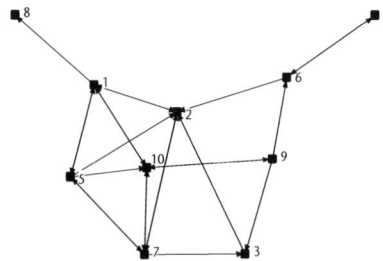

Figure 9–1. Illustration of data re-shaping for maximum pseudo-likelihood estimation (MPLE) analysis. A hypothetical network of 10 people with sex and age attribution.

of data. For example, one might want to estimate whether the two people are in a transitive triad in addition to any triadic relationship. Or the researcher might want to estimate the effect of in-degree nominations. And of course with longitudinal data on the same people over time many types of interactions can be created. The conceptual point to understand is that the relationships naturally viewed as a matrix can be converted to dyadic relationships and variables indicating aspects of those relationships are then associated with each one. These challenges led to the development of exponential random graph models (ERGM).

Exponential Random Graph Models (ERGM)

ERGMs provide a statistical analysis of a network that can serve two functions: (1) to determine whether network structural properties such as transitivity occur in a network more than expected by chance and (2) to determine whether there is an association between network links and behavior. It should be stressed that ERGMs are used for cross-sectional data. The statistical test measures the likelihood that the observed network could have emerged by chance. Specifically, it can be determined whether this observed network is a function of properties based on the algorithms and materials presented in Chapters 5 through 8. The algorithms and indicators presented in Chapters 5 through 8 are used to calculate the density, degree of reciprocity, transitivity, clustering, and so on that exist in that network. They do not, however, empirically assess the extent to which these properties exist, given the density and other lower-order dependencies. For example, in any network, there is likely to be some reciprocity just by chance, and in a network with more links (greater density) there will be more reciprocity just by chance. To determine if there is a tendency toward reciprocity in a network, a statistical model should control for the density of the network. ERGM provides a way to determine whether network properties occur by chance as a result of other network properties or whether the properties so measured are unlikely given other parameters of the network.

The second primary use of ERGMs, and perhaps the more substantive, is the ability to incorporate nodal attributes in model estimation. Nodal attributes are characteristics that might influence the formation or dissolution of a tie, such as whether adolescent boys are more likely to form friendships with boys than with girls. The node attribute's sex then is an important determinant of network structure and ERGMs can determine whether this tendency is exhibited in the friendship network. In addition to antecedent characteristics such as sex, researchers will often want to include a behavioral outcome variable such as smoking. For example, ERGMs can determine whether friendships are more likely to form among teens when they have similar smoking status.

In sum, ERGM analysis can be used for (at least) three functions: (1) describe a network in terms of its structural properties; (2) determine if individual attributes (or node characteristics) are associated with network structural properties; and (3) determine if individual attributes are associated with behaviors controlling for items 1 and 2. So, for example, an ERGM can be estimated to determine if ties are reciprocated, if that reciprocation is greater than expected by chance, and if it is associated with sex (boys more likely to reciprocate friendships with boys). We might then include a behavior in the model to determine if smoking is more likely among friends controlling for sex and reciprocity.

Simulation

The MPLE approach has been shown to lead to biased estimators (van Duijn, et al., 2009) and thus reflects an approximation. When the dependence among networks ties is not strong, then the pseudo-likelihood estimates will be more accurate. However, recent efforts using maximum likelihood approaches to estimate the structural tendencies in the observed network leads to more accurate estimation. This approach is based on Markov chain Monte Carlo (MCMC) techniques by which a distribution of networks are simulated, parameter estimates are obtained by comparing the observed network with the simulated networks, and this process is repeated until there is little change in the parameter estimates (Robins et al., 2007).

The simulations are run thousands of times to generate a distribution of networks based on the characteristics of the empirical networks. This distribution indicates the possible networks given the characteristics of an empirical one. For example, the distribution indicates the degree of reciprocity in a set of randomly generated networks that have the same density as the observed network. The structural properties of interest are parameters of higher order structure than those used to generate the distribution. Each parameter estimated from the randomly simulated networks is compared to the parameters found in the empirical network. If the empirical network parameter is different than the average calculated from the simulated networks then the researcher can conclude that the empirical network has the property, or more accurately, exhibits a tendency for the property.

So, for example, suppose an empirical network has 100 nodes and 500 links for a density of 5%. We might wonder if there is a tendency for reciprocity in the empirical network (if A named B, was B more likely to name A?). To determine if there is a tendency for reciprocity, hundreds or thousands of networks are generated with 100 nodes and 500 links. The mean of the simulated distribution of reciprocal ties are calculated and then compared to the value in the real network. If the reciprocity of the empirical network differs from the mean reciprocity in the simulated networks more than it would be expected to by chance, then it can be concluded that there is a tendency for reciprocity in the empirical network. Figure 9–2 diagrams some of the parameters calculated during the ERGM simulation process. Researchers may optionally elect to include more parameters to guide the simulation. The network properties that generate the simulation are matched (e.g., density and reciprocity) and then higher order structural properties are compared to determine if they occur at a rate greater than expected by chance given these lower-order parameters.

It is important to realize that structural properties of networks, such as density, reciprocity, transitivity, and so on, are considered hierarchically. A test for transitivity also needs to test for density and reciprocity. In other words, a test for transitivity also generates simulated networks based on the empirical density and reciprocity. The simulated networks will have an average density and reciprocity similar to that of the empirical network because that was the basis for the simulation. The analysis then answers the question: Does the amount of transitivity in the empirical network match that of the

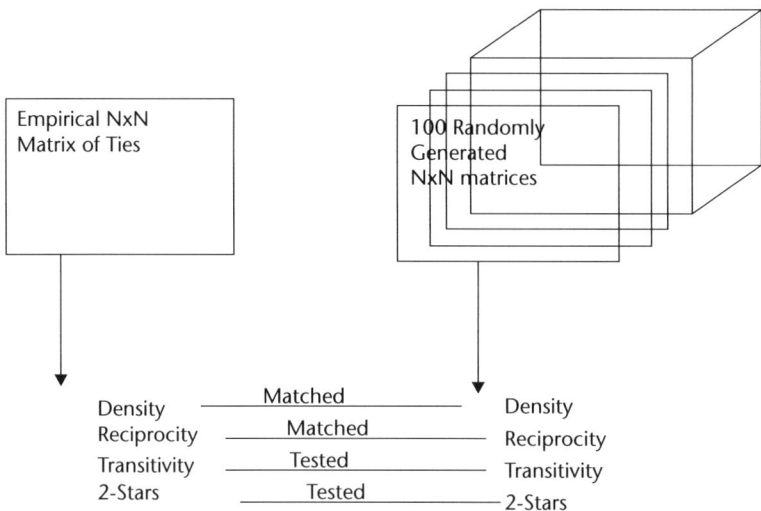

Figure 9–2. The empirical network is described by its density, reciprocity, transitivity, and other structural indicators. Random networks are generated which have these same structural characteristics for the control structures and those which are not generated explicitly in the simulation are tested.

simulated networks, or are they different? If different, then the observed network can be characterized as having transitivity above or below what would be expected by chance in networks of this size, density, and reciprocity.

Of course, things can get more complicated than this for several reasons. First, it is hard to know how many networks need to be generated to get a valid distribution of parameters. Second, as networks get bigger, it becomes increasingly difficult to generate lots of networks and calculate multiple structural properties. Third, as node attributes are added to the analysis (e.g., gender, drug use), the computational effort increases further. To address these difficulties, statisticians have devised ways of generating the simulated distributions without creating whole simulated networks.

Returning to the hypothetical example of 100 nodes and 500 links, the analysis would need to generate 1,000 networks of 100 nodes and 500 links and calculate reciprocity on all of them to create a distribution of reciprocity values for networks of 100 nodes and 500 links. Rather than generate an entire matrix of random links spread among the 500 nodes, we might randomly choose links to be on or off (connected or not). Now the procedure generates random networks based on the size and density parameters of the empirical network, but rather than generate entire networks, only a sample of each network is created. This sample is then used to calculate network parameters of interest. In this way, a large distribution of network parameters can be obtained based on randomly generated networks in an efficient manner.

One issue is how to generate the random networks. In the ERGM framework, the simulated networks are created by randomly generating networks based on the structural parameters of interest (density, reciprocity, transitivity). These simulated networks are referred to as dependence networks because they specifically indicate the nonindependence that exists between cases in the network. Unlike randomly selected samples, cases in a network dataset are specifically linked to one another as indicated by the network links and the structures in that network. So the dependence graph describes the dependencies indicated by the network based on the structural model. For example, if the structural model specifies that a network is characterized by transitivity, then two nodes linked in a transitive relationship are dependent on one another according to this structure. The dependence network is the connections in a network implied by a structural model. In other words, the dependence network indicates what links would exist in a network if the structural model explained the specific set of relationships.

In sum, ERGM is used when there is an empirical network in which we want to know whether there is a tendency for some structural relations, such as transitivity. A large sample of random networks is generated (actually sampled networks because it is too time-consuming to generate the entire network), which is based on the dependence graph implied by the structural model, transitivity, plus lower-order dependencies (density and reciprocity). The empirical network's transitivity is then compared to the transitivity of the simulated sample. If the simulated sample's average and empirical values are different (where a *t*-value greater than 1.96 indicates statistical significance at the 0.05 level), the researcher concludes that the empirical network exhibits a tendency toward transitivity. Note that this analysis does not prove the network is transitive because the analysis has not been able to longitudinally model the underlying processes implied by the transitivity.

One other element needs to be added to make the story complete, and that is how to seed the simulated networks to create the distribution. The structural model indicates whether links should exist, given the implied dependencies in the model. But how do we know how to start the creation of the random networks? The "burn-in phase" of network generation refers to the initial seeding of links in the simulation of randomly generated networks. Initial links are selected at random and then the rest of the network is filled in according to the structural models specified. One of the challenges facing ERGMs is discovering ways to build these networks that provide reliable parameter estimates for the simulated networks. Some earlier techniques, Bernoulli graphs and Markov random graphs, were based on simple rules that did not provide satisfactory simulated network distributions. Recent developments in model specification have resulted in programs that generate better simulated networks in the sense that they are structurally similar to the empirical networks.

New Specifications

The approach outlined thus far had been used for some time with mixed success. One problem was that simulating networks with higher-order properties (such as transitivity) degenerated. *Degeneration* refers to the scenario when the simulation parameters lead to very non-normal networks that are either too connected or too disconnected. Specifically, transitivity is a key structural feature of networks and so researchers often wanted to control for transitivity in a network. Growing simulated networks that are transitive was problematic, however, because such networks tend to have highly connected subgroups with no bridges between them. The simulated networks often resulted in completed connected subgroups or completely null networks no links at all. Thus, the simulated networks did not resemble the empirical one on which they were based.

As Harrigan (2009) points out, two recent specifications have helped to solve these earlier problems and made it possible to estimate ERGMs (Robins and Pattison, 2005; Robins, et al., 2007; Snijders et al., 2007). These two advances were (a) the introduction of the four-cycle and (b) the use of a "rubbery ceiling" on structural parameters, which limited the number or density of certain specifications such as transitive triangles. The most prominent model parameter that incorporates these changes is the alternating k-star configuration (Snijders, 2005).

The alternating k-star parameter is critical to model estimation and has three features. First, all star configurations (those that involve an ego's direct ties) are incorporated into one parameter estimate. Rather than count the number of 2-stars, 3-stars, 4-stars, and so on, the k-star configuration estimates how many of all kinds of stars there are in a network. Second, the probability of a star of a particular order is inversely proportional to its order. So 2-stars are more likely than 3-stars, which are more likely than 4-stars, and so on. This makes sense, of course, because in most networks, 2-stars are more common than 3-stars, which are more common than 4-stars, and so on. A parameter estimate for k-stars captures in one estimate the distribution of stars in the network. Finally, the sign, positive or negative, for the probability of higher-order stars alternates so that if a 2-star has a positive sign, the 3-star will be negative, the 4-star will be positive, and so on.

Researchers also introduced the alternating k-triangle parameter, which is similar to the alternating k-star. The alternating k-triangle incorporates a four-cycle and so relies on the conditional independence assumption mentioned earlier. Finally, researchers introduced the alternating k-two paths parameter, which estimates the probability that two nodes share another node (i.e., two people are connected by an intermediary). In sum, estimating traditional Markov models was problematic for some time until these alternating k-star, k-triangle, and k-two path parameters were introduced. Once they were incorporated into the simulation of the distribution of networks, comparisons between empirical and simulated networks could be made and parameter estimates generated. Some progress has also been made at estimating the simultaneous effects of multiple networks (Koehly & Pattison, 2005).

Obesity Example

For example, Valente and others (2009) collected data from sixth-grade students in four schools in 17 classes. Students were asked to name their five closest friends in the class. Height and weight measurements were taken of all the students and their body mass index (BMI, in kg/m^2) was calculated. BMI is typically used as an indicator of body composition, with adult BMI values greater than 30 signifying obesity.

An ERGM model was used to test the probability that friendship ties existed (relative to no tie) as a function of the network change statistics of the structural properties density, reciprocity, and so on. The network change statistics refer to the difference in the count of various network configuration types when the tie from node i to node j is absent to when the tie is present. This study used the latest specification for ERGMs as discussed earlier (Robins et al., 2007). A common model was applied to all 15 classes and parameter estimates and their standard errors were aggregated as in a meta-analysis to determine if the effects generalize across classes (Snijders & Baeveldt, 2003).

After controlling for structural effects, weight status similarity had a strong and statistically significant effect ($T^2 = 53.73$, $df = 15$, $p < .001$) with a mean effect size of 0.22 ($p < .001$), indicating friendships were more likely to exist between students of the same rather than different weight statuses. The estimated between-classroom standard deviation of this effect size was 0.06 ($p = $ NS). The study also tested whether weight status was associated with naming more friends or being named as a friend. For naming friends, there was a significant main effect of weight status ($T^2 = 27.93$, $df = 15$, $p < .05$) with a mean effect size of 0.13 ($p < .05$), indicating that overweight adolescents named more friends than nonoverweight ones. The estimated between-class standard deviation of this effect size was 0.13 ($p < .05$), indicating the estimated effect size was different between classes.

Note the ERGM results do not show which direction the association occurs. That is, there is an association between friendship and weight status, which also means that nonobese students are also more likely to be friends with one another. The ERGM parameter estimate is not particularly informative as the researcher does not know how strong the association is. The ERGM analysis, however, does assure the researcher that the association between weight status and friendship is not a function of being connected to the same others in the class or other structural characteristics of the network. This study (Valente et al., 2009) also used regular random effects logistics regression to estimate the association between being at risk for obesity and having obese friends. The regression results indicated an approximate two-fold increase in obesity for those with obese friends.

In sum, ERGMs are the first building blocks of statistical estimation of network structural effects. Researchers wishing to know whether an empirical network is significant can use ERGMs to generate simulate (random) networks derived from the features of the empirical networks. Higher-order structural effects can be compared, between the empirical and simulated distributions, provided the lower-order structural effects are matched. For example, transitivity can be tested provided size, density, and reciprocity are matched (or at least the analysis is conditioned on density).

The statistical analysis conducted to test whether a network exhibits the proposed structural features is conducted by estimating how well the ties in the empirical network match those generated by the simulations. The networks are simulated, a matrix representing the links implied by the structural model is constructed, and then this matrix is converted into a vector that indicates who is linked to whom if the structural model were true. This vector can then be regressed (logistically since its binary) on the actual vector of who is linked to whom to determine if the empirical data fit the model.

Actor-Oriented Model

To this point, ERGMs have been described as ways to determine whether an empirical network exhibits structural tendencies (e.g., amount of transitivity) and whether individual attributes may be associated with a link between two people. For example, do the actors tend to form reciprocal or transitive relationships, and are obese students more likely to be friends with other obese students? Researchers, however, have been interested for some time in how networks evolve and whether there are individual (or node) characteristics associated with network evolution. Testing whether there are certain properties that drive network changes associated with network evolution is often referred to as the *actor-oriented model*. The estimation procedure allows researchers to identify whether behaviors are associated with the formation and/or dissolution of a tie between actors and whether network ties lead to changes in behaviors.

The actor-oriented model follows similar logic to ERGMs except that rather than generating 500 simulated networks to compare against an empirical one, the researcher specifies the way the network at time one *evolves* to become the network at time 2. Identifying the evolution of social network preferences over time uses what have been called stochastic actor-oriented models (Burk et al., 2007; Snijders, 2001; Snijders et al., 2007). Instead of calculating frequencies of various types of social configurations as is done in ERGMs, actor-oriented models simulate dynamic processes using what is essentially a form of agent-based modeling. Current software programs used to estimate actor-oriented models require the researcher to specify the parameters that are thought to govern how the network evolves from time 1 to time 2 and then generates a simulation of networks to determine whether imposing those rules will generate networks similar to the observed network at the later time point. The challenges for the researcher are to specify the structural and behavioral tendencies in the network (this is known as the *objective function*).

Currently, there are three computer platforms used to test longitudinal network and behavior models: SIENA (Simulation Investigation of Empirical Network Analysis) STATNET, and PNET. The rest of this section is written somewhat from the SIENA perspective. Specification of a SIENA model entails specification of the objective function and rate function. The objective function is the specific network structural properties thought to drive the evolution of the network, and the rate function is the estimated number of changes each actor can make between observed time points. The objective function indicates the tendency or preference for the current state of the network. Practically, the researcher specifies in the software the structural and attribute-based factors thought to affect social and behavioral evolution and does not write out the objective function. For the rate function, the researcher typically allows the software to estimate the rates without imposing a rate function.

To test an actor-oriented model using SIENA, the researcher needs to specify the data, the network matrices, and the attribute vectors. If the researcher has multiple networks, such as several schools or organizations, then he or she needs to decide whether to estimate each network separately and conduct a meta-analysis to aggregate the results, or combine the networks into one large file and insert "structural zeros" for links between separate networks. Once the data are imported, SIENA provides separate windows to conduct data transformations and/or selection (subset of the population, for example).

The heart of the evolutionary analysis occurs with the model specification. Researchers can specify the networks of relations as independent or dependent variables, and attributes can be constant or change over time. In addition, the researcher can specify relationship covariates that change over time (e.g., whether two individuals are married, or how far they live from one another). Finally, the researcher indicates the parameters to be estimated— structural parameters such as density, reciprocity, and transitivity—as well as the attributes that interact with these structural parameters. For example, a basic SIENA model might test whether students tend to reciprocate ties, to make transitive ties, and to make ties with others of the same gender (boys more likely to name boys and girls more likely to name girls). *Great care should be taken when specifying the model parameters as these should be guided by the theoretical model being tested.*

Once the model has been specified, the simulation runs by generating networks based on the model specifications. The model will converge if the simulation can generate networks that resemble the empirical ones. Often models do not converge because the parameter specification cannot generate networks that resemble the empirical ones, due in part to the empirical data (e.g., the networks are too sparse or too dense; see Chapter 8) or the model specification contains inherent contradictions.

t-Tests are provided to determine if the model converged. Here the researcher looks for non–statistically significant *t*-tests because we want the simulated networks to be similar to the empirical ones. SIENA then provides estimates and standard errors to determine whether the analysis has produced significant *t*-values. Like in regression statistics, *t*-values greater than 2 signify significant estimates and the researcher can conclude that there is a tendency for the corresponding phenomenon in the data. A useful way to understand the various parameter settings to fit actor-oriented models is to diagram the parameter in terms of its relation from a focal actor and its neighbors.

Table 9–1 provides a diagram of some of the different structural properties tested in the actor-oriented evolution analysis. Each row represents a different structural parameter, which is a pattern of network relationships. The first row shows out-degree, which is an indicator of the density (the number of links) in the network. Out-degree is always included in an actor-based model to control for density. Out-degree parameter estimates are almost always negative, which suggests that ties are structured and nonrandom (a positive out-degree would indicate that network structures would tend to become decentralized with a density of 50%). The second row shows mutuality (reciprocity), where

Table 9–1. Structural Parameters Typically Estimated in ERGMs

Parameter	Illustration of Social Process	Description	Example
Out-degree (density)		The overall tendency to have ties	Actors increase their connectedness
Reciprocity		Tendency to have reciprocated ties	Actors prefer others who have selected them.
Transitive triplets		Tendency towards triadic closure of local ties	Actors prefer others who are friends of their friends
Balance effect		Tendency to have ties to structurally similar others (structural balance)	Actors prefer to have ties to others in their circle
Attribute alter		Main effect of alter's behavior (covariate determines in in-degree)	Alters are nominated based on having an attribute or not nominated based on not having the attribute
Attribute ego		Main effect of ego's property on tie preference	Actors make ties based on having an attribute or do not make ties based on not having the attribute
Attribute similarity		Tendency to be connected to similar others	Actors prefer ties with others who are the same on an attribute.

Based on Steglich et al. (2007).

a positive estimate would indicate that given an incoming tie from B to A, there is high chance for A to reciprocate that tie to B. The other rows in the table are structural tendencies that can be tested after these first two.

WINCART

To illustrate the co-evolution model, a study was conducted to evaluate the effects of a Community-Based Participatory Research (CBPR) intervention designed to increase linkages between community based organizations and university researchers around issues of cancer education, training, and research (Israel et al., 2000; Wallerstein & Duran, 2006; Valente et al., in press). This study reports the results of the Weaving an Islander Network for Cancer Awareness Research and Training (WINCART) initiative designed to reduce cancer disparities among Pacific Islanders in Southern California (Tanjasiri & Tran, 2008). WINCART was created as a forum for community groups to meet and establish connections between various Pacific Island community groups and involved both a scientific advisory board and a community advisory board to guide WINCART's education, research, and training activities. A stated objective of the WINCART initiative is to create linkages between community-based organizations (CBOs) and academic institutions conducting cancer research (Tanjasiri et al., 2007). These linkages would enable community organizations to disseminate information about cancer research and treatment developments to their constituents. At the same time, WINCART was designed to create connections from academic institutions and cancer researchers to CBOs so that cancer research, education, and training would be more community informed

WINCART conducted many activities to bridge the gap between community and academia such as retreats, events, symposia, and relationship building. An actor-oriented model was used to determine if WINCART was effective in integrating these groups. There were 19 organizations in the study: 11 CBOs, 5 universities, and 3 national cancer-related organizations (e.g., American Cancer Society). Fourteen network questions were asked with regard to (1) communication, (2) formal agreements, (3) client referrals to, and (4) client referrals from; non-cancer communication or interaction regarding (5) education, (6) outreach, (7) training, (8) advocacy, and (9) research; and cancer communication or interaction regarding (10) education, (11) outreach, (12) training, (13) advocacy, and (14) research. Respondents were presented with a roster of all 19 organizations and invited to check those with which they interacted.

Electronic invitations and surveys were sent to 121 individuals in 16 organizations in June 2005 and 113 individuals in 17 organizations in July 2007.

Ninety-one respondents completed the survey at time 1 (75.2%) and 56 at time 2 (49.5%). At time 1, the three national organizations were not solicited to participate but invitations were sent to representatives of CIS working in the community at time two. These responses were not included in the study since these data were only available at time 2. All linkages to these three national organizations were removed from the data for this analysis because they did not make any nominations (were not invited participate in the study). At least one individual from every participating organization responded. The lower than expected response rate may have been a function of individuals within the same organization telling each other they responded for the organization. Follow-up conversations with some nonresponders also indicated that they mistook the time 2 solicitation for a reminder of the time 1 survey they already completed. The data were aggregated to the organizational level so that individual responses are unknown.

Because the number of respondents from each organization varied, links between organizations were summed and then divided by the number of respondents from each organization. The dependent variable in this case is the percent of links from one organization to another and the guiding research question is whether connectivity increased over time and became more heterogeneous on status (CBO versus university).

There was a decrease in respondents per organization from 4.79 and 2.95 at time 1 and 2, respectively. Most respondents were female, 87.9% and 81.4% at time 1 and 2, respectively. Respondents were experienced working in their organizations, averaging approximately 7 to 8 years working with their current organization. Most had participated in WINCART activities, 58.6% to 67.9%, averaging 1.71 to 2.38 activities in the past year. There were 1,426 links reported in response to the 14 network questions at baseline, and despite the fewer number of respondents, there was an increase to 1,617 links at time 2. There were 146 and 159 links within the organizations at time 1 and 2, respectively.

The linkage rate (percentage of respondents in the organization who nominated another organization) was 30% at time 1 and increased to 43% at time 2. At both time points, organizations were nominated by the most respondents in response to the question, "Which organizations have you communicated with in the past year" (44% and 54%, respectively). At time 1, the number of connections was lowest for receiving clients (19%), but at time 2 it was lowest for non–cancer-related research (34%). Figure 9–3 illustrates the cancer education network at times 1 and 2 with organizations depicted as CBOs (circles) or universities (squares).

As in the ERGM example, initial analysis consisted of estimation using ordinary least-squares regression of the connection percentage as a function of time; follow-up response rate; network question (general, noncancer, or

(a)

(b)

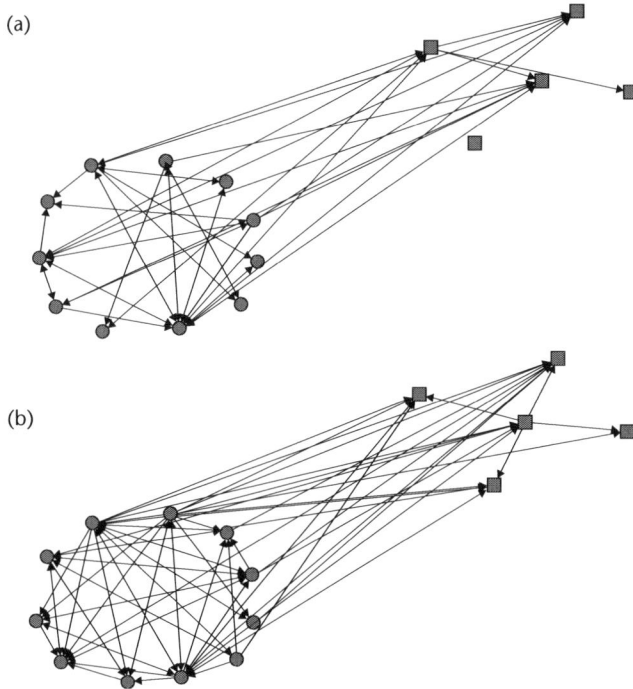

Figure 9–3. (a) Cancer Education Network at time 1. (b) Cancer Education Network at time 2. Links indicate which organization nominated which other dichotomized on the median value. Circles are CBOs and squares are universities. There is an increase in linkage from CBOs to universities but not from universities from CBOs. Figures created with Netdraw (Borgatti, 2005).

cancer); organization type; and a time-by-type interaction term. A positive and statistically significant time-by-type interaction effect indicates that linkages increased over time between and/or among types. The regression model was also reestimated using a random effects probit model to control for clustering of responses within organizations. For both of these models, the regression analysis showed a statistically significant interaction terms in which links from CBOs to CBOs and links from CBOs to universities increased over time (see Valente et al., in press).

In the statistical evolution model, parameters were included that tested whether there were tendencies for linkages between organizational types to occur after controlling for the network structural effects of density, reciprocity, and transitivity. Specifically, the objective function specified whether (1) there were more outgoing links based on organizational type, (2) there were more incoming links based on organizational type, and (3) organizations of the same type link with one another more than they link with other types (similarity effects of the organizational type). The joint contribution of these organization-type effects to the objective function is (Snijders et al., in press) presented as follows:

$$\beta_e \sum_j x_{ij} v_i + \beta_a \sum_j x_{ij} v_j + \beta_s \sum_j x_{ij} I\{v_i = v_j\} \tag{9-1}$$

where β_e is a parameter for the ego effect, β_a is a parameter for the alter effect, β_s is a parameter for the same effect, x_{ij} is a tie variable from organization i to j, v_i is an ego's value of the organizational type, v_j is an alter's value of the organizational type, and $I\{v_i = v_j\}$ is an indicator function of the similarity coded as 1 if $v_i = v_j$ and as 0 otherwise. The equation representing the contribution to the objective function of the single tie from organization i to organization j (x_{ij}) that takes only the effects related to organizational type is as follows (Snijders et al., in press):

$$\beta_e(v_i - \bar{v}) + \beta_a(v_j - \bar{v}) + \beta_s I\{v_i = v_j\} \tag{9-2}$$

where $\bar{v}$ is a mean value for the centering.

The 14 networks were analyzed separately and combined using meta-analysis (Snijders & Baerveldt, 2003). Each network was dichotomized on median values of the proportion respondents nominated for each network across waves (ranged from 0.20 to 0.33). The same objective function specifications were applied to each network and the results were combined to produce vectors of parameter means and standard errors across networks (with specification of the upper bound of 5). Based on these results, ego-alter selection values were created using Equation 9-2 for the two values of organization type, v_i and v_j. Organization type was coded as 0 for the five universities and 1 for the 11 CBOs yielding a global mean $\bar{v} = 0.69$. The centered value for university was -1.69 (= $0 - 1.69$) and 0.31 (= $1 - 0.69$) for CBOs. All estimation was done using SIENA (Snijders et al., 2007).

For the SIENA results, all 14 networks attained convergence with t-ratios being less than .1 in absolute value. The results of the meta-analysis across all networks indicated there was a significant ego effect for CBOs indicating they increased their outgoing linkages more rapidly than universities ($T^2 = 69.00$, df = 14, $p < 0.001$; mean effect size = 1.15, $p < 0.001$). The alter, or incoming, effects ($T^2 = 20.02$, df = 13, $p = 0.10$; mean effect size = -0.64, $p < 0.001$) and similarity effects ($T^2 = 14.49$, df = 13, $p = 0.34$; mean effect size = 0.55, $p < 0.01$)) based on organizational type were not significant indicating no difference in nominations received by organization type and no difference in the likelihood of linkage between organizations of the same type. The estimated between-network standard deviation for the ego effect (outgoing) parameter along with those for incoming and similarity parameters were negligible indicating similar effects across networks. The estimated mean effect sizes for each covariate were entered into equation (3):

$$1.15(v_i - 0.69) - 0.64(v_j - 0.69) + 0.55I(v_i = v_j) \qquad (9\text{-}3)$$

Substituting the values 0 for Universities and 1 for CBOs into v, yields the following results for ego-alter selection tendencies as in Table 3: university to university, 0.20; university to CBO, –0.99; CBO to university, 0.80; and CBO to CBO, 0.71. Consequently, CBOs exhibited a tendency to prefer relations with universities (0.80) or other CBOs (0.71); whereas universities tended to prefer connections to other universities (0.20) and not to CBOs (–0.99). In sum, these results show that there was a tendency for CBOs to connect to one another and to universities, but universities did not demonstrate a preference for connecting to CBOs or themselves.

These results illustrate how the actor-oriented co-evolution model can be applied to a substantive public health problem, evaluating CBPR as a means to bring evidence-based public health to communities and to enable researchers to conduct community-informed research. The statistical analysis showed that linkages from CBOs to other CBOs and from CBOs to universities increased during the study. In contrast, university faculty did not increase their ties to other universities or to CBOs. This suggests that WINCART was successful at motivating network change among the community partners but not among university researchers (Valente et al., in press).

There are many other applications in public health that are just being tested. SNA provides a framework for understanding the structural processes that give rise to a specific network. The regression approach treats social relations as antecedents to behaviors. Usually in public health, we are more concerned with how a specific network structure affects the spread of disease or risk behavior, not in the mechanisms that created a specific structure. However, to the extent that attributes are included in the analysis, SNA can be useful for understanding how certain attributes interact with network structure. So for example, it can be determined whether smokers are more likely to associate with other smokers, thus testing for homophily on smoking behavior, which is critical for understanding peer influence.

Summary

This chapter has attempted to provide a nontechnical introduction to techniques used to conduct statistical analyses on networks. The ERGM was introduced as the building block for statistical estimation. ERGM is a technique in which an empirical network is compared to randomly generated ones to determine if structural properties in the empirical network occur greater than expected by chance. The critical element is to understand that structural properties are hierarchical so that density is nested within reciprocity, which is nested with triadic structures, and so on. The simulated networks match on the lower structural properties and are used to statistically assess the higher ones.

The chapter also emphasized the innovation of testing structural properties against the presence of a link in the network. Initial statistical analyses of networks involved converting the matrix of links to a vector representing each tie and regressing this on structural elements in the networks. Recent developments of new specifications for the generation of simulated networks has created the capability to test co-evolution models that simultaneously test for network and behavior changes in one statistical model. The chapter included some empirical examples. As Snijders notes, "The statistical modeling of social networks is difficult because of the complicated dependence structures of the processes underlying their genesis and development" (Snijders, 2005, p. 215). In spite of these challenges, considerable progress has been made and many new discoveries regarding network effects and processes are imminent.

Acknowledgments: The author thanks Laura Koehly, Kayo Fujimoto, and Kate Coronges for help with this chapter.

10

Diffusion of Innovations

This chapter reviews the diffusion of innovations theory, which has been the theory that has used network principles and perspectives most extensively. An introduction to the theory and a review of its principles are provided. The chapter then covers the major models used to understand how diffusion through networks occurs. Empirical data illustrating network exposure effects are presented as well as the calculation and interpretation of network thresholds. The chapter closes with a brief critique of the theory. Many concepts related to diffusion have been interspersed throughout this volume, but this chapter delves deeper into the issues.

Behavior change theories are used to understand how social change occurs (Valente, 2002). The most prominent behavioral application of network analysis is the study of the *diffusion of innovations,* which explains how new ideas and practices spread within and between communities. Diffusion of innovations theory has provided the theoretical underpinnings to research how networks affect behavior and behavior change. Diffusion theory is one of the most widely used theories in public health (Glanz et al., 2002). It has its roots in anthropology, economics, geography, sociology, marketing, among other disciplines (Brown, 1981; Hägerstrand, 1967; Katz, 1962; Katz et al., 1963; Robertson, 1971; Rogers, 2003) and has in some ways been adapted from epidemiology (e.g., Bailey, 1975; Morris, 1993). The premise, confirmed by empirical research, is that many new ideas and practices spread through inter-personal contacts largely consisting of interpersonal communication (Bass, 1969; Beal & Bohlen, 1955; Katz et al., 1963; Ryan & Gross, 1943; Rogers, 2003; Valente, 1995, 2005; Valente & Rogers, 1995).

A new idea or practice may originate in another community and be trans-ported to the host community, or it may originate, be invented in, the com-munity where it diffuses. Ideas and innovations enter communities from external sources such as the mass media, via labor exchanges, technological innovations and shifts, cosmopolitan contact, and many other sources. The critical element for diffusion is that information about the new idea or prac-tice spreads through interpersonal contact networks. (Many diffusion stud-ies have not measured social networks and how information flows through networks and a purist might argue that these studies fall into the realm of behavior or social change studies and not diffusion.)

In their pioneering study, Ryan and Gross (1943) laid the groundwork for the diffusion paradigm by showing that, among other things, social factors rather than economic ones were important influences on adoption (Valente & Rogers, 1995). Hundreds of diffusion studies were conducted in the 1950s and early 1960s to examine the diffusion process in more detail across a variety of settings (Rogers, 2003). Many studies sought to understand how information created in government or otherwise sponsored programs could be disseminated more effectively. Diffusion research peaked in the early 1960s but has been reinvigorated recently with the advent of more sophisti-cated network models and technology, making it possible to study the diffu-sion process more explicitly.

Most diffusion studies focus on trying to understand the factors that lead some members of a population to adopt a new idea, while others do not. Further, studies try to understand why some people adopt the behavior early while others wait a substantial amount of time before accepting the new practice. For example, Ryan and Gross (1943) wanted to know why some farmers purchased hybrid seed corn almost immediately upon its availabil-ity while others waited until almost all the farmers purchased it before they were willing to do so. Similarly, Coleman and others (1966) wanted to know why some physicians began prescribing tetracycline as soon as it was avail-able, while others waited until most physicians prescribed it before they were willing to do so.

The five main elements of the diffusion model are (Rogers, 2003) that (1) perceived characteristics of the innovation affect its rate of adoption; (2) diffusion occurs over time so that rate of adoption often yields a cumu-late adoption S-shaped pattern, and individuals are classified as early or late adopters; (3) individuals pass through stages during the adoption pro-cess typically classified as knowledge, persuasion, decision, implementation, and confirmation; (4) people can modify the innovation and sometimes discontinue its use; and (5) mathematical models can be developed to measure the rate and character of diffusion curves (Mahajan & Peterson, 1985; Valente, 1993; Young, 2006).

Some scholars have treated the rate of new adopters as normally distributed, and in such cases adopters can be classified in terms of their innovativeness or how early or late they are in the diffusion process relative to the population. By treating the new adopters, the incidence curve, as normally distributed, adopters are classified as early adopters (first 16%), early majority (17% to 50%), late majority (51% to 84%), and laggards (85% to 100%). Diffusion is usually a very slow process, taking years and decades for many significant innovations. For example, the telephone took decades from its invention to widespread acceptance.

The prototypical diffusion study was Ryan and Gross' (1943) study of factors that influenced rural Iowa farmers to adopt the use of hybrid seed corn (Box 10–1). Hybrid seeds took decades to be developed and perfected

---

Box 10–1. Ryan and Gross and the History of Diffusion

Bryce Ryan studied sociology and economics at Harvard University and obtained his first faculty appointment at Iowa State University. He was assigned a doctoral student named Neil Gross. Ryan was casting about for a study topic and noticed that there was a lot of corn in Iowa. Throughout the early part of the twentieth century, scientists had been creating various hybrid corn seeds, which replaced open pollinated varieties. Hybrid seeds were a radical departure for farming since they required the purchase of seeds each year, that the farmer then planted in contrast to using his or her own crop to provide the seeds for each year's planting.

Hybrids had higher yields and were more drought resistant than open pollinated varieties, so they were a seemingly advantageous innovation. Yet it took decades for hybrids to be adopted by farmers in the United States and internationally. To spur diffusion, the U.S. Agricultural Extension Service was created to publish information on hybrid seed productivity, and private seed companies often distributed free samples to farmers.

Ryan launched a study in two Iowa communities to determine factors associated with the adoption of hybrid corn seed (Ryan & Gross, 1943). They contrasted economic variables (e.g., size of farm) with social ones (e.g., readership of farm bulletins). The Ryan and Gross study became a classic as it was a model for the study of behavior change and how new ideas and practices within and between communities (Crane, 1972). The diffusion of hybrid corn seed among the 257 farmers Ryan and Gross was textbook diffusion in action.

in experimental lab stations. Once the hybrids were ready, it then took years, and in some cases decades, for these innovative seeds to diffuse among famers. In the Ryan and Gross (1943) study, there was a 14-year time span between the first and latest adopters even though the innovation was patently advantageous.

It should also be noted that diffusion typically takes a long time. Hybrid seed corn was under development for decades before it became commercially viable and seed companies had to give away samples for years before farmers would pay for it (Crabb, 1947). The telephone took decades to diffuse widely in the United States, and the VCR, while seemingly an innovation that diffused rapidly, took decades to reach a majority of households. To be sure, some innovations diffuse rapidly, but only rarely, and usually only under extraordinary conditions. The slow pace of diffusion is often a result of network structures that often inhibit diffusion. The advent of computer communications seems to have accelerated the spread of information and in many cases adoption of technologies and other products. Facebook, for example, spread to hundreds of millions of users in a few years (*http://www.facebook.com/press.php*).

The second element of diffusion theory is that adoption does not occur immediately after someone first learns about a new product; rather people pass through stages in the adoption process from becoming aware, to learning more information about it, making a decision to adopt it, trying it, and eventually confirming their use. These stages can be used for market segmentation as well as measuring progress toward behavior change. Most behavior change models describe stages in the adoption process (Valente, 2002; Valente et al., 1998). Diffusion of innovations is studied in many different fields, but here the discussion is primarily concerned with how social networks affect adoption and diffusion of disease and/or associated risk behaviors. The starting point is referred to as the homogeneous mixing model.

Homogeneous Mixing

Homogeneous mixing can be demonstrated with a simple spreadsheet exercise illustrated in Table 10–1. Assume a hypothetical population of 100 people at time 1 (year 1, for example), and 5 people adopt a new idea or practice. These 5 initial adopters may adopt because they are persuaded by the mass media to adopt or because they are willing and perhaps eager to try new things. These 5 initial adopters have random interactions with the 95 who have not yet adopted and they persuade them to adopt at a rate of 1%. The product (5 × 95 × 0.01) yields 4.75 new adopters at the end of time 1. At the start of time 2, there are 9.75 (5 + 4.75) adopters interacting randomly with

Table 10–1. Homogeneous Mixing Sample in Excel

Adopters	Rate	Nonadopters	New Adopters
5.00	1%	95.00	4.75
9.75	1%	90.25	8.80
18.55	1%	81.45	15.11
33.66	1%	66.34	22.33
55.99	1%	44.01	24.64
80.63	1%	19.37	15.62
96.25	1%	3.75	3.61
99.86	1%	0.14	0.14
100.00	1%	0.00	0.00

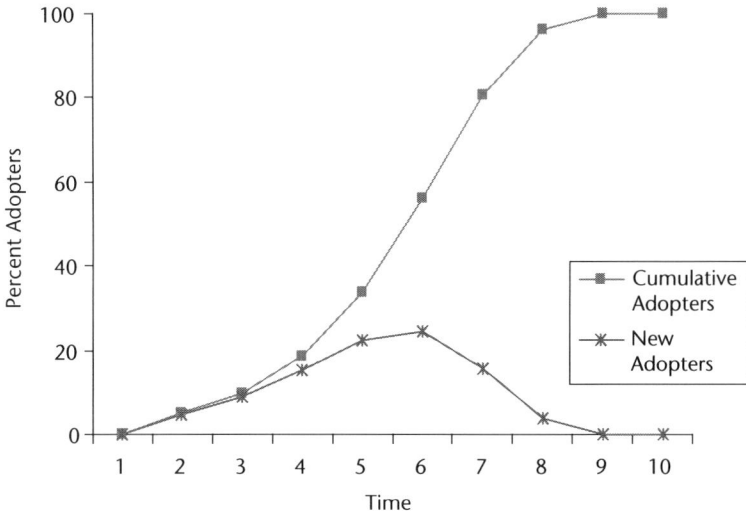

Figure 10–1. Typical diffusion and adoption curves (generated from hypothetical data). In this hypothetical scenario, five initial adopters interact and convince the remaining 95 nonadopters at a rate of 1%. The subsequent adoptions and interactions result in a cumulative growth curve resembling a logistic function with everyone converted by 10 time periods.

the 90.25 left in the population, and they convince them to adopt at a rate of 1% and we get 8.8 new adopters, or 18.55 total adopters.

Figure 10–1 shows the incidence and prevalence graphs for this hypothetical scenario. The growth in adoption occurs gradually at first and then accelerates toward the middle of the diffusion process and then tapers off as the pool of nonadopters shrinks. The model assumes no one dis-adopts (quits using) and assumes uniform conversion rates (1% throughout the process).

One can change the conversion rate to generate different curves. The model also provides an example how an epidemic can spread in a population.

Unfortunately, or fortunately depending on the setting, diffusion is not as simple as the homogeneous model implies. For one, people do not interact randomly as noted in the sections on homophily, reciprocity, transitivity, and so on. Two, conversion rates are not likely to be uniform for everyone; some people have more resistance than others. Three, the media and other external factors influence perceptions about appropriate behaviors and may differentially affect people's adoption decisions. In particular, there has been some research on how media influences and social networks interact to collectively bring about behavioral and societal change (Box 10–2 on two-step flow hypothesis). Diffusion network scholars have developed a set of approaches and theories

---

Box 10–2. Two-Step Flow Hypothesis

During the 1940s and 1950s, Paul Lazarsfeld (often with his colleague Robert Merton) had established a tradition of research studying the effects of the mass media on many behaviors including voting patterns and consumer behavior. Lazarsfeld and Merton were based at Columbia University and were joined by Elihu Katz in the mid-1950s. The team pioneered many research innovations with their primary focus being research on how radio and TV influenced mass audiences.

Although the prevailing view was that the mass media influenced people directly, Lazarsfeld thought that media effects were mediated by interpersonal influence. People who were exposed to media messages did not automatically believe them and did immediately accept the information provided to them. Instead, people digested media information within the context of their social networks. One specific hypothesis of theirs was the two-step flow hypothesis. The two-step flow hypothesis stated that the media influenced opinion leaders who in turn influenced others. Opinion leaders paid attention to the media at a greater rate than others and were thought to be more informed on many topics than opinion followers. Opinion leader use of media and other sources of information enabled them to be more knowledgeable and hence influence others.

Opinion leaders were found to receive more media and were more aware of current events than were nonleaders. To persuade others to follow their opinions, opinion leaders used media communications to buttress their arguments. Gladwell (2003) writes, "These mavens make extensive use of the media to stay expert on their favorite subjects and become trusted sources of information for others." It may be that media influence opinion leaders who influence others that influence others—a three-step or even multistep flow. Furthermore, it may be that some

(Continued)

Box 10–2. Continued

opinion leaders influence one or a few others, whereas others have much higher multiplier effects, influencing five, ten, or hundreds of others. These opinion leader models, however, neglect to consider a number of other factors regarding the media influence process.

First, it is likely that opinion leaders are influenced by others as much as others are influenced by them and that media shape their messages in accordance with what they think the audience wants to see or hear. In summary, to say that media communications can influence person A who influences person B may be an oversimplification. Second, individuals are embedded within complex social network structures. Some people have small networks, whereas others have quite large ones. Some social networks are integrated (their friends know each other), whereas others are radial (their friends do not know one another). What follows are three ways in which social network structures can affect media processes First, Potterat and others (1999) proposed that network structure, especially the cohesiveness of an individual's network, is associated with STD/HIV risk for the individual. The authors report that lower cohesiveness of network members is associated with lower STD/HIV transmission, even in a high-risk population. Second, the norms held within social networks alter the media influence process. For example, if a social network composed of young adults has negative safer sex norms, a media campaign designed to target and change these norms may increase condom use (Friedman et al., 2001). Third, as mentioned earlier, homophily affects the flow of ideas and behaviors. Information flows and persuasion occur more readily among homophilous dyads, that is, people who are like one another, rather than among heterophilous ones. Consequently, diffusion tends to occur along sociodemographic lines because social networks are contoured by sociodemographic characteristics. Finally, the media influence process may vary by the degree of risk taking and risk avoidance in the population, their personal network thresholds.

These four factors, and perhaps others, suggest that the relationship between mass media and interpersonal communication is complex. Unlike the simple opinion leader model, it is more likely that people attend to media communication, and then interpret and discuss it in unanticipated ways. For example, an antitobacco campaign may be parodied by the intended audience, resulting in boomerang (opposite) effects rather than antitobacco effects. This boomerang effect has also occurred with HIV campaigns. Some members of the gay community have begun to refuse participation in safer sex behaviors because of the widespread access to antiretroviral drugs, believing the risk for HIV to be diminished (Bertrand et al., 2004). In other words, the effect of media communications on individuals is a function of how the messages are interpreted within the context of people's social networks—how, with whom, and in what ways the messages are discussed.

about how social networks influence diffusion of innovations. There are four classes of models for network diffusion: (1) integration and opinion leadership, (2) structural models, (3) critical value models, and (4) dynamic models.

Integration and Opinion Leadership

Early diffusion network studies noted that those people who are integrated into a community generally adopt behaviors earlier than those who are less integrated. For example, Coleman and others (1966) in their study of network influences on physician adoption of a new drug showed that physicians who received three or more nominations as advice and discussion partners had a faster diffusion than those who received none. Figure 10–2 illustrates the diffusion curves for integrated physicians compared to nonintegrated ones. Coleman and others (1966) concluded that the new drug spread through the connections among the physicians in a snowball process (also see Coleman et al., 1957).

Other studies also confirmed that people who are well integrated into the community were likely earlier adopters than those on the margins (Rogers & Kincaid, 1981). In general, it was discovered that opinion leaders, those who

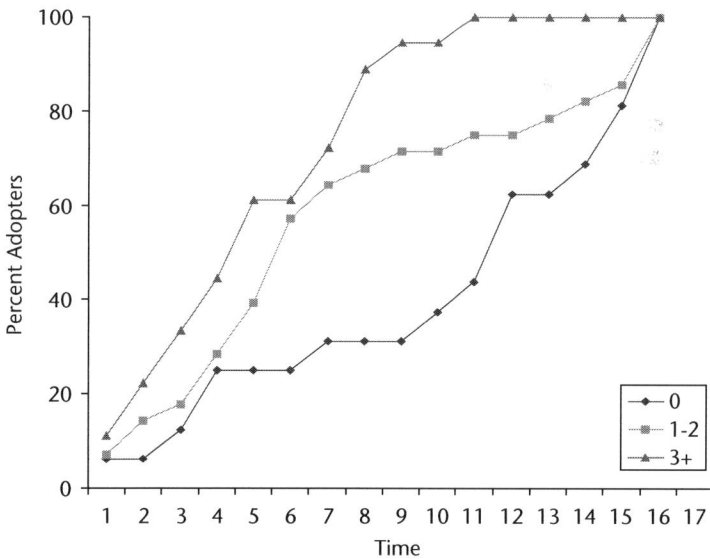

Figure 10–2. Diffusion of tetracycline among physicians by their integration in social networks. (Data from the classic network diffusion study of medical innovation by Coleman, Katz, and Menzel [1966].)

received many choices as discussion partners from their colleagues, were earlier, but not the earliest, adopters of new ideas and practices. Rogers and Kincaid (1981) also discovered that study villages could be characterized by specific contraceptive methods which became widespread within each village. For example, in some villages, the IUD would be the most prevalent method whereas in others the pill or withdrawal would predominate. Opinion leaders seemed to play a role in this process since oftentimes the most prevalent method in a community was also the one being used by those women most frequently nominated as discussion or advice partners. Research of course is needed to determine whether these opinion leaders merely reflect the normative practices of their communities or whether their behavior is being imitated by others in the community. The role of opinion leaders is also likely to vary based on characteristics of the innovation.

Becker (1970) questioned whether opinion leaders would always be earlier adopters of innovations. Becker (1970) hypothesized that opinion leaders would be earlier adopters of innovations that were compatible with the community norms but later adopters of innovations perceived to be incompatible. He studied public health officers' adoption of two behaviors: measles immunization, which was compatible with the mission of public health officers, and diabetes screening, which was not. Becker (1970) showed that opinion leaders, measured with in-degree centrality, delayed their adoption of diabetes screening because they perceived it to be incompatible with the norms of public health at that time.

The importance of opinion leaders is hard to overstate. It is also important to note that opinion leaders are not necessarily the earliest adopters of innovations. Opinion leaders need to reflect the norms of their community and they cannot deviate too much from what is accepted in the community or they will lose their privileged position in the network. Thus, they can lead but not too far ahead of the group. Typically, the earliest adopters are innovative and often on the margins of the community; they innovate because they are different. The opinion leader then translates this innovation for the rest of the community. Translation is one of the skills associated with being a good opinion leader. Opinion leaders are admired by many and are good at scanning the environment because they are connected to lots of people.

Once opinion leaders embrace a new idea, diffusion can accelerate. Leaders are connected to many others; hence, once they embrace the idea, the number of relationships involving adopters and nonadopters increases dramatically. Not all adopters are equal, so while the earliest adopters may be the first to adopt, their behavior does little to influence the rest of the system because they are not role models for many others. The leaders, however, represent a shift from adoption on the margins of the network to the center and accelerate the behavior change process.

Structural Models

Opinion leadership and integration have obvious implications and effects on diffusion—as those who occupy prominent roles in a community adopt, the balance of information and persuasion in the community tilts toward the new idea. Granovetter (1973) focused on a different aspect of the diffusion problem by showing that other people in a community can occupy critical positions in the network that affect diffusion at the macro level. Granovetter's (1973) strength of weak ties argument has both micro and macro levels of analysis and implications for both.

Granovetter (1973) noted the tendency for homophily and stated that two people who are friends are also likely to be friends with a third person (see Chapter 8 for information on triads). The tendency for triads to be closed is an important property used in the study of network evolution (see Chapter 8 and Kossinets & Watts, 2006). Networks thus tend to close in tightly formed pockets since friends tend to introduce people to one another. Granovetter argued that because of this triadic closure tendency, only some people will have networks that do not close around them but instead are open and connect different groups in the network. Granovetter presented the example in Figure 10–3 and argued that nodes A and B constitute a weak tie because they connect two different groups in the network.

Granovetter's central insight is that the friends of my friends typically know the same people I know and have access to the same information. Consequently, information received from my close personal networks tends to be redundant. New information comes from weak ties, people one sees

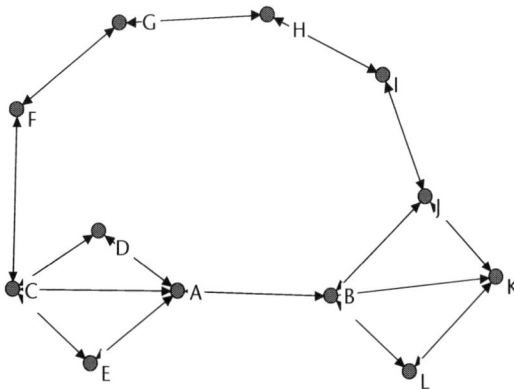

Figure 10–3. Granovetter's (1972) illustration of weak ties, in which the link between A and B creates shorter path lengths connecting others in the network.

only occasionally or who are connected tangentially through acquaintances. The original data Granovetter collected for this thesis came from interviews with people who had recently obtained new jobs, and many of them reported weak ties as the source of information about the new job (Granovetter, 1974). Weak ties are strong in information because weak ties connect people to others to whom one is not normally connected.

The applicability of the weak ties argument was widespread. Weak ties clearly had implications for diffusion since the presence of weak ties would create bridges connecting different segments of a network and hence enable diffusion to traverse group boundaries. Weak ties were also instrumental in learning new information because, as stated, weak ties are connections to people different from one's usual conversation partners and so they have access to novel information. Finally, the identification of weak ties has implications for community mobilization and performance since organizations (and individuals) need to maintain a diverse set of contacts to be able to access resources and information critical to survival and success (Burt, 1992; Valente & Foreman, 1998; Valente et al., 2007a).

Granovetter's (1973) strength of weak ties article is one of the most widely cited articles in social science research, but it is important to be clear about what it says. For one, the main argument is that weak ties have implications for diffusion at the macro level, not the micro level. That is, weak ties enable diffusion to traverse bridges and connect otherwise disconnected or distally connected groups. It does not imply that weak ties are more persuasive adoption influences at the micro level, for individuals. Second, the main argument for the strength of weak ties is with information diffusion, not necessarily behavioral adoption. Weak ties may be very effective at communicating information but may be less effective at persuasion. Precisely because weak ties are weak and because they may contain less trust and reinforcement than strong ties, they are less likely to be conduits for behavior change.

Finally, weak ties are often measured in two different ways: structurally and relationally. Structural measures of weak ties are derived from sociometric data and can be measured as links between individuals connected in different triads. A structural measure of a weak tie would be a bridge that spans otherwise disconnected, or distally connected subgroups. Chapter 11 provides an explicit measure of bridges based on the weak tie concept. Relational measures of weak ties are derived from individual reports of frequency of interaction or emotional/affective closeness. Weak ties are those with whom one is less close and interacts with less frequently.

The weak ties argument was developed further by Ron Burt with his measures of structural holes and constraint (Burt, 1992, 2005). Burt noted that weak ties were ties that spanned structural holes in the network. This directed researchers to look at the white space in the network diagrams and find those nodes or people who had links that spanned the holes in the network. People who occupy structural holes occupy critical positions in the network that enable them to excel. Burt created a measure called *constraint,* which calculated how well a person's ties reached out into the network and provided access to novel sources of information. Burt (2005) has shown how people who score high on constraint, span structural holes, have received higher pay, and gained better promotions in organizations.

The structural basis of diffusion and the role of weak ties were also developed by Duncan Watts (1999) in his analysis of the small world introduced in Chapter 1. Watts and Strogatz (1998) introduced a measure called the clustering coefficient (CC) defined as:

$$CC = \frac{2T_i}{k_i(k_i - 1)} \tag{10-1}$$

where T_i is the number of connections between the direct ties of each node, and $k_i(k_i - 1)$ is the maximum number of possible connections between each node's direct ties. A high (closer to 1) clustering coefficient indicates that a person's friends know one another, whereas a low coefficient indicates that a person's friends are unlikely to know one another. The clustering coefficients for all nodes in a network are averaged to calculate the overall clustering in the network.

As shown in Chapter 8, clustering provides a measure of network structure somewhat independent of its size (the number of nodes), the density (the number of links), and its centralization. Clustering provides a measure of "clumpiness" of the network. A random network will look the same everywhere, but one that is clustered has pockets of interconnectivity, with some nodes having more clustering and others less. Clustering and centralization give rise to the small world phenomenon because they increase the likelihood that two people who meet will have friends in common.

Critical Levels

The Nobel Laureate Thomas Schelling published *Micromotives and Macrobehavior* (1978), in which he coined the term "the tipping point." Schelling showed that seemingly rational and obvious behaviors by individuals can create unexpected outcomes for the system. For example, while most individuals in a community might be considered tolerant with regard to living in mixed ethnic communities, the individual actions by everyone can create strongly segregated communities. Schelling found tipping points in the distribution of behaviors such that once a certain level of the behavior was reached, it had ongoing momentum that kept it going and was hard to reverse.

Tipping points (Gladwell, 1999) have subsequently been discovered to apply to many different phenomena and seem nearly ubiquitous. Gladwell showed how opinion leaders can have a strong influence on others' behavior and can make the difference between a product having no sales or taking off. Gladwell's contribution to diffusion network models was to show how the concepts can be scaled up to a population level. While many scholars had been focusing on behavior within small self-contained communities, Gladwell generalized these principles on a large, national, and international scale, and to a wider range of behaviors.

A number of researchers have developed diffusion models that emphasize the importance of critical levels or tipping points. These tipping points exist at both the micro (individual) and macro (system or community) levels (Valente, 1995). Scholars had long recognized that the diffusion curve (any growth curve for that matter) contained *inflection points*, times where the curve accelerated or decelerated dramatically (Hamblin et al., 1973; Mahajan & Peterson, 1983). Marwell, and others (1988) wrote persuasively about the importance of the critical mass for achieving collective action. Once critical mass was reached, momentum toward achieving collective goals would propel the social movement forward. Markus (1987) argued that interdependent innovations (telephone, fax, e-mail, Facebook, and so on) were particularly prone to critical mass effects because once a technological medium was adopted by a large enough number of people, it would be too difficult for them to defect to another medium and there were inherent advantages to subsequent adopters to adopt the technology.

Identifying critical values at the individual and system levels provides an understanding for how diffusion occurs. Individual tipping points, *thresholds,* enable researchers to identify different types of adopters, low- and high-threshold ones, who might have different motivations to adopt (Valente & Saba, 1998). Similarly, individual influences and motivations on adoption behavior are likely quite different before and after a system has reached its tipping point. Adoption before the tipping point carries more risk than after it.

Dynamic Models

All of the models presented in this chapter are dynamic in that time is specified—diffusion occurs over time, the structural characteristics (weak ties, holes) have consequences for how diffusion occurs over time, and the critical levels occur at a point in time. There have been a series of models created that treat time more explicitly in the sense that they model what happens at the micro (individual) level at each point in time during diffusion. The basic building block of these models and for much diffusion research is network exposure (Burt, 1987; Marsden & Friedkin, 1993; Marsden & Podolny, 1990). Network exposure is the influence of a person's social network, measured with the following equation:

$$E_i = \frac{\sum W_{ij} y_j}{\sum W_i}$$

(10-2)

where W is the social network weight matrix, and y is a vector of adoption behavior. For a person with five friends in a network, network exposure (E_i) is the proportion of those friends who have adopted a behavior. Figure 10–4 provides a graphical display of how Equation 10-2 works. The network is represented as "W" because it is conceived as a weight matrix. For now, the W network will represents direct contacts, a person's five closest friends. Later, we show how W can represent different kinds of network properties, or weights (W), such as the degree of similarity between two nodes (alluded to in Chapter 4). To calculate network exposure, the network (W) is multiplied by y_j, which is a vector (column) of behavior scores.

If y_j represents smoking, for example, the numerator is a calculation of the number of one's friends who smoke. To control for the number of friends named, we divide the numerator by the number of friends to get a percent. Network exposure, then, is the proportion of friends who smoke, friends being those people with whom the respondent indicated he or she was a friend.

Figure 10–5 displays network exposure for one person who has three friends at three points in time. This person has one adopter at the first time point, so exposure is 33%. At the next time point, there are two adopters,

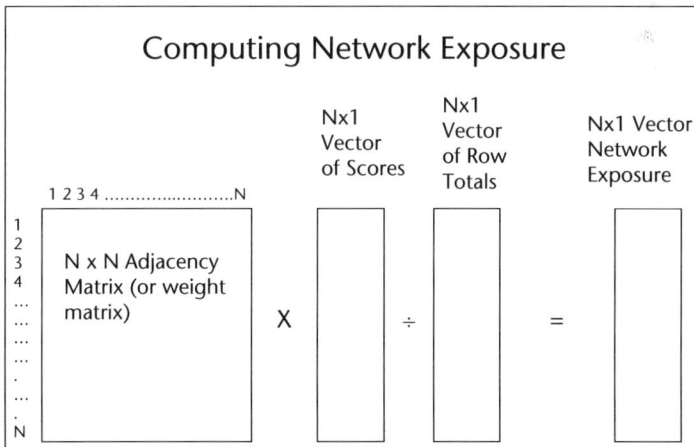

Figure 10–4. Illustration of network exposure calculation. The $N \times N$ adjacency matrix is multiplied by a binary vector of behavior and then divided by the number of people each person named to get a percentage of personal network exposure to the behavior.

Network Exposure

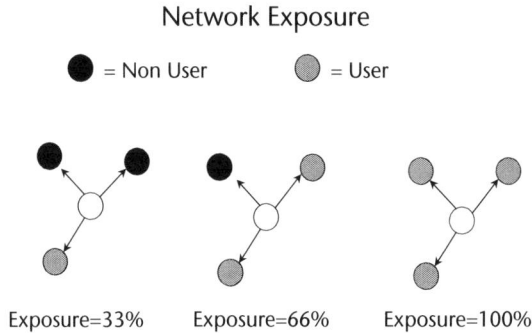

Figure 10–5. Network exposure is the proportion of a person's personal network who have adopted the behavior.

so exposure increases to 66%, and then after all three friends adopt, it is 100%. As diffusion occurs, everyone's network fills with adopters. For each person in a community, we can track the percentage of their contacts who have learned about the new product or adopted the behavior based on those persons' self-reports. If diffusion for 30 people occurs over 10 time periods, say 10 months, then at each month, the percentage of each person's network who adopted is calculated.

Calculating a person's adoption status at each time period is referred to as *event history analysis* (Allison, 1984). Event history analysis is the process of constructing data for each person at each point in time. So in diffusion studies, we can analyze for each person whether he or she has adopted the innovation and how many of his or her network partners have adopted it. The data are not measured at each time period in the study; rather the existing data are reshaped to replicate what happened over time. For example, suppose data were collected at the end of the year on whether each person in a school heard a rumor and the month they heard it. Suppose further that network data were collected in the school. How the rumor spread through the network can be replicated by reshaping the data and constructing the network exposure model. (Multiple measures of the network would be necessary to determine the network structure and how it varied over the year.)

To model the rumor spread, the information on which month each person heard the rumor would be converted to a set of vectors (columns) with a 0 for not heard, and a 1 for heard at each month. The network would be multiplied by each of these vectors and divided by the number of friends each person reported. Any updates or changes to the network can be incorporated in the network over time. This will provide a measure of the percent of each person's personal network who heard the rumor for each month. So if there are a 100 students and 12 months, the new database will have 1,200 cases, 100 students at each month, and at each month we know how many of a student's friends were aware of the rumor. Chapter 12 shows how rumor spreading in the school can be simulated by using this network exposure model.

Empirical Estimates Using Diffusion Network Data

The network exposure model in the event history framework has been used to calculate empirical estimates for social influence in diffusion. Three datasets have collected social network data and time of adoption (Valente, 1995). These three datasets are quite varied in where they collected the data and the behaviors of study, but they all have the common features of measuring the network and the time of adoption. The event history framework was used to reshape the datasets and calculated the percentage of adopters in each person's personal network at each time point. Adoption behavior was then regressed on the percentage of adopters in each person's personal network. These estimates then determine if being exposed to the innovation through the network affected adoption in a dynamic way, one that considers each person's social network at each point in time.

Table 10–2 reports the regression results. The associations between network exposure and adoption varied across the thre datasets. In the medical

Table 10–2. Event History Analysis of Factors Associated with Adoption for the Three Diffusion Network Datasets

	Medical Innovation	Brazilian Farmers	Korean Family Planning
No.	947	10,092	7,103
Time	132.7**	5.14	4.34
Cumulative adoption	0.03	2.27	0.32
Number sent	1.04	0.99	1.02
Number received	1.05	1.01	1.05**
Cohesion exposure	1.05	1.93**	2.08**
Structural equivalence exposure	1.04	5.01**	1.34
Science orientation	0.65**		
Journal subscriptions	1.67		
Cosmopolitan-ness		1.00	
Income		1.14**	
Number of children			1.23**
Media exposure			1.03*

Coefficients are adjusted odds ratios for likelihood of adoption. Estimates adjusted for clustering within community.
$*p < .05$; $**p < .01$.

innovation data, network exposure via cohesion (direct ties) and structural equivalence (SE) were not associated with adoption. This result is consistent with analysis reported elsewhere (Van den Bulte & Lillien, 2001). Adoption was associated with exposure via SE in the Brazilian farmers' dataset, indicating that farmers who occupied similar social network positions were more likely to adopt hybrid-seed corn at the same time than those who occupied different social network positions. Adoption was associated with exposure via cohesion (direct ties) and SE in the Korean family planning dataset, indicating that family planning adoption was associated with both types of network influence in the Korean family planning data.

These results should be interpreted as suggestive rather than definitive. There are many choices made to build the model, all of which can be varied to derive different empirical results. First, in all three studies the networks were measured only once, assuming they are static, when evidence would indicate that people's networks change. Second, time of adoption was assumed to occur at monthly or yearly intervals so that two people who adopted in different months in the same year were given the same adoption time (in the medical innovation study, the data were collapsed into months). These broad time intervals forced calculating exposure contemporaneously rather than as a lagged effect. Most models regress adoption on exposure in the prior time period, the last month. Third, there are missing data, and no provision was made for the behavior of those not interviewed. Finally, there might be errors in people's recall of adoption (the Korean family planning and Brazilian farmer data used recall for time of adoption) or their specification of the networks.

In one sense it is surprising that the association between adoption and network exposures is not stronger. The diffusion model has long specified, and logic has long dictated, that the more people in a person's social network, the greater is the likelihood of adoption. Diffusion and most behavior change models believe that the greater the exposure, the greater is the likelihood of adoption (Gross et al., 2002; Valente et al., 1997). For example, many studies have shown that students who smoke are more likely to have friends who smoke (Alexander et al., 2001; Urberg et al., 1997). Recent studies of a large social network over time has shown that obesity and smoking cessation are more likely once one's social networks become obese or quit smoking (Christakis & Fowler, 2007, 2008). One would expect this result to be replicated in these three datasets, which measured time of adoption and social networks.

Interestingly, the failure of exposure to predict adoption in the medical innovation could have been discovered as early as 1957 when the data were first analyzed. The inability of computer programs to analyze network data prevented diffusion scholars from discovering this lack of association between exposure and adoption, which might have created a crisis in the diffusion field, giving it new life. If exposure does not lead to adoption in some or many cases, what is the role of social networks?

Extensions to Exposure

The network exposure model is very flexible, as mentioned in Chapter 4. With egocentric data, network exposure model provides a measure of social influence based on ego's perceptions. Network exposure model may be weighted by many factors including the frequency of interaction or the similarity between ego and the named alters. With sociometric data, however, many types of social influence weights can be used and estimated. Virtually any theoretical mechanism of social influence can be modeled.

Network exposure model can be calculated on outgoing or incoming ties. Using outgoing ties models the influence of the people whom the focal individual names, who he or she thinks are his or her friends. For most analysis, using outgoing ties is probably the most appropriate way to calculate network exposure model because people are probably more strongly influenced by those they perceived to be their friends rather than by those who name them as a friend (incoming ties). Network exposure model is calculated on the named friends' self-reports.

Network exposure model can be calculated on incoming ties to model the influence of those who name the focal individual. Hall and Valente (2007) referred to incoming ties as *influence* and outgoing ties as *selection*, as the incoming ties are the ones who want to influence the focal individual. Incoming behavioral exposures may represent pressures to conform directed to the focal individual or the potential for the focal individual to access information and behavior from adopters. Further research is needed to understand how outgoing and incoming exposures compare.

Other network measures can be used to calculate social influences based on network concepts of position and influence. For example, suppose it is hypothesized that central members are more influential than peripheral ones. Exposure can be weighted by the centrality scores of friends in the network or even the difference in centrality scores. To weight exposures by centrality scores, the adjacency matrix (the matrix of direct connections) is multiplied by the centrality scores, which is then multiplied by the behavioral indicator (and optionally divided by the row sum to normalize).

As mentioned in Chapter 4, exposure can also be calculated on structural equivalence and other measures of role equivalence (see Chapter 7). Recall that structural equivalence measures the extent to which two people occupy the same position in the network. Exposure calculated on structural equivalence models the influence on the focal person of those who are similarly located in the network. Structural equivalence exposure can be a good measure of competitive influences on adoption because people who occupy the same position but are not directly connected to one another are often competitors. This is particularly true, for example, in networks of firms and organizations.

Exposure can also be calculated on any attributes, attitudes, or behaviors of the people in the network. For example, a researcher who has measured ethnicity can construct a network based on ethnic similarity and this multiplied (element-by-element multiplication) by the friendship network to calculate network exposure indicating being exposed to the behavior by those of the same ethnicity. Measures of positive attitudes toward a behavior can also be used to construct exposure by friends with positive attitudes.

One of most promising ways to calculate network exposure is using affiliations to construct two-mode data. Fujimoto and others (submitted) have conducted affiliation exposure analysis among in-school adolescents using joint membership in clubs and sports. The analysis showed the utility of affiliation exposure and showed that adolescent smoking was associated with belonging to extracurricula groups that had a lot of smokers. Wipfli and others (in press) used membership in an online community over time to construct a weight matrix, which varied over time.

Infection and Susceptibility

The simultaneous inclusion of behavior and network structure in the modeling of diffusion dynamics has considerable appeal given the rich variety of theoretical processes that can be modeled. As mentioned so far, many theoretical influences can be included to construct the exposure term. One significant advance in this regard is the ability to model the extent to which individuals are infectious or susceptible to behavioral influence (Myers, 2000; Strang & Tuma, 1993). [As a side note, Strang and Tuma (1993) also proposed that time intervals can be included in these estimates so researchers can estimate short- or long-term infectiousness and susceptibility.] Infectiousness and susceptibility constitute two specific mechanisms that have public health analogs.

Infectiousness and susceptibility are measured as the extent many others adopt after or before the focal individual adopts the behavior. The researcher can specify whether there is some characteristic associated with infectiousness or susceptibility. For example, the researcher might specify that people who are popular are infectiousness in high schools. Popularity is often measured as the number of nominations received, in-degree, and analysis conducted to determine if the number of adoptions increases after high in-degree individuals adopt. Any individual characteristic can be used to determine its association with infectiousness and/or susceptibility. From a network perspective, however, in-degree and out-degree are the logical candidate attributes to use.

Valente (1995) introduced a critical mass index that is a network-weighted adoption score. Not all adoptions are equal, and the critical mass index captured the notion that high in-degree adopters might contribute disproportionately to the diffusion process. The critical mass index is the ratio of adopter-nonadopter dyads in the network. Rather than measure diffusion as the number or percentage of individuals who have adopted, the critical mass index focused on the dyads or interactions and measured the percent of interactions which have the potential to result in further adoptions (those between adopters and nonadopters).

Thresholds

It may be naïve to think that exposure leads to adoption the same way for everyone. If everyone required a majority of their network to adopt before they were willing to, diffusion would never get started. Some people need to be willing to take risks and adopt new behaviors before their peers are willing to do so. These early adopters relative to their peer group are labeled low-threshold adopters. Granovetter (1978) proposed that the distribution of thresholds in the community affects the likelihood of diffusion. If no one is willing to adopt before their peers, diffusion will never get started. Further, if there is a discontinuity in the threshold distribution, diffusion can fail to take off.

Granovetter (1978) used the example of rioting. If the distribution of those willing to riot is distributed such that the number of people required to see rioting before a person is willing to do so was distributed as 0, 1, 2, 3, 4, ... N, then a riot can occur because the person with a 0 threshold initiates a riot and the person with a threshold of 1 see this and riots, and so on. However, if there is discontinuity in the distribution such as thresholds distributed as 0, 1, 2, 4, 4, ... N, then the first three people begin rioting because their thresholds are reached, but no one else does because their thresholds are not reached. Thresholds can be calculated relative to social networks as well by determining for each person the number or percent of adopters in his or her personal network required for him or her to adopt.

The trouble with calculating network thresholds is that it is hard to refute it. That is, if diffusion occurs completely irrespective of networks, one can still calculate how many people were in everyone's network when they adopted, regardless of whether those people had any influence on a person's adoption. Yet, the concept has appeal, mainly because it resonates as true; we know people who are eager to be early adopters among their peers so they can show others how something works or be the first to use it. We also know people who wait until they see all of their peers adopt before they are willing to do so. So the network threshold concept has appeal. Disproving network thresholds may be difficult, but they can be calculated and the resulting variable used in subsequent analysis. (It might also be possible to measure network thresholds using a Likert-type scale and treat it as an attribute.)

Network thresholds were calculated for the three empirical diffusion network datasets. Figure 10–6 plots the thresholds for one village of the Korean family planning study (village 24). The y-axis is the threshold, the proportion of each person's network who adopted before or at the same time the focal person adopted, and the x-axis is time, the year each person adopted. A cumulative adoption curve was overlaid on the graph to show the average expected exposure at each time period. For example, at year 5, about 50% of the community will have adopted family planning, so exposure at that time will be 50%, on average. We can see, however, that many people have thresholds above and below this expected value indicating that they adopted after 100% of their network adopted (person 59) or when 20% of their network adopted (person 19).

The average threshold values for the three datasets were MI, 55%; BF, 62%; and KFP, 63%. These values are inflated somewhat by the recoding of nonadopters to the last time period. For example, all nonadopters in the medical innovation data were recoded to 18 (the last month of data collection). Average thresholds excluding nonadopting cases were MI, 49%; BF,

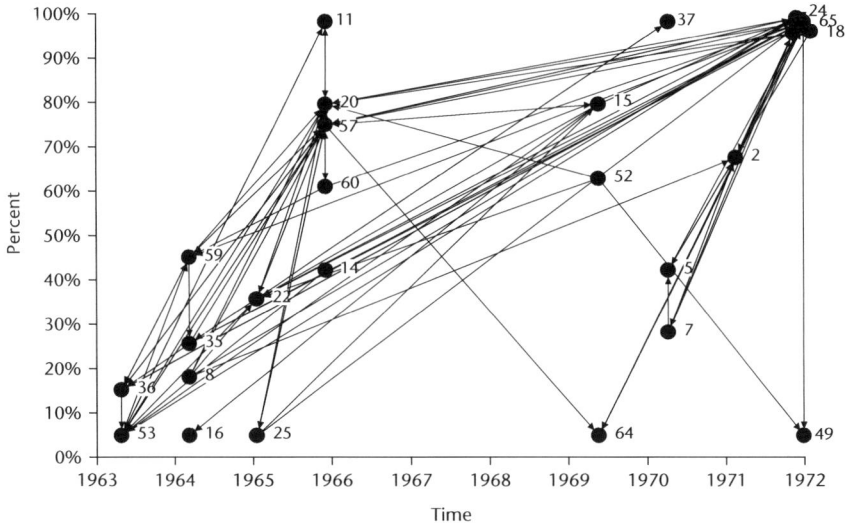

Figure 10–6. Graph of thresholds for one village in the Korean Family Planning study. The x-axis indicates year of adoption, and the y-axis, thresholds, the percentage of network contacts who adopted before each individual. Woman 31 was an early adopter and earlier than her peers, whereas person 59 was an early adopter but late relative to her peers.

51%; and KFP, 46%. Not surprisingly, thresholds are strongly correlated with time of adoption, with earlier adopters much more likely to have very low thresholds than later adopters.

If thresholds exist, we might expect people with low thresholds to turn to the media or other outside sources of information to learn about these new ideas. This occurs in part because low-threshold adopters have had few peers to turn to for advice about the new idea before deciding to adopt. Diffusion scholars have postulated change occurs when individuals come into contact with others outside their normal sphere of influence and learn about new ideas and practices from these other communities. They then transport the ideas to their host community, acting as bridges. Media theories propose that the mass media and other focused communications can act as the agent of change as well, disseminating information about new idea and practices. Change agents then are the people willing and/or able to accept these new ideas in the media and transmit them to others in their communities.

This hypothesis was tested in an evaluation of the Bolivia National Reproductive Health media campaign in which interviews were conducted with two samples of urban Bolivian residents. One sample consisted of three waves of independent (cross-sectional) residents in seven cities, and the other was a panel (following the same people over time) in one city (Valente & Saba, 1998). Low- and high-threshold adopters were calculated. Low-threshold adopters were Bolivian women who adopted a contraceptive method during the time of the study with a minority of their peers who had adopted previously, whereas high-threshold adopters had a majority of their peers who had adopted previously. We found that low-threshold adopters, in both the urban cross-sectional and panel samples, reported more media campaign exposure than high-threshold adopters (Table 10–3).

Calculating thresholds enabled measuring the two-step flow hypothesis of media influence. Katz (1957) had proposed that the media do not influence everyone, but rather they influence opinion leaders who in turn use

Table 10–3. Association between Campaign Exposure and Adoption for Low- and High-Threshold Adopters, Bolivia Media Campaign

| | Cross-Sectional Data ($n = 611$) | | Panel Data ($n = 141$) | |
	Low-Threshold Adopters	High-Threshold Adopters	Low-Threshold Adopters	High-Threshold Adopters
Campaign Exposure	2.36**	1.92	1.71*	1.26

$*p < .05$; $**p < .01$.
Note: Regression controls for education, age, income, and number of children.

the information in the media to persuade others. Thus, media influence, and diffusion of new ideas and attitudes, spreads in a two-step process: first the media influence leaders and these leaders in turn influence others. The leaders that will be influenced by the media are those with low thresholds, and once they adopt, these low-threshold leaders can influence many others. Thresholds explain how diffusion jumps from innovators to early majority opinion leader adoption. If the thresholds of opinion leaders remain high for a particular issue, then diffusion is delayed.

Limitations to Diffusion Theory

Diffusion of innovations has been a theory with considerable explanatory power and predictions extend beyond available data at this time. There are several limitations to the theory, however. First, as just stated, the data required for complete testing of diffusion postulates and hypotheses are quite high. It requires data at multiple points that include behavioral adoption decisions as well as social network contacts. This can be further complicated by the long time span required for most innovations to diffuse. Further, a comprehensive study will require multiple communities studied simultaneously so the results span beyond a simple case study. Thus, it is difficult to get data over time on behavior and social networks.

A second limitation is that diffusion theory has focused more on system-level properties of diffusion at the expense of studies designed to understand individual decision making. For example, it is easier to hypothesize that diffusion occurs more rapidly in dense or centralized networks than in sparse or decentralized ones. How these postulates influence individual decision making, however, is much less often explored. For example, do individuals increase their resistance to social influence in dense networks? A third limitation is that diffusion theory to date has not hypothesized how the network changes as a consequence of innovation diffusion. For example, does adoption change one's status in the network, thus affecting the network structure? Most diffusion studies investigate how networks affect diffusion rather than how diffusion affects networks. New research in actor-oriented models may shed light on the dynamic interplay between networks and behavior.

Summary

This chapter reviewed diffusion of innovations theory which use social network analysis as a major causal mechanism. Diffusion of innovations theory is the most prominent network theory, as diffusion explains how new ideas and practices spread through social networks. The chapter presented the five elements of diffusion: (1) perceived characteristics of the innovation affect its rate of adoption; (2) diffusion occurs over time so that rate of adoption often yields a cumulate adoption S-shaped pattern, with individuals are classified as early or late adopters; (3) individuals pass through stages during the adoption process typically classified as knowledge, persuasion, decision, implementation, and confirmation; (4) people can modify the innovation and sometimes discontinue its use; and (5) mathematical models can be developed to measure the rate and character of diffusion curves.

The chapter then reviewed the four major classes of diffusion models: (1) integration/opinion leadership, (2) structural models, (3) critical levels, and (4) dynamic models. All four models explicitly account for network diffusion dynamics but vary in their mathematical rigor and complexity. Dynamic models using the network exposure model were explained. Network exposure influences can be varied to model different social influence mechanisms. The chapter also introduced the calculation of infectiousness and susceptibility which dynamically account for adoption behavior and in-degree and out-degree, respectively. Infection is measured by examining the degree to which others adopt the innovation after the focal person has adopted, and susceptibility is the extent to which a person adopts after others adopt. The chapter closed with a presentation of network thresholds and limitations of diffusion theory.

11

Network Interventions

The preceding chapters have provided many measures and models useful for understanding networks and how they influence human behavior. The most useful application for network data, however, might be using network data to accelerate behavior change and/or improving organizational performance. Network interventions consist of behavior change programs that use social network data to identify specific people or groups to deliver and/or receive the behavior change program. Network interventions can take many different forms and have many different implementation considerations.

At least six different network interventions have been developed, tested, or considered:

1. Identification of opinion leaders or key players
2. Identification of groups
3. Identification leaders within groups or creation of leader-learner pairings
4. Snowball sampling or recruitment
5. Rewiring (changing) networks
6. Networks and attributes

Before discussing specific techniques, however, it must be stressed that the behavior change theory guiding the program's development should play a critical role in determining the type of network intervention. Programs designed to change cultural norms or opinions should probably rely heavily on identifying and recruiting opinion leaders whereas programs aimed at disrupting communication or disease flow should probably identify bridges. Qualitative and ethnographic information about the community or organization's existing structures and history is also likely to be important elements in successful deployment of network interventions.

It should also be stressed that network interventions have the potential to create empowered communities and organizations by stressing the importance of community members. Rather than relying on outside change agents, network interventions underscore that capacity to change lies within the community and that a learning organization identifies people and structures best suited for making change recommendations.

Opinion Leaders

The most typical network intervention is using opinion leaders to be advocates or champions for a new behavior. Opinion leaders are present in all types of organizations, communities, and/or settings. Opinion leaders are people who influence the opinions, attitudes, beliefs, motivations, and behaviors of others (Rogers & Cartano, 1962). The roles and activities of leaders and leadership span numerous political, social, economic, medical, as well as public health issues. Opinion leaders have been used in public health to gain support for and implement community health programs.

Opinion leaders have several functions and responsibilities critical for the implementation of successful behavior change efforts. First, they provide entrée and legitimize behavior change programs. Second, they provide communication from their communities back to agencies that implement programs. Third, they can act as role models for behavior change within the community. Fourth, they can be the conveyors of health messages. Finally, they may act as the "capital" left after the agency has withdrawn from the community or organization thus institutionalizing program goals. Opinion leaders are critical to program implementation and success. As shown in Table 11–1, at least 10 different techniques for identifying opinion leaders have been used in public health programs (Valente & Pumpuang, 2007).

Network data can be used to identify opinion leaders by finding individuals at the center of the network. We conducted computer simulations to determine the potential effectiveness of opinion leader interventions. Randomly generated networks were created, and diffusion through those networks was simulated by selecting 10% to be the initial adopters. Network exposures were created and thresholds set to 15% adoption. Three conditions were

Table 11–1. Methods for Identifying Opinion Leaders (Methods 8, 9, and 10 Constitute Social Network Methods)

Method	Technique
1. Celebrities	Program recruits well-known people, either mass-media or "local" celebrities (such as school athletes), to promote behavior
2. Self-selection	Volunteers are recruited through solicitation and subsequently selected and trained.
3. Self-identification	Surveys are administered to the sample, and questions measuring leadership are included. Those scoring highest on leadership scales are selected.
4. Staff selected	Program implementers select leaders from information they have gathered about the community.
5. Positional approach	Persons who occupy leadership positions such as clergy, elected officials, media and business elites, and so on are selected.
6. Judge's ratings	Knowledgeable community members identify leaders to be selected.
7. Expert identification	Trained ethnographers study communities to select leaders.
8. Snowball method	Index cases provide nominations of leaders who are in turn interviewed until no new leaders are identified.
9. Sample sociometric	Randomly selected respondents nominate leaders and those receiving frequent nominations are selected.
10. Sociometric	All (or most) respondents are interviewed and those receiving frequent nominations are selected.

See Valente and Pumpuang (2007) for a complete discussion.

simulated: initial adoption by opinion leaders, random nodes, and marginal nodes (those who receive only one nomination). Each model was run 100 times and averaged. Figure 11–1 graphs the diffusion trajectories for the three conditions. The study shows that when diffusion starts with opinion leaders, diffusion occurs more rapidly than when diffusion starts with randomly selected network members or those on the margins.

Identifying opinion leaders is the most typical of network interventions in part because it is easy to implement and in part because it is intuitively appealing as a mechanism to create change. Further, logic dictates that opinion leaders, by definition, should have a strong influence on program success. If the leaders of a community will not support a new program, it is unlikely regular members are going to do so. At least 20 studies using social network data to identify opinion leaders for behavior change have been conducted (Valente & Pumpuang, 2007). Most of these studies have demonstrated that using opinion leaders for behavior change is an effective tactic.

Opinion leaders can be identified with network data by selecting those who receive the most network nominations. For example, you might ask

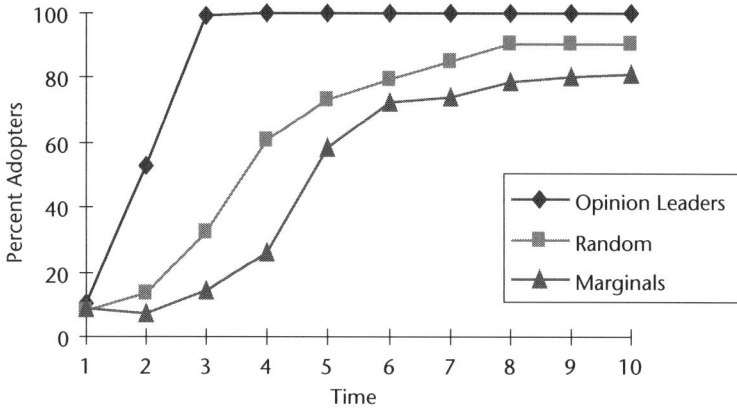

Figure 11–1. Hypothetical diffusion in randomly generated networks when the initial adopters are (1) leaders, (2) randomly selected, or (3) marginals.

who in the organization respondents go to for advice about X (where X is the topic of interest such as new administrative procedures, technology, or behaviors). The people within the organization or community who receive the most nominations are identified as the opinion leaders and used as change agents (in degree centrality). Typically the people who receive the top 10% to 15% of nominations are identified as opinion leaders, but one can vary that threshold based on the program or data. If there is a tie in the number of nominations received, another centrality measure such as closeness or betweenness can be used as a tie-breaker. In some cases, the opinion leader may be one person.

Lomas and others (1991) conducted a classic study testing opinion leader effectiveness by recruiting four hospitals to participate in the study: two were intervention sites and two were control. The study sought to determine whether opinion leaders could be identified and recruited to promote vaginal birth after C-section (VBAC). Medical guidelines had been introduced in the late 1980s recommending that women who had had a C-section in their first child delivery attempt a vaginal birth on their subsequent pregnancy. Prior to the guidelines, most physicians recommended a C-section for the second birth if the first had been a C-section. Using social network techniques, physicians in the two intervention hospitals nominated others they would turn to for advice about obstetric or gynecological issues. These leaders were then recruited and instructed to promote VBAC to their colleagues during general hospital activities. Follow-up data showed a decrease in C-sections for second deliveries in women who had C-sections on their first births. (VBAC is still somewhat controversial as some have questioned the guidelines and recommend that second births be C-sections if the first was.)

In a similar study, Soumerai and others (1998) used network analysis to identify physician opinion leaders in 20 hospitals while 17 hospitals acted as controls. These leaders promoted the use of aspirin as a beta-blocker for patients who presented in the emergency department with acute myocardial infarction (AMI). Chart review of eligible patients showed that physicians in the opinion leader hospitals were more likely to use aspirin in the treatment of AMI than were physicians in the control hospitals.

Studies have also been conducted among other providers such as substance abuse treatment counselors. Substance abuse treatment counselors in six clinics were asked to nominate peers to whom they would turn for advice when treating co-occurring disorders (mental health and substance use). One person was identified in each of the six clinics and this person became the coach within the clinic for the deployment of a manual on how to treat co-occurring disorders (Peters et al., 2005). Moore and others (2004) showed that these opinion leaders were similar to other counselors in terms of age, education, and experience but were more knowledgeable about treatment of dual diagnoses. Comparison clinics in another city were given the same intervention, but it was delivered by professional trainers who did not work in the clinics. At 3-month follow-up, counselors in the opinion leader clinics were more likely to diagnose co-occurring disorders and spent more time discussing co-occurring disorders with their clients.

The opinion leader model has also been implemented at the community level. Latkin (1998) recruited street opinion leaders to communicate safe injecting practices and showed that these opinion leaders adopted the safe injecting messages themselves and effectively communicated it to others. Sikkema and others (2000) used network nominations to identify opinion leaders to promote HIV risk reduction techniques among women living in a low-income housing development. These studies indicate that the opinion leader is a very general approach to behavior change that can be implemented in many settings among many different populations.

These opinion leader studies attest to the ability to identify opinion leaders in communities and have them act as change agents for behavioral change programs. These communities can be organizations, geographic locales, schools, and so on. The population may be physicians, other health professionals, drug users, lay community members, and so on. Opinion leaders have natural abilities at being role models for others. They take to the task of leadership and behavior change promotion like fish to water because they know they function as opinion leaders and welcome the opportunity to be given tools and techniques enabling them to lead more effectively.

There are many implementation issues that arise when conducting an opinion leader intervention. First, how much training do opinion leaders need? In many adolescent school-based studies, opinion leaders are provided at least a 1-hour-long training session. These sessions teach students how to manage groups, mediate conflicts, and act as leaders. As a rule of thumb, leadership training should consume about 10% to 15% of the total time of the behavior change program. For example, if physician change program is expected to take 6 months and require about 30 hours of promotional time by the change agent, then the leadership training should be a ½-day training session, or 3 to 4 hours.

Second, how should leaders contact others? In organizations and some school studies, leaders are expected to engage in conversations with others as a part of their day-to-day activities (Bloor et al., 1999; Lomas et al., 1991). Since leaders are highly visible in their community, they can be expected to have many contacts. In many cases the leaders might wear buttons, hats, or other devices that prompt conversations about the behavior change issue. In other settings, the program may specifically create promotional events or programs to provide a forum for leaders to persuade others. Although it may be preferable to have specific events that create opportunities for promotion these events can detract from the spontaneous and natural-occurring interactions that may be more conducive to behavior change.

One limitation to opinion leader interventions is that effectiveness may depend on the leaders' abilities to persuade their peers. A second limitation is that one or a few leaders may resist the innovation or not embrace the new behavior wholeheartedly. More subtly, the leaders may be less than enthusiastic about the change program. A final limitation is that the opinion leader strategy requires leaders be identified and new training conducted repeatedly. Aside from its intuitive appeal and logistical simplicity, the opinion leadertactic can also be beneficial because it creates a learning organization. Training indigenous or local opinion leaders creates the norm that the community looks to within itself to change and grow.

Key Players

Generally, opinion leaders are identified as those individuals receiving the most nominations in response to a network question such as "who do you go to for advice?" Leaders are often identified as those people who receive the most nominations, those with the highest in-degree scores. One limitation to using in-degree centrality is that nominations received may be redundant. For example, Figure 11–2 shows a network in which the people who received more than five nominations are all connected to mostly the same others. Consequently, the leaders that are identified are likely to be leaders

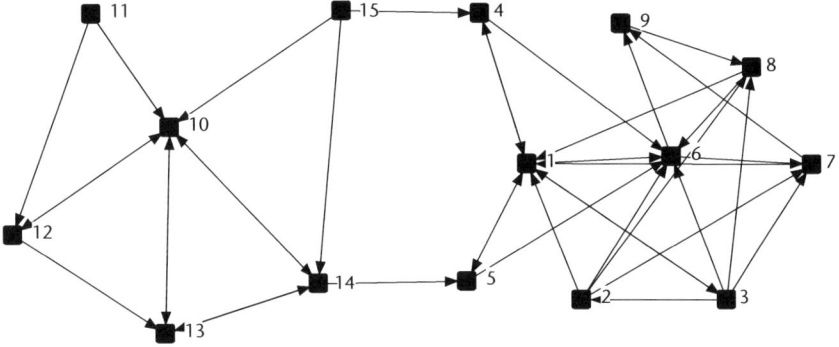

Figure 11–2. The two nodes who received the most nominations are numbers 1 and 6 each being nominated six times. If two leaders were chosen only by considering in-degree then 1 and 6 would be chosen but their links are mostly to the same others. Node 10 received nominations but these nominations are unique and so 1 and 10 or 1 and 6 span the network more effectively.

for the same people and so do not span the network efficiently. Borgatti (2006) addressed this limitation by developing a method to identify key players in the network as those individuals who optimally reach others in the network.

Borgatti (2006) showed that traditional measures of centrality (see Chapter 5) are inadequate for finding nodes optimally positioned to spread information for diffusion or to be removed from a network to disrupt spread. Borgatti developed "Key Player," a computer program (which comes with UCINET) that can identify the optimal set of nodes for diffusion and/or containment. Key Player can also be used to vary the desired number of key players to be identified and provides a metric showing how many others in the network can be reached by the key players in one, two, or more steps (Borgatti, 2006).

Key player identifies the nodes best selected to accelerate diffusion and those best select to inhibit spread through a network. As Borgatti (2006) shows these two processes are not necessarily symmetric in that some nodes are ideal for spreading behaviors while others are most optimally removed to retard diffusion.

Groups

In many cases, it may be beneficial to identify groups in the network and create behavior change programs implemented by or in groups. For example, suppose a new software program was introduced in an organization. It might be desirable to have social network groups identified and trained together in the new software. By learning together, the group can reinforce the new behavior and support each other with implementation issues. In this way, individuals can rely on one another for help and advice as they learn the new behavior. Further, when the group adopts the new behavior, it reduces the risk for each individual.

Moreover, many innovations and behaviors are suited to group-level adoption rather than individual behavior. For example, interdependent innovations such as fax and email are useful only if at least one other person uses them and they increase their utility as more people use them. Facebook, for example, is most gainfully adopted when an entire group uses the technology to share information and experiences.

Many methods for identifying groups in networks were presented in Chapter 6. Different intervention approaches may suggest different group identification approaches. Probably one of the more useful network definition algorithms is the Girvan and Newman (2002) algorithm because it creates mutually exclusive groups. Having every person assigned to one and only one group may facilitate implementation. On the other hand, having assignments to multiple groups may make is easier for people to attend a group meeting that is convenient to their schedule.

In addition to finding groups, one may want to identify specific hierarchical positions in the network. For example, a change program in a large organization might recommend certain behaviors for employees who are frequently sought out for advice and different behaviors for those who frequently seek advice. In such a case, the change agents might want to identify positions, rather than groups (see Chapter 7). Two critical implementation issues for group- and position-level interventions are whether the groups need to be constrained to be the same size and whether groups need leaders. Some programs may be content to have groups of varying sizes while others may need to have groups the same size. For example, a school-based curriculum with a workbook specifying the number of group members will want to have all groups of the same size. Other interventions may be content to specify a group range, say from 5 to 10 people. To date, group-based interventions have assumed that groups need leaders and at least two techniques were developed to identify leaders and groups simultaneously.

Identifying Leaders and Groups

Some researchers have identified groups and then selected leaders from within those groups. For example, Wiist and Snider (1991) pilot-tested a study in which groups were formed using social network data, and then leaders were selected from within those groups. Wiist and Snider (1991) showed this to be an effective method for preventing tobacco use. Buller and colleagues (2000) used network data within a worksite to create mutually exclusive groups and then identified leaders as those who received the most nominations within groups. Buller and others (2000) showed that this intervention was effective at improving fruit and vegetable consumption. Amirkhanian (2005) also identified groups via network nominations and selected leaders who received the most nominations. These leaders then acted as change agents to promote safe sex practices among a group of Roman gypsies who are traditionally at high risk for HIV.

Valente and Davis (1999) proposed a model in which leaders are identified first and groups are formed based on the network nominations. Leaders can be identified using in-degree centrality (or other measures) and then others are assigned to the leaders they nominated. If a person did not nominate one of the chosen leaders, he or she is assigned to the leader to whom he or she is closest to sociometrically. One can also add weights to the links in the network (e.g., first choices ranked higher than second ones, which are ranked higher than third ones, etc.). These weights can then be incorporated into the leader-follower matching to create groups.

Valente and others (2003, 2006) tested this technique in a school-based smoking prevention program delivered to sixth-grade (middle school) students in 16 southern California schools. The study randomized three conditions—random, teacher, and network—at the classroom level nested within an evaluation of two curricula—a social influences one and a culturally tailored one. Results showed that students in the network condition reported higher antitobacco attitudes and greater friend support for antismoking norms immediately postcurriculum. Analysis also showed that students in the network condition had a 56% reduction in susceptibility to smoke, which is a known precursor of smoking.

At 1-year follow-up, the two curricula and three network implementation methods were compared on changes in smoking (Figure 11–3). The data show (Unger et al., 2004) that the culturally tailored curriculum (FLAVOR) was more effective than the social influences one (CHIPS). The greater effectiveness was dependent on who and with whom the curriculum was delivered. When groups were formed using the network approach recommended by Valente and Davis (1999), the culturally tailored curriculum, FLAVOR, was more effective (by reducing the increase in smoking). When teachers defined leaders and groups, the FLAVOR curriculum was the most effective. When analysis was restricted to only students who had complete data on all survey items, the network condition with FLAVOR was the most effective (Valente et al., 2006).

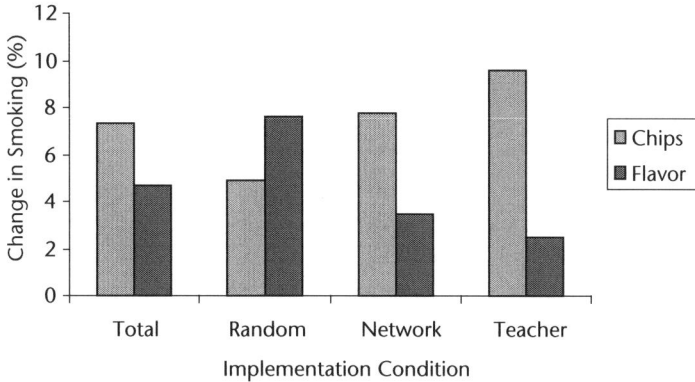

Figure 11–3. Change in smoking at 1 year for middle school adolescents by curriculum (Chips v. Flavor) and implementation method, the manner in which leaders were selected, and groups formed (random, network, teacher) determined effectiveness.

There are several reasons the network method might not have been the most effective. First, the algorithm used to minimize network distances between leaders and followers was not optimal and has since been improved. Second, the algorithm did not include link weights so that closer ties would be given preference over less close ones. Third, teachers may have been very good at identifying students who worked well together because they were given specific worksheets for this task and because they had been in the classroom for 8 months (data were collected in March). The important consideration here is that the type of intervention is not independent of how or by whom it is implemented.

Snowball Sampling or Network Recruitment

Epidemiologists and public health officials have used contact tracing and snowball methods to combat infectious disease for decades. When individuals present at healthcare facilities with an STD, for example, public health officials will ask for the names of the person's sexual contacts to contact those people and inform them they were potentially exposed to an STD. Such procedures are critical for adequate public health protection, but the data have usually not been analyzed using network data and techniques.

Some researchers have used snowball sampling to develop respondent-driven sampling (RDS) methodologies useful for recruiting subjects into health promotion programs (Broadhead et al., 1998; Heckathorne, 1997, 2002; Latkin, et al., 2009). Heckathorne (1997) referred to this system as RDS and the website provides software and tools for its implementation. In RDS, existing clients are given vouchers to go out and recruit new clients to come to the clinic, and these new clients are in turn used to recruit new clients. Research has shown that the respondent-driven approach provides a more diverse and more cost-effective means of reaching "hard to reach" populations than traditional outreach methods (Salganik & Heckathorn, 2004). RDS uses coupons to track who refers whom and to provide monetary incentives to make the referrals and have people visit the data collection and intervention sites. The RDS website provides sample implementation programs and instruments.

One application of snowball sampling is to recruit participants for vaccines. For example, research has been under way for decades to develop an HIV vaccine. Such a vaccine, should it become available, will probably not be appropriate for the general population because not everyone is at risk for HIV. Consequently, a study was conducted to determine whether social network data could be collected from HIV-positive patients to recruit a sample of high-risk HIV-negative adolescents who might be at risk for HIV infections (Valente et al., 2009). The study used snowball sampling and recruitment in order to reach high-risk populations.

Recall Figure 4–4, which displays the networks collected in this study. Index cases (HIV-positive patients) are displayed as squares, their first-degree enrolled alters are triangles, and nonenrolled alters are circles. Links are coded by willingness to invite alter to participate in vaccine preparedness activities: solid arrows represent willing, dashed arrows represent not willing; dash-dotted arrows represent absence of a response, and dash-dot-dot indicates enrolled but not named first-degree alters. The data illustrate three remarkable things about this snowball recruitment. First, there is considerable variation in the number of people named by the respondents. Second, there is variation across relationships regarding who people are willing to invite to participate in the study. Respondents are willing to invite some of their network members, but not others. Third, there were some cases in which a respondent indicated they were not willing to invite a social network member, but they recruited the person anyway.

The results of this study showed that index cases were willing to invite their social network members to participate in the vaccine preparedness study if they were older and thought the person knew his or her HIV status. Awareness of HIV status varied by network member; thus, this factor was a relationship variable. Index cases were also less willing to invite network members with whom they used drugs, but this was a small fraction of the overall sample. Adolescents were less willing to invite network members to participate, but they named considerably more adolescents than adults, thus providing a greater yield of potential adolescent vaccine participants.

There are several implementation challenges to using snowball techniques. First, keeping track of which persons recruited which ones specifically can be a challenge. The coupons have the index person's ID number but it is possible for participants to share coupons. A second challenge occurs when a person named by one index is the same someone nominated by another index. Consequently, knowledge of the population can be critical when conducting snowball sample studies so the research team recognizes the study participants. Finally, researchers are challenged in the data management since individuals named by one respondent also become respondents in the study. Keeping track of the unique identifiers and making sure they are consistent across cases require considerable attention to detail.

Rewiring Networks

One of the most powerful yet untested approaches to network interventions would be to change networks by deleting or adding links; or deleting or adding nodes. Clearly this type of change happens in organizations when new teams are formed or colleagues introduce people to one another. Organizations may at times purposively rearrange offices to facilitate network change, but such activities are not often created or measured in systematic ways. Rewiring or changing links is not done randomly rather links are added or deleted to maximize some network property.

It is important to first decide which property one wants to maximize when rewiring networks. For example, in many cases the researcher may wish to create networks that are more cohesive where cohesion is defined as follows (Borgatti, 2006):

$$C = \frac{\sum \frac{1}{d_{ij}}}{n(n-1)}(i \neq j) \tag{11-1}$$

where d_{ij} is the geodesic distance between dyads and $i \neq j$ indicates distances are not calculated between persons i and j. The goal then is to determine how much adding or deleting a link in the network changes cohesion. It is simple though tedious to calculate cohesion and then delete each link and add each nonexisting link and calculate change in cohesion for each link deletion and addition. This produces a change matrix with each cell entry indicating the amount of change in cohesion due to link deletion or addition. Of course, the matrix could be calculated for any network property discussed in Chapter 8 such as change in centralization, clustering, or transitivity, for example. Cohesion (or fragmentation) is probably the most relevant metric, however. With the change matrix, the researcher can easily report the link changes most critical to the network.

Bridges and Potential Bridges

Table 11–2 reports the 10 links that decrease cohesion the most when deleted and the 10 links that increase cohesion the most when added. *Bridges* are the links that decrease cohesion when deleted, and *potential bridges* are those that increase cohesion when added. Researchers wishing to disrupt communications or inhibit organizational performance should concentrate on removing the bridges, severing the links that decrease cohesion. Removing bridges disrupts

Table 11–2. Top 10 Bridges and Potential Bridges Scores for the Network in Figure 1–1

Bridge Links		
From	To	Change
27	29	−0.04
29	26	−0.01
2	37	0
7	8	0
29	31	0
3	2	0
37	22	0
20	3	0
19	27	0
21	27	0

Potential Bridge Links		
From	To	Change
31	35	0.08
10	35	0.08
14	35	0.07
29	35	0.07
28	35	0.07
5	35	0.07
16	35	0.07
12	35	0.07
15	35	0.07
22	35	0.07

Bridges are link deletions that increase average path length the most, and potential bridges are the link additions that decrease average path length the most.

network performance and forces communications to travel longer paths to reach each other. Like real bridges, network bridges provide a path connecting one location to another, and like real bridges, they are critically important.

Identifying bridges as those that decrease cohesion is an idea derived directly from Granovetter's (1973) insight, and that of many other network scholars—that links that connect otherwise disconnected groups are important structural bridges in the network. "Any given tie may, hypothetically, be removed from a network; the number of paths broken and the changes in average path length resulting between arbitrary pairs of points (with some limitation on length of path considered) can then be computed" (Granovetter, 1973, p. 1366). Perfect bridges that connect otherwise disconnected subgroups represent only a special case of the bridging phenomenon. By calculating all the link deletion changes, every tie can be assigned a bridge score.

These bridges may be important for diffusion of information or behavior from one group to another. Bridges represent potential bottlenecks to the flow of information within the community and in some cases may need to be strengthened to keep the community from fragmenting. Bridge links might also represent links useful to delete to create a more fragmented network if one wishes to slow diffusion such as trying to slow the spread of HIV/STDs.

Potential bridges are those links that, when added to the network, increase cohesion the most. Each hypothetical link is added to the network, and the resulting increase in cohesion is calculated. In some settings, these would be the links most advantageous to add to the network. For example, if an organization joined two departments, this analysis will show which links would be best to create to maximally increase organizational cohesion.

Other measures may be used to calculate bridges and potential bridges. Recall that in Chapter 5 centrality measures were introduced for nodes that can also be calculated on the links. Specifically, betweenness centrality has been proposed as an important link-based centrality measure (all links have degree scores of less than 3). Potential bridges may be calculated by taking the complement of the network (0s become 1s and 1s become 0s) and calculating bridging or link centrality on the complement network. Also recall from the simulations reported in Chapter 8 that changes in cohesion due to link deletions and addition were greatest when network density was in the 15% to 25% range, suggesting that this technique is most appropriate when networks fall within this range.

Links versus Nodes

The previous section discussed bridging as a link phenomenon, and here the discussion reverts back to the node. Most interventions have focused on identifying leaders and those at the center of the network. Although often more difficult to find but potentially more important are identifying bridges. The methodology just described shows how to identify bridging or potential bridging links; it may be useful to identify the nodes (people) who occupy these bridging positions.

Technically, bridges are links and the anchors for the links are bridge nodes. People are often referred to as bridges when they connect two separate groups. Of course we want to identify a measure of bridging which indicates every node's degree of bridging. We often want a measure of bridging at the individual level so we can determine correlates of bridging. For example, we might think that bridges have certain personality characteristics such as being open to new ideas or that bridges are at higher risk for substance use. Individual bridging is calculated by using the change scores created for all of the links by calculating each person's average change score. Thus, we define individual bridging as:

$$B_i = \frac{\sum_{j=1}^{k}\left[C - C'_{ij}\right]}{k} + \frac{\sum_{j=1}^{l}\left[C - C'_{ji}\right]}{l}, \left(i \neq j\right) \tag{11-2}$$

where C is cohesion for the observed network, C'_{ij} is cohesion when the link from i to j is removed, C'_{ji} is cohesion when the links from j to i are removed, and k and l represent the number of ties sent and received, respectively. B_i is average change in cohesion when the links incident to each node are deleted. The measure can be disaggregated into its two components, bridge-from and -to, respectively, calculated as the average change in cohesion when links *from* and *to* each node are deleted. The measure can also be used to measure potential bridges calculated as the average change in cohesion when nonexistent links from and to each node are added. The one difficulty with this measure is that it does not control for network size so calculations across networks cannot be compared. Box 11–1 shows this bridging measure applied to the hypothetical network Granovetter (1973) used to illustrate the strength of weak ties.

Bridges can be used to find critical nodes in a network that should be strengthened or supported to retain a cohesive network. Betweenness centrality is often used to identify central nodes in bridging positions. Valente and Fujimoto (submitted) have shown that bridging and betweenness are only moderately correlated. That correlation, however, depends on the network structure, when there are few absolute bridges the correlation is high. As the network structure becomes more amorphous, the correlation decreases and bridging and betweenness identify different nodes. The bridge measures enable the identification of important nodes in a network that are not peripheral or

Box 11–1. Granovetter's Strength of Weak Ties Revisited

Granovetter (1973) wrote an influential article titled the strength of weak ties (SWT) that emphasized the importance of network bridges for diffusion of information and innovations. The basis of Granovetter's argument was that people's friends are also likely to be friends. Consequently, it was not common for people to be connected to others who do not know one another. These connections between people whose friends do not know one another are more likely to be bridges connecting un-connected groups. Figure 11–4 shows Granovetter's original diagram showing the link between nodes A and B as a bridge. According to Granovetter (1973), bridges reduce the overall distance between individuals in a network where distances were conceived as the number of steps between people. Reduced distance enables information to spread more rapidly throughout a network. Granovetter linked the micro-level tendency for transitivity to translate into the macro-level property of weak ties being bridges.

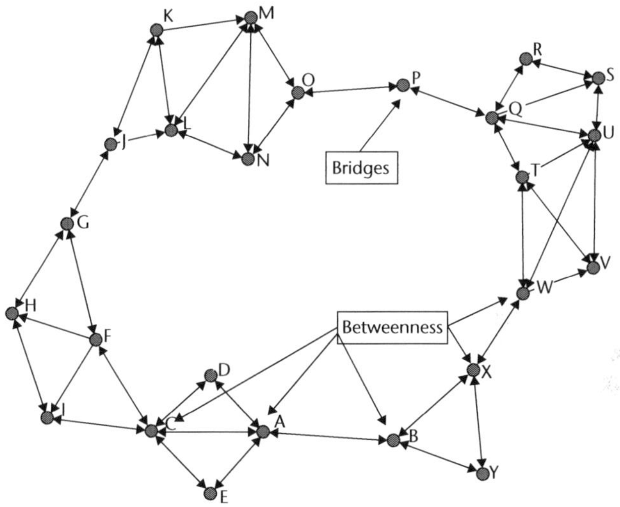

Figure 11–4. Graph used to illustrate weak ties in Granovetter's (1973) strength of weak ties paper.

Traditionally, social network researchers have used centrality betweenness (see Chapter 5) to measure bridging in networks. The bridging measure (p. 210) as well as centrality betweenness were calculated on this network. The analysis shows that bridging, when conceived of as a node or person, is the node P at the top of the network, not nodes A or B. Nodes A, B, C, X, and W all have high and nearly equal betweenness scores. P is unique, however, in that P has only 2 links and thus the average change in distances when P's links are deleted is greater than for other nodes.

central, but reside in an intermediate position within the network. These nodes might function as important intermediary relays in the diffusion process.

The bridge and potential measures may have particular application to the prevention of disease transmission. To prevent diseases from spreading within communities, researchers advocate immunizing central nodes as that would have the greatest effect on preventing further spread. To prevent disease from spreading between communities, however, bridges should be immunized. From a local perspective it makes sense to focus on central nodes, but from a global or macro perspective, bridges are critical.

In sum, the rewiring methodology has provided several insights. First, it indicates specific links that should be deleted to slow diffusion or those to be added to accelerate diffusion based on changes in network cohesion. Second, other network properties (see Chapter 8) can be maximized so that link changes can be proposed that maximally (or minimally) affect network centralization, transitivity, clustering, and so on. Third, the average link changes can be aggregated to the nodes (take the average) to identify critical nodes in the network that occupy bridging positions. These nodes may be essential to network performance.

It should be acknowledged that purposively changing networks, in many cases, is likely to be very difficult since people have the relationships they have for very good reasons. People are attracted to one another for many reasons and may not want to create new affiliations that a management or advocacy team recommends. For example, organizations often have divisions that need to be merged. It may be relatively straightforward to identify the people who should communicate more frequently to make the newly merged organization more cohesive. Members of the two subgroups, however, may have functions, activities, beliefs, and norms that inhibit communication between the groups. Still, having a set of rewiring network tools available may be very useful.

Networks and Attributes

The intervention techniques presented so far have used network data only, without regard to the characteristics of the people involved. It makes more sense to consider the characteristics (age, sex, attitudes, behaviors, etc.) of the people in the network along with the network data. For example, an intervention designed to promote adoption of a new technology in an office may need to consider the skill levels of individual members of the group before creating groups based on network data alone. Or it may be necessary to check the gender of all group members so that no groups are formed that have less than a certain percent of each gender.

Network-attribute interventions will logically be of two types. First are those in which personal attributes such as gender, ethnicity, age, and education status are considered after the network data have been used to design the intervention. In these the researcher may simply inspect network groupings or assignments to verify that there is an appropriate distribution of the attributes in groups or assignments. For example, one may want to create groups of the same gender or ensure that all groups have at least two members of either sex. An intervention designed to reduce racial tensions in a school may want to create ethnically heterogeneous groups but also inspect those groups to be sure there is a reasonable and appropriate distribution of ethnicities within groups.

Interventions may also be designed that adequately and appropriately distribute knowledge and skills within groups. For example, a school-based curriculum may wish to use network data for identifying leaders and groups but also guarantee that each group has people of varying abilities. So a math game could be constructed based on friendship patterns but also guaranteeing that equal numbers of low, medium, and high math performers are represented in each group.

The second type of network-attribute intervention considers attributes first and segments the population on the attribute. For example, in the field of substance use prevention, nonusers can be grouped together to discuss ways to continue resisting peer influence on use, while users can be grouped together to discuss ways to quit or support nonuse. Future interventions may want to explore novel ways of harnessing the positive effects of social influence. For example, Killeya-Jones and colleagues train "deviant" peer leaders to devise and spread antidrug messages to younger peers (Killeya-Jones et al., 2007).

Regardless of how implemented, considering networks and attributes simultaneously seems a reasonable approach to intervention procedures since many interventions are designed to change behaviors. Network influences on behavior must be seen in the context of the attitudes and behaviors of the population and the specifics of how behaviors interact with the network structures. Just as network analysts may criticize research conducted devoid of context, behaviorists may criticize network research's overreliance on structure absent the attitudes and behaviors that define people. A further caution is warranted: Because networks are often homophilous, using network data to define intervention groups can sometimes create overly homophilous structures, thus increasing barriers to change. Consequently, interventions may also be designed to purposively separate people based on existing attitudes and behaviors or purposively structured to sever existing friendships.

For example, network data on friendship links may be used to purposively construct groups in which the members do not know one another. This might be done to break down existing communication and influence paths or to experiment with how groups composed of (near) strangers perform. It might also be done because a classroom or organization had been experiencing negative actions and performance and so something is needed to "shake things up."

Iatrogenic Effects

One concern with using network data to construct interventions has been the possibility of iatrogenic effects. Even the most well-intentioned health promotion programs may have negative or unanticipated consequences, referred to as *boomerang* or *iatrogenic effects*. Negative effects occur when an intervention's design exacerbates the problem behavior it is supposed to improve. Dishion and others (1999) conducted a series of studies among high-risk youth evaluating interventions designed to address their problem behavior. Results showed that participation in peer groups with other high-risk youth resulted in a greater prevalence of the problem behavior. Dishion and others (1999) refer to this as deviancy training: "youth with moderate levels of delinquency, and who had deviant friends, were those who escalated to more serious forms of antisocial behavior" (Dishion et al., 1999, p. 761). Students who receive a prevention curriculum in groups of friends who favor drug use may be more likely to subsequently favor drug use and the method of curriculum delivery would have negative effects. Indeed, such an occurrence is plausible since adolescents may take curriculum content and use it to promote substance abuse by parodying scripts in a pro-use manner.

Deviancy training can occur both when problem adolescents are grouped with other problem adolescents and when problem adolescents are grouped with previously "good" adolescents. Dodge and others (2007) reviewed several large-scale natural experiments in which student mixing resulted in an increase in the number of regular students in settings with poor performing or "deviant" students. For example, some school districts may change their policy putting six-grade students in middle schools, with seventh- and eighth-grade students, rather than a kindergarten through sixth-grade arrangement. The prevalence of problem behaviors (smoking, substance use, detention) increased dramatically for sixth-graders in schools with seventh- and eighth-graders compared to sixth-graders who remained in elementary schools (Dodge et al., 2007).

Iatrogenic effects might be expected in a network-delivered substance abuse prevention program. Valente and others (2007b) used leader/matching methodology to create TND Network, a network-tailored version of an existing substance use prevention program. The study was designed to prevent and reduce substance use among high-risk high school students who attend continuation (alternative) high schools in southern California. An earlier study using networks to prevent tobacco use showed that the network performed as well, and in some cases better, than teacher-defined leaders and groups (Valente et al., 2006). A significant research and practice question emerging from this prior study was: To what degree is any network tailoring effect dependent on the program within which it is embedded? Consequently, TND Network was created as a network-tailored version of an existing evidence-based curriculum, Towards no Drug Abuse (Sussman et al., 1993). The network version used network data to construct groups and make the material more interactive, keeping program content constant. Of interest was whether TND Network was more effective than TND and whether TND Network might create peer aggregation that has deleterious effects on substance use outcomes, deviancy training, or iatrogenic effects.

Results showed that TND Network was associated with monthly reductions in current use of marijuana, cocaine, and a composite substance use score at 1-year follow-up (Valente et al., 2007b). The effects on current use were strongest when the regression included an interaction term composed of peer use (network exposure) and being in the TND Network condition. This indicates that, for some students, being in the network condition increased their use if they had a friendship network composed mostly of users.

The reduced substance use came at the expense of increasing use among some students with existing networks of substance using peers. Substance use was reduced mainly for those students who nominated as friends other students who reported low levels of substance use. If a student received the network curriculum and had friends in the class who reported using substances, he or she was likely to increase his/her substance using behaviors over the 1-year interval. Thus, the network curriculum seemed to achieve its goal of increasing peer influence, yet that peer influence, in the context of an alternative high school, was potentially negative for adolescents with drug-using friends.

Reducing substance use in a high-risk sample such as alternative high school youth is challenging at best. The TND Network curriculum was able to achieve relatively long-term behavioral effects on marijuana and cocaine use and on a composite use index when all substances were considered together. This success, however, came at some cost to students at elevated risk due to their having friends who use drugs.

Future studies will no doubt explore how to use social networking sites such as Facebook, MySpace, LinkedIn, and others to learn how networks evolve and how they influence behavioral choices. Many people now use these services and are familiar with their properties. These or similar systems may be developed to understand how individuals or organizations create, manage, and change their social networks and how these dynamics influence attitudes and behavior. There is considerable potential for using these sites as intervention loci.

A Pharmaceutical Marketing Example

Many of the studies reviewed thus far were conducted among small isolated communities or in laboratory-type settings. Network techniques can be used to accelerate marketing in real-world applications such as among physicians practicing in communities. Survey data were solicited from 188 medical doctors in the San Francisco Bay Area who treat or potentially treat patients with a type of viral infection. The survey was mailed twice and a reminder postcard was sent. The final response rate was 43%. Physicians were asked with whom they discuss the management and treatment of the condition and to whom they refer patients. Surprisingly, respondents wrote names primarily from the list provided for the mailing. It was as if the respondents consulted the list in their selection of discussion and referral partners rather than being asked open-ended questions. Some additional names, not on the list, were provided.

Figure 11–5 graphs the network of discussion in the San Francisco Bay Area. The network showed two large subgroups with one group anchored by physicians numbers 12, 18, 58, and 160. This group turned out to have predominantly European surnames. In contrast the second group was smaller, a bit less densely connected, with number 175 receiving the most nominations. This second group had primarily Asian surnames. Clearly two different groups of physicians constituted the treatment community in this region. To be successful at marketing its products, a pharmaceutical firm would be wise to understand this and similar underlying structures. Notable findings from this research were that a marketing strategy that did not include number 175 would have a hard time being successful in the Asian and Asian-American community in the Bay Area. Further, marketing efforts directed at numbers 12, 18, 58, and 160 are, to some extent, redundant. These four physicians are prominent and important opinion leaders, but they are influential within the same group (recall the key player section). It is more efficient to find opinion leaders in different groups rather than leaders all in the same group. We also measured self-reported opinion leadership among this group with an opinion leadership scale (King et al., 1999). We found a modest correlation ($r = 0.43$, $p < .01$) between self-reported leadership and receiving nominations as a discussion partner (Iyengar, et al., in press).

Another outcome from this study was to test how well the identification of leaders would perform if the sociometric study was conducted using only a subsample of the 188 physicians on the original list. In this experiment,

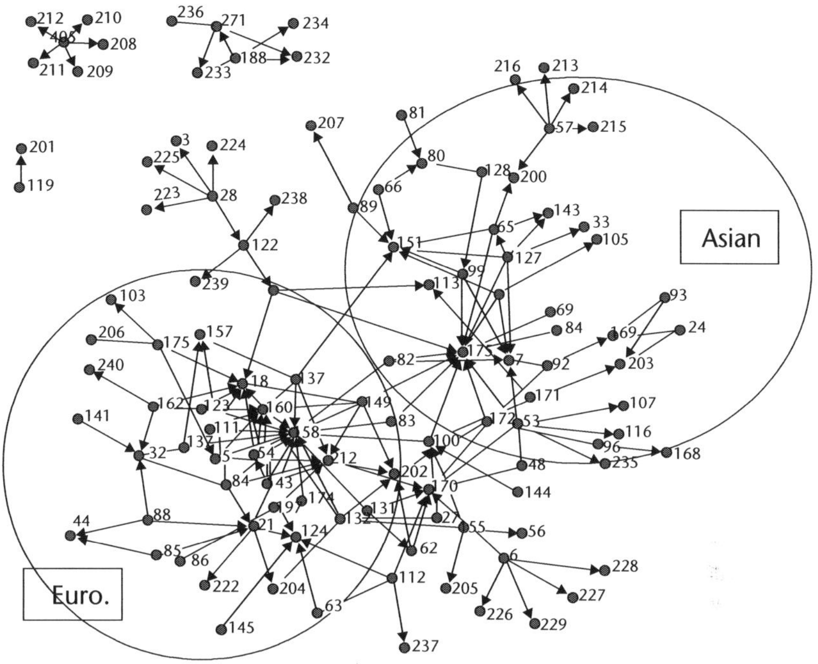

Figure 11–5. Discussion and referral linkages among physicians in one metropolitan area. The cluster on the left was composed mostly of physicians with European surnames, whereas the one on the right was composed mostly of physicians with Asian surnames.

a 20% random sample of the mailing list was selected and the data from responding physicians within that sample were analyzed. Essentially, the study asked the question: what would have happened if surveys were sent to 20% of the entire list of 188 physicians? The results showed a markedly different network structure with considerably more isolates, not surprisingly. The sample survey failed to capture the network structure that was so apparent from the full dataset.

These procedures can be scaled up somewhat. In a national survey of dermatologists who treat patients with psoriasis, respondents were asked to indicate other dermatologists with whom they discuss patient treatment and go to for advice regarding treatment options. The data showed a remarkable degree of local clustering such that over 90% of the discussion relationships were within the same geographic region as the respondent. The geographic regions were large, dividing the United States into four areas: northeast, south, midwest and west. Advice-seeking was slightly less geographically bound, with about 80% of contacts being within region.

The techniques proposed in this chapter have considerable utility for interventions in many domains across many settings. It may be, however, that the most effective network intervention is simply collecting the data and reporting it back to the interested communities. Seeing their own network data, in a way no individual could see it without collecting data from everyone, can be a powerful motivator for energizing change. Thus, assessments of network intervention effects should consider that simply asking network questions can have an effect on behavior and simply providing network feedback can stimulate change.

Summary

This chapter introduced the concept of network interventions, using network data to implement behavior change programs. Six classes of methods were reviewed: opinion leaders, groups, leaders matched to groups, snowball methods, rewiring networks, and crossing network data with attributes. Many cautions were expressed about the importance of theory and ethnography to ensure the research team has sufficient knowledge of the community. Caution was also expressed regarding the potential for iatrogenic effects and that interventions may purposively attempt to divide existing networks.

The chapter closed with a community example illustrating the capability of network data collection from physicians practicing in a broad geographic area. Most, if not all, behavior change programs ignore social networks and thus lack the capacity to know whether program success or failure was dependent in part on who delivered the message. The messenger is the medium in the sense that who delivers the intervention and the social context within which it is received may be as, if not more, important than the message itself. The potential for network interventions to accelerate behavior change is great, but the application of these methods is likely to be challenging at first as both researchers and communities learn how best to apply networks and networking in the most effective ways.

12

Summary

This book has introduced the many theories, procedures, techniques, methods, measures, and applications of social network analysis to health topics. In Part I, Chapter 1 provided an overview of the major models and concepts used to understand social networks. Major models and research areas include understanding the importance of homophily, scale-free or centralized structures, social capital, algorithms, dynamics, diffusion of innovations, and interventions. These models have focused the research attention of many scientists and produced a rich body of research.

Chapter 2 provided a history of the network analysis field and reviewed some of the major areas of application. Early network studies were derived mostly from data collected in small groups and often entailed in-depth observation and study. The field was slow to grow in part because social science researchers were trained to collect random samples from populations and make inferences based on sampling properties. This preoccupation slowed the development of appropriate statistical and computational tools for social network analysis.

The growth of the Internet, the ubiquity of computer communications, and an increased appreciation of social context helped spur growth in network analysis by the 1990s. The medical and public health fields expanded network applications from risk behaviors to infectious and eventually chronic diseases. Public health applications also included the study of community coalitions, interorganizational relationships, and systems approaches to policy and social change. Modeling and analysis of large contact network structures provide insight into potential epidemic threats. Today, network analysis represents a full-grown paradigm of research and constitutes a perspective that is increasingly difficult to ignore.

Many theoretical approaches have been used to understand how networks influence behaviors that affect health and the provision of health services. Most behavior change theories include a role for social influence, norms, and peer influences. The network approach provides specific methodologies and theories for modeling and testing such influences. The traditional approach has been the study of the diffusion of innovations, a perspective that attempts to understand how new ideas and practices spread within and between communities.

Studies of the diffusion of innovations and behavior change have consistently shown that the behavior of peers and close personal networks has a strong influence on people's adoption behavior. If a person's closest friends do something, the focal individual is approximately twice as likely to do it also. Strong ties have a strong influence on people's behavior. There are people who are not influenced by their friends but instead have lower personal network thresholds to behavior. These individuals are innovative with respect to their peers and so innovate before their friends do. Low-threshold individuals turn to the media or peers outside the immediate peer group for influences on their behavior.

Given the importance of close, strong ties on behavior, numerous methods have been developed to measure social networks. Chapter 3 presented the many different network approaches including egocentric (local), snowball (partial), and census (complete) approaches as well as general and specific approaches for each. Understanding how network data are collected is critical to understanding how to manage, analyze, and interpret network data. All the approaches provide more contextual information than independent random samples, yet the approaches vary in how, where, and when they can be applied.

Egocentric data can be collected with random samples and typically involve the measurement of a person's close contacts. For example, many surveys ask people to name the people they talk to about important matters and then ask the respondent to provide information on the person's named such as their gender, education, religion, and any health behaviors under study. Egocentric techniques have been used to demonstrate homophily: the tendency for people to have close friends and contacts who are like themselves (being of the same ethnicity, socioeconomic status, religious persuasion, and so on). Egocentric data have also been used to show that people are influenced in their behaviors by their social networks.

Census approaches are in some ways more powerful than egocentric techniques as they provide a full map of the network and require the researcher to specify the network boundary. Respondents are asked to name others within the boundary (or check their name from a list) and the network is then mapped and analyzed. More powerful computing has also enabled researchers to map networks from archival records or communications systems such as telephone or e-mail logs. Census network data can be used to derive many measures that indicate a person's position in the network, whether central or not, for example. Census techniques have enabled researchers to measure group properties, positions, and network-level measures.

Part II of this book consisted of Chapters 5 through 8, which provided a review of methods and measures calculated with census (complete) network data. Chapter 5 reviewed centrality measures, which indicate the degree a person (or node) is in the center of the network. Many centrality measures have been proposed, the three most common being degree, closeness, and betweenness. The calculation of these measures and their application to health behaviors was detailed. Many studies have shown that leaders, those who occupy central positions in the network, often adopt innovations early but not necessarily the earliest. Leaders, and those who occupy critical positions in the network, can have a large influence on many processes hypothesized to occur on networks.

Chapters 6, 7, and 8 provided measures for assessing groups, positions, and network-level properties, respectively. Each chapter provided the methods historically used for these topics and how health behaviors have been studied with these techniques. There are many different algorithms available to measure groups and positions in a network depending on how one defines what it means to be in a group. Attention was paid to the Girvan-Newman (2002) algorithm as a widely available technique to sort nodes into mutually exclusive groups and at the same time getting a measure of how well the grouping fits the data. As with groups, several position algorithms were also presented, with attention being paid to CONCOR and structural equivalence, which sorts nodes into equivalent positions based on how similar the ties are between nodes. Chapter 8 provided algorithms and interpretations for the most common network level indicators: size, density, diameter, average path length, transitivity, clustering, and centralization.

Part III of this book covered applications of network analysis to areas of substantive interest by explicitly considering how ideas, attitudes, and behaviors are embedded in networks. Chapter 9 provided an introduction to exponential random graph or P* models that provide a means to conduct statistical tests on network properties, network evolution, and the interaction between networks and behavior. The exponential random graph model (ERGM) framework has generated considerable excitement among network researchers as it links network dynamics to a statistical model in a manner similar to the evolution of inferential statistics. Chapter 9 illustrated the main components of testing the actor oriented co-evolution model used to test network influences while controlling for network dependencies.

Chapter 10 reviewed the theory and literature on diffusion of innovations. The four main eras or diffusion models were reviewed: (1) opinion leaders and integration, (2) structural influences such as weak ties, (3) critical levels or tipping points, and (4) dynamic, event history models. Analysis of the classic diffusion network datasets was provided. The chapter shows the many ways researchers have investigated how networks influence the spread of new ideas and practices within and between communities. If networks do influence diffusion, then perhaps networks can be used to accelerate positive behavior changes. As Christakis and Fowler (2007) wrote, "The spread of obesity in social networks appears to be a factor in the obesity epidemic. Yet the relevance of social influence also suggests that it may be possible to harness this same force to slow the spread of obesity" (p. 378).

Chapter 11 reviewed network interventions, techniques for using network data to accelerate behavior change or enhance community/organizational performance. Several approaches to network interventions were presented, including opinion leaders, groups, leaders and groups, snowball designs for recruitment, and rewiring or network reconfiguration. Several studies have tested network interventions with results generally showing that network interventions are effective but also can create unintended consequences. Caution regarding the application of network interventions was voiced as well as the importance of including individual attributes along with the network data.

As this summary suggests, the network analysis field is large and expanding in many ways. Like most research endeavors, choosing the appropriate methodology for answering one's research questions is a critical challenge. Inappropriate methodology frustrates the researcher into trying to fit a round peg into a square hole. Network analysis compounds this problem by providing a research methodology that is intuitively appealing and, on the surface of it, appropriate for many settings, and is remarkably easy to do. The researcher need only ask one question: Name your closest friends (in a school, say), and the researcher has a dizzying array of standard measures available to him or her to comprehensively understand the individuals, groups, hierarchies, configurations, systems, liabilities, and assets contained with that school.

Once an attribute is added such as gender or ethnicity, the researcher can determine if these attributes affect how the network is formed. Are adolescent boys more or less likely to name other boys as friends? The tendency for ties to be reciprocated among people who share attributes is referred to

Table 12–1. Network Data Provide an Almost Unlimited Number of Variables in the Analysis

Individual level: Centrality degree; closeness; betweenness; group member; isolate; pendant; reciprocated ties; density; constraint; exposure on attributes; exposure to behaviors

Network level: Density; reciprocity (%); transitivity; triad census; core-periphery; average path length; diameter; positions; block model; image matrix

Symmetrize original data (repeat above)

Compare and combine two or more networks

Exponential random graph modeling

Actor-oriented co-evolution model

Network diffusion

as homophily and the tendency of homophily creates network structure. Just a few attributes (age, sex, ethnicity, marital status, and religion) can create complex effects on networks. Table 12–1 illustrates the array of variables and analyses that can be constructed from a few simple network questions.

Of course, in many studies, researchers ask multiple network questions to compare them. For example, one might ask adolescents in schools who are their best friends and whom they would like to lead a project in class. Although there is some overlap in these two networks, the questions will elicit different names. Researchers can compare these networks by studying their correlation and test hypotheses at both the individual and network levels regarding the role these networks might play in academic performance and other behaviors.

In the case of school-based adolescent research, it is quite common to collect network data in multiple schools, thus permitting comparisons of network structures across settings. For example, one can study the variation in friendship network density, transitivity, and clustering across schools. It might be hypothesized that network structural properties vary in part based on the ethnic distribution of the students in the schools. A school with a large majority of one ethnicity may be characterized as having high transitivity and a relatively cohesive and stable network structure. Conversely, a school with considerable ethnic diversity may be characterized as having restricted transitivity such that triangles are more likely to be closed when the people share the same ethnic background. These variations in structure may have implications for behavioral diffusion, normative beliefs, and the potential for change.

While network analyses, and the procedures and algorithms for doing so, are of interest to network scientists, the research hopefully adds some benefit to the participants and policymakers who fund the research and have an interest in the outcome. In such cases, it is quite common to track student performance and determine whether network factors are associated with, perhaps causally linked to, this performance. For example, researchers might want to know whether students who get poor grades are more likely to have friends who get poor grades. There may be many reasons for the association between individual and friend grades some more plausible and amenable to change than others. Locating this relationship, however, unlocks the grade performance problem for many parents who can now take remedial action. It is quite possible the friends spend too much playing video games and not enough time studying, so the parent might insist the student study with his or her friends first before they can play their games.

The techniques covered in this book help researchers understand how to analyze social network data including analysis of a single network, comparing networks, and including individual attributes. An additional dimension to network analysis of behavior change occurs when researchers have data on time of adoption, when individuals initiated a new behavior. In cases where researcher knows when individuals initiated behavior change, the dynamic process by which a new idea or practice spreads through a network of contacts can be modeled and analyzed.

Often, this time of adoption has been measured retrospectively, after diffusion has occurred. In this case, respondents are asked to recall when they first used a new product or changed their behavior. In some studies, time of adoption is measured with some recording system such as when people first accessed a website. The challenges inherent in recording time of adoption, especially since diffusion often takes quite a long time, has meant that there are few studies that have measured social networks and time of adoption. Consequently, much of the literature on diffusion networks is derived from computer simulation.

Interpersonal influence is a leading cause of behavior change. Individuals cite friends and social networks as the primary influence on their behavior, so using social network analysis to understand behavior change is critically important. Amazingly, given a bounded setting, asking a simple question that is very easy for the respondent to answer (e.g., Who are your friends?), yields an embarrassingly large array of measures. In some cases, the data are available unobtrusively (e.g., who sends e-mail to whom) and so even easier to collect. The challenge is to understand how to analyze the data and select the appropriate algorithms and models to capture the researcher's substantive interest. One way to illustrate and test the complexities of network science is by using agent-based modeling (ABM).

Agent-Based Modeling

ABM is a computational technique used to investigate theoretical issues by use of computer simulation. Agent-based models are a specific type of simulation used to model network effects. Agent-based models typically start with a hypothetical community that is composed of agents that may be thought of as people but can also represent organizations, agencies, or other entities. A set of rules the researcher may be interested in understanding are proposed and these rules become the actions that dictate agent behavior in the model. The researcher then posits variations on the rules or a range for some parameters to vary. The computer simulation then runs through the various configurations of the model to understand how the system behaves under these hypothetical conditions.

ABM has many advantages and, with the growth of computational capabilities in the past decade, has become an increasingly useful research tool. One advantage is that it can help the researcher specify the variables, rules, and models that are of theoretical interest. Developing a model helps the researcher think about his or her problem of study. For example, the hypothetical random mixing model presented in Chapter 11 to show how diffusion occurs via random interactions between adopters and nonadopters helped clarify one way in which the diffusion process works. A second advantage is that ABM allows the research to investigate issues of theoretical importance without collecting data. Since data collection can be time-consuming and expensive, being able to do research without having to collect data can be very beneficial.

The disadvantage to ABM is that the results are only as good as the set of rules, assumptions, and procedures built into the model. If the assumptions and rules of the model do not reflect situations found in the real world, then the model will not provide useful results. Calibrating ABM parameters to empirical data is a requirement for building useful models for them to reflect real-world settings and processes.

To illustrate, agent-based models were created to simulate behavioral diffusion varying three parameters: (1) initial adopter characteristics, (2) network structure type, and (3) the adoption threshold. These simulations demonstrate the effects of network structure and initial seed adopters on diffusion. Four different initial adopters (seeds) were simulated: (1) opinion leaders (those receiving the most nominations), (2) randomly selected ones, (3) highest centrality betweenness (see Chapter 5), and (4) marginals, those receiving the fewest nominations. Four different network structures of the same size and density were modeled: (1) a real network derived from data collected in a high school, (2) a random network, (3) a centralized (scale-free) network, and (4) a clustered (small world) network.

Contact diffusion was simulated first, which occurs when adoption happens by simply coming into contact with an adopter. This is also known as *knowledge awareness diffusion* or *rumor diffusion*. in which there is very little cognitive effort required for a person to be an adopter. People (or agents) thus change their status from being nonaware to aware when one of their connections is aware. The simulation is created by starting with an initial set of adopters and an initial network at time 1. At time 2, network exposure is calculated for each person using the network exposure model (see Chapter 4). The threshold is set to just above 0 (0.01), so any person with exposure becomes an adopter at time 2. The process is repeated for 18 time periods, keeping track of the number and proportion of adopters at each time period. Each combination of parameters is run 100 times so that any anomalies that may arise from a particular simulation run are accounted for by taking the average across many runs. By chance, for example, a random network may have been generated that is quite centralized, and this would perturb the results of the simulation. By averaging across many runs, this possibility is accounted for since it is unlikely that as many as 100 randomly generated networks were centralized (for example). It is usually recommended to simulate each scenario at least 100, 500, or 1,000 times to account for these chance events. The number of iterations is determined by the degree of certainty needed in the results.

Of course, any randomly generated network, even with specified properties such as being centralized or clustered, may have variations within it that skew the simulation results. To guarantee that these results were not a product of any chance occurrences within any one of the networks, the procedures were repeated 100 times. In total, there were 4,800 possible permutations, four network structures, four different starting seeds, three thresholds settings, and 100 runs each ($4 \times 4 \times 3 \times 100 = 4,800$). The 48 possible permutations were simulated 100 times and the average within these 100 stored as the model results.

Table 12–2 depicts the parameters studied in this ABM. The average of the 16 scenarios (4×4) for the three threshold settings provides model results. Each scenario consists of simulated diffusion over 18 time periods. A diffusion rate was calculated for each scenario providing a single parameter estimate to compare across scenarios. Table 12–3 reports the rate of diffusion

Table 12–2. Average Rate of Diffusion across 16 Different Hypothetical Scenarios by Varying First Adopters (Seeds) and Network Structure

Seeds	Network Structure			
	Real	Random	Centralized	Clustered
Leaders	0.16	0.42	0.41	0.27
Random	0.18	0.43	0.41	0.27
Between	0.20	0.45	0.47	0.27
Marginals	0.20	0.44	0.45	0.27

Table 12–3. Selected Network-Level Indicators for the Four Network Structures within which Diffusion Was Simulated

	Size	Density	Centralization	Clustering	Reciprocity. %
Real	150	1.46%	3.28	15.4	43.0%
Random	150	1.46%	3.25	1.85	1.05%
Centralized	150	1.46%	7.67	1.63	1.01%
Clustered	150	1.46%	2.81	15.5	10.3%

for the 16 conditions. The principle analytic tool is a graph of the diffusion curves providing a visual comparison across conditions.

Figure 12–1 shows the diffusion curves comparing network structures between different seeds (comparing the columns in row one of Table 12–2). Figure 12–1a depicts diffusion across the four network structures when the first adopters are leaders. Diffusion occurs fastest in the random network when the first adopters are opinion leaders. Diffusion is nearly as fast in a centralized network when the first adopters are leaders but not quite as fast as in the random networks (compare rates 0.42 to 0.41). Leaders are those with the most nominations, and once they adopt, they spread the innovation to many others rapidly. In a random network, the spread happens most quickly because the leaders are randomly spread throughout the network and so their connections are not redundant. Further, the people connected to the leaders are not necessarily connected to other leaders. Consequently, there is little redundancy in the leader communications with the nonleaders, and so the idea spreads quickly. In a centralized network, there may be some redundancy in the connections between leaders and nonleaders, so at any one time period there is a greater likelihood that a nonadopter will be in contact with two leaders who both are adopters than in a random network. Therefore, diffusion is slightly slower in the centralized network than in the random one when the first adopters are leaders.

Figure 12–1b reports diffusion curves when the first adopters are randomly selected. Here diffusion is again fastest in the random network, followed closely by the centralized networks and then much slower in the clustered and real ones. Notice also that in all four seeding conditions the clustered network has slower diffusion, and the real network is the slowest.

Figure 12–1c shows diffusion curves when the first adopters are those with the highest centrality betweenness scores. Here diffusion starts off faster in the centralized networks and remains faster than in the random networks. The betweenness seeds have a slightly larger impact on diffusion in the centralized network than the random one because, on average, their initial persuasive connections reach more nonredundant people. Consequently, diffusion reaches the leaders rapidly and diffusion accelerates. The centralized

(a) Leader Seeds by Network Structure

(b) Random Seeds by Network Structure

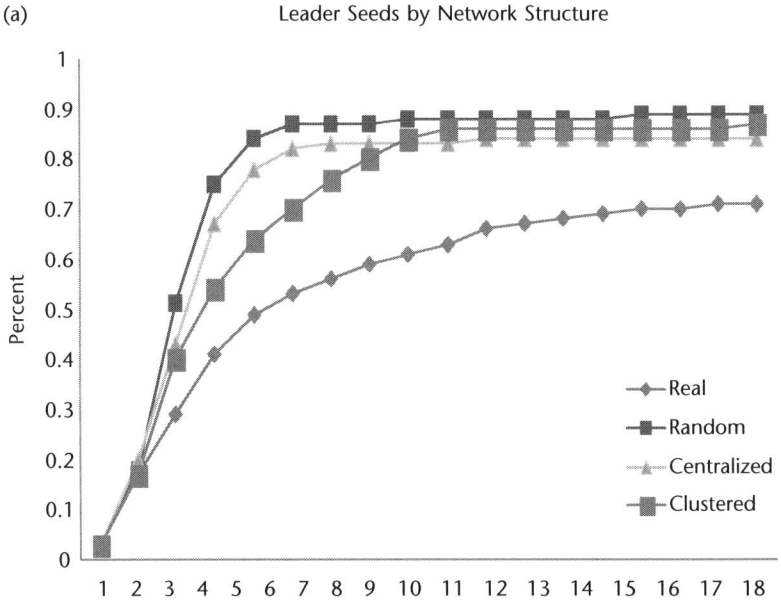

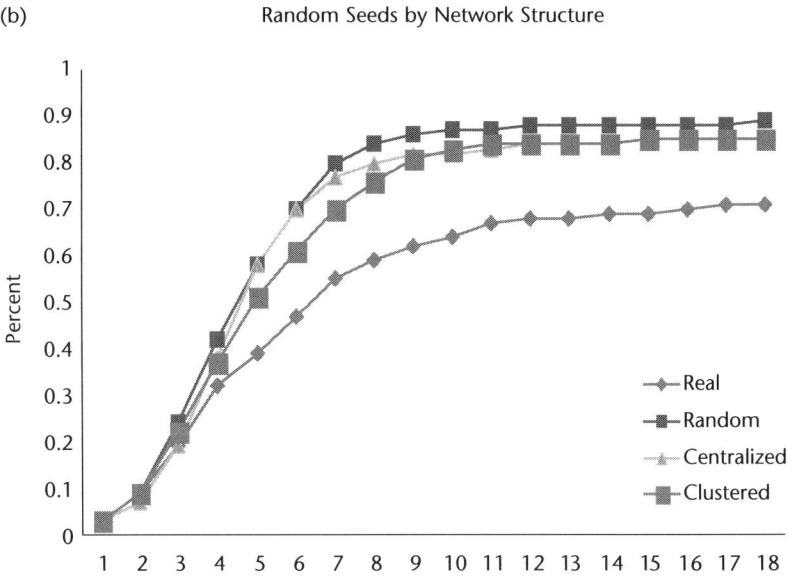

Figure 12–1. Simulated diffusion varied across four network structures—(1) real, (2) random, (3) centralized, and (4) clustered—and four different initial adopter (a) highest in-degree, (b) random, (c) highest betweenness, and (d) marginals.

Betweenness Seeds by Network Stucture

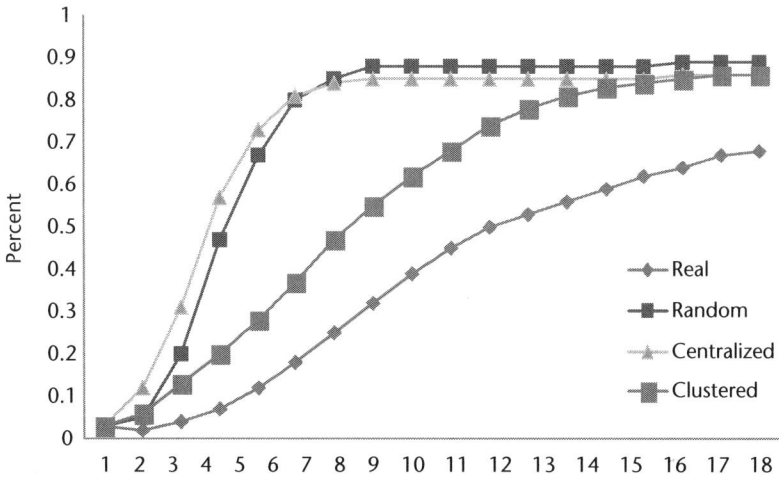

(d)

Marginal Seeds by Network Structure

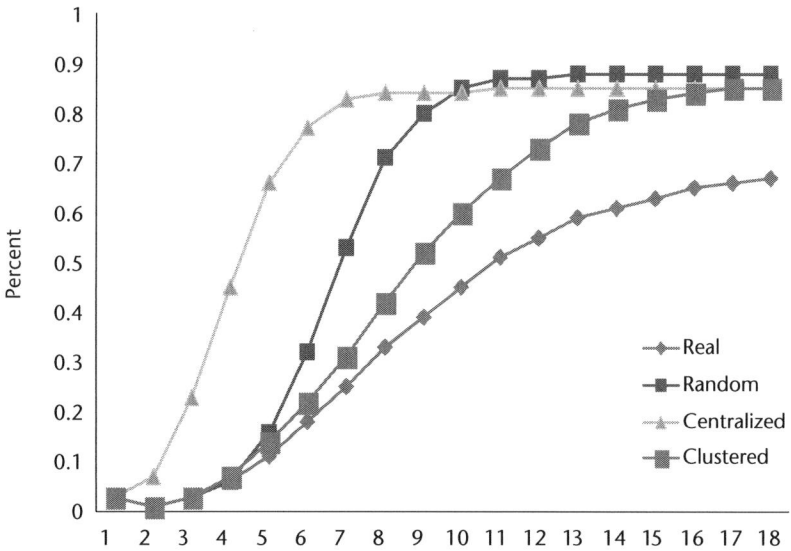

Figure 12–1. Continued.

229

network accelerates diffusion when initial seeds have high betweenness. This is also true, but to a slightly lesser extent with the random networks.

Figure 12–1d shows the results when initial seeds are on the margins of the network and provides the clearest results of any of the conditions. Here diffusion is fastest in the centralized network, followed by the random networks, then the clustered one, and the real one had the slowest diffusion. When initial adopters are on the periphery of the network, receiving only one nomination, for example, then diffusion will be slowed except in a centralized network. In a centralized network, marginal people may still only be one step away from the leaders and so the innovation can travel quickly to them and be quickly spread to everyone else. In contrast, in a random or clustered network, innovations starting on the margins take some time to percolate through the network and reach everyone else.

Figure 12–2 aggregates the data across different network structures to compare the influence of different seeds, or initial adopters, on diffusion trajectories. Diffusion is faster when initiated by opinion leaders or randomly selected seeds than when initiated by those high in betweenness or marginals. High betweenness and marginal members have few connections and therefore their adoption behavior does not spread to many others. In some cases using people high in betweenness as initial adopters may be a

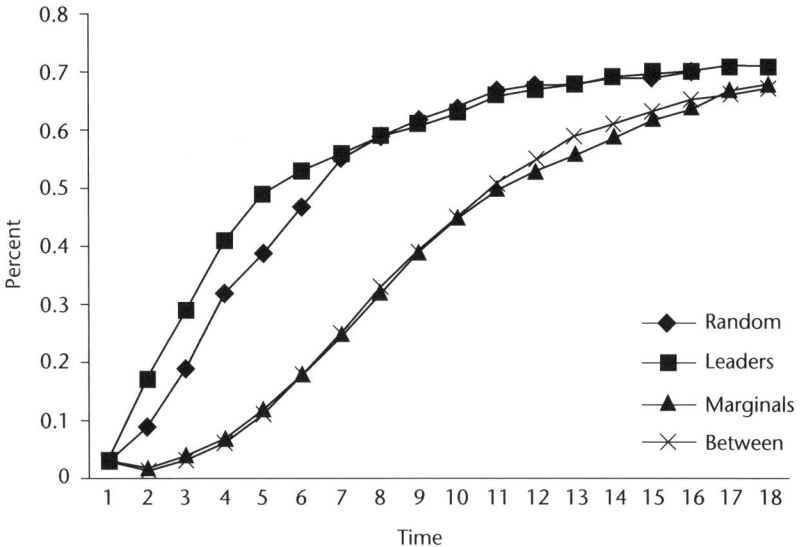

Figure 12–2. Hypothetical diffusion curves averaged across the four network structures. Diffusion is faster when initiated by opinion leaders or randomly selected nodes rather than those high in betweenness or marginals (in part because high betweenness initial seeds have slow simulated diffusion in the real network).

wise strategy but in these simulations diffusion is slow in both the clustered and real networks when initial adopters have high betweenness. Surprisingly, randomly chosen initial adopters are almost as effective as leaders.

Several overall conclusions may be gleaned from these models. First, random networks have more rapid diffusion than one might naively expect. Random network structures provide short overall paths in the network and little clustering which creates bottlenecks. Thus, overall random networks perform very well. Second, centralization, in general, speeds diffusion. Once the idea reaches the central members in a centralized network, it can spread rapidly. Centralized and random networks compete for the fastest diffusion in all conditions, but centralization clearly outperforms random networks when initial seeds are marginals. Third, clustering retards diffusion. The clustered networks have slower diffusion than the centralized or random ones, and only consistently outperform the real network when initial seeds are high betweenness nodes. Clustering can accelerate diffusion within pockets of interconnectivity but slows diffusion when it has to cross bridges that connect the clustered pockets. Finally, the real network had the slowest diffusion under all initial conditions. This may be explained in part by the relatively high clustering in the real network.

Table 12–3 reports the average centralization and clustering scores for the four networks. The real network had a clustering coefficient considerably higher than the random or centralized networks. Further, the real network had a much higher percentage of reciprocated ties than any of the other networks. Consequently, once a person adopted the new idea, one of his potential converts would have been the person who just converted him or her. So diffusion would be slowed in a symmetric network compared to asymmetric ones.

This analysis indicates, in one sense, why rumors can be so wrong and so destructive: Communication is not reflected back to the source of the information but instead transmitted to someone else, someone who has not heard the rumor. That someone is not likely to be connected to the source of the rumor otherwise he or she would have heard the rumor. So rumors spread unchecked and never are revalidated for accuracy. A rumor will spread most efficiently in a random network, particularly one with low clustering or reciprocity.

Increasing the Threshold

The simulation models were also run setting the adoption threshold to 25% and 50% to determine its effect on diffusion. Increasing the threshold to 25% had no effect on diffusion because this low threshold was essentially the same as the first contact threshold. Since the networks are constrained to have no more than five out-degree choices and an average out-degree of 2.2 choices, a 25% threshold amounts to being connected to one adopter in order to adopt. When raising the threshold to 50%, however, diffusion is slowed considerably, although the overall results remain the same. Of considerable interest, and further complexity, would be to vary thresholds by network properties such as the degree of centrality, or group or position membership. For example, it might be hypothesized that central members have lower or higher thresholds than less central members and simulate diffusion. This would contrast compatible versus incompatible innovations such that central members would be expected to have lower thresholds for compatible innovations than for incompatible ones. Thresholds might also be varied by time, expecting that thresholds will lower over time since the risk to adoption decreases as more people adopt. The ABM approach enables the testing of these various theories and scenarios with simulation rather than empirical data. The models help clarify scholarly thinking and often provide surprising results.

Statistical Analysis

It is possible to use the simulated data in statistical tests to determine the relative magnitude of different factors associated with model properties such as diffusion rates. For example, in this exercise diffusion rates for the first contact model were regressed on network structure and seeding type. The results showed that, relative to the real network, diffusion was accelerated in the random, centralized, and clustered networks. The *t*-values and associated regression coefficients were similar for the random and centralized networks and lower (but still significant) for the clustered networks. Seeding had a marginal and limited effect on diffusion rates, with only betweenness seeding showing a slight marginally positive effect on diffusion rates once network type was controlled for.

Network Scale

The diffusion simulations were calculated on networks of 150 individuals based on the empirical data collected in one grade of a U.S. high school. This number (150) also happens to be size postulated as optimal for human groups to retain stable relationships (Dunbar, 1992). At the same time, many of the examples presented in this book have been from smaller networks, school classrooms averaging 30 or so students, communication coalitions ranging in size from 4 to 41, and single coalitions with multiple organizations and multiple respondents per organization. The advent of online communities such as Facebook and mobile communications has created the potential to study single very large networks of tens of thousands and even millions of nodes.

Given these variations in network and data scale, it seems relevant to reiterate the variations in these data sources and means to manage and analyze the data. Network data may be derived from the following settings:

1. One group of three or more nodes, one network
2. One group of three or more nodes, multiple networks (e.g., advice, discussion, and friendship)
3. Multiple groups with one network (e.g., friendship within school classrooms)
4. Multiple groups of multiple networks (e.g., friendship and advice within classrooms)

These variations are compounded by the need to have data on node and relationship attributes. For example, nodes may be people of varying ages who do and do not practice particular behaviors; relationships may be valued indicating the strength or intensity of the relationship. A single small network or several small networks may be comfortably managed in an Excel spreadsheet, but most researchers will have much larger databases.

Consequently, it is usually recommended to store the data in link list format in a statistical program such as SAS, SPSS, or STATA. The node attributes can be stored in a statistical package making sure each case has a unique ID. If the data are nomination data, the nominations can easily be stored with the attribute data as well. Roster data, however, and most data collected via archival methods from computer systems will need to be stored in link list format. Each row will need to contain the unique ID numbers of the sender and receiver as well as information denoting the group (if there are multiple networks) and any information on relationship characteristics (such as frequency of interaction).

Future Research Questions

Despite the tremendous progress in network research and application, there are still many fundamental questions and research topics to be explored. For one, there is still interesting research to be conducted to understand the most appropriate network questions to ask respondents to generate the network. Different questions will yield different people named. Researchers have conducted studies comparing network generators (Bernard et al., 1990; Campbell & Lee, 1991) but more research in this domain is urgently needed.

In a related vein, research on the validity and reliability of network data is also needed (e.g., Coromina & Coenders, 2006). Behavioral research often advances quickly when valid and reliable measures are made available to a community of researchers. Such measures enable researchers to easily include them in other studies and see how they perform in different research contexts. The network approach may require different sampling methods and sometimes extensive questioning of the respondent on each network alter. Consequently researchers often think network research is difficult to do. Making valid and reliable measures easily available will help accelerate the field.

Once networks are measured, further research is needed on the characteristics of relationships that influence information exchange and personal influence. It was argued in Chapters 4 and 10 that close, strong ties are more likely to influence behavior than weak ones but that weak ones were important bridges between communities and may be effective at sharing new information or transmission of things that do not require much cognitive engagement. The research questions that spin out from this observation include studies designed to determine how best to measure tie strength and whether the association between tie strength and behavior change varies by topic. For example, Valente and Vlahov (2001) argued that alter rank was a proxy for tie strength, but is this true? Are alters named early in a response to a network question closer than those named later? Do different measures of tie strength correlate differently with different behaviors?

Of course, interpersonal influence may be a function of ego's perception of his or her alters behavior. Several studies have compared respondent perceptions of their friends' behaviors and those friends' self-reports (Iannotti & Bush, 1993; Rice et al., 2003; Valente et al., 1997). The evidence seems to indicate that respondents are not accurate in their estimates of friends' attitudes and behaviors. It also seems that people are more likely to be influenced by their perceptions of their friends' attitudes and behaviors rather than their friends' actual attitudes and behaviors. It would be interesting to know the factors associated with the discrepancy between perceived friend attitudes and behaviors and self-reported friend attitudes and behaviors. The discrepancies may be associated with social distance, observability of the behaviors being studied, tie strength, or respondent projection of their beliefs among other factors.

If social influence occurs through direct social networks, can it occur through indirect ones? Can social influence be transmitted by others who are two or more steps removed from ego? If indirect influence does exist, is it dependent on the attitudes and behaviors of the intermediary person? Few studies have investigated indirect influences and researchers are constantly challenged in their interpretation between network tie weights, indirect influences, and network thresholds.

Research into network sampling continues to be needed. In Chapter 5, issues surrounding missing data from complete networks were discussed. It was concluded that some centrality measures hold up quite well under conditions of missing data. Researchers can still identify central nodes from a closed population or list even when as few as 20% or 30% of the list responds. As researchers deploy network methods for outreach and recruitment (see Chapter 11), it is of increasing importance to understand the number of indexes and the number of degrees to sample into the network necessary for projects to be successful. In other words, what combination of indexes and alters is required to confidently measure community networks?

For mathematically inclined researchers, there is still considerable research needed in designing and testing different algorithms for network measures. New measures for newly created concepts may be needed as increased understanding and further exploration of networks evolve. In some cases, it may be desirable to create more efficient algorithms for existing measures so they can be calculated on larger networks.

Finally, new research on the basic association between network indicators is needed to understand how network measures correlate. For example, many network indicators explicitly control for size in their calculation. Density, the proportion of links in a network, is calculated by dividing by the number of links by the total theoretically possible. Yet evidence indicates that size and density are negatively correlated; density is low in large networks (see Chapter 8). Understanding why this occurs and how size and other network indicators correlate might shed light on how individuals, groups, and networks are interrelated.

In terms of behavior, the most significant area for future research is the collection of new data on the diffusion of innovation through a social (or other) network. Few studies have collected data on when individuals (or other nodes) adopt an innovation and the network contacts among the potential adopter units. The three datasets reviewed in Chapter 10 are publicly available but are less than perfect for testing diffusion hypotheses. New data that trace the diffusion of an idea or a practice through multiple communities complemented with social network data on who talks to whom or who is connected to whom is desperately needed to test diffusion models. Examples might be diffusion of a new process, procedure, or idea in organizations or branches of an organization or adoption of policies or programs among teachers, administrators, or managers.

One potentially fruitful source of diffusion data is switching the unit of analysis to states or nations and studying the adoption of policies. Data were obtained on when countries ratified the framework convention for tobacco control (FCTC) and showed that diffusion of this legislation occurred over a 5-year period. Approximately 82.9% of 193 countries ratified the FCTC from May 2003 to December 2008. Network data were derived from registrations to GlobaLink, an electronic list service created for individuals to share information about the FCTC. The analysis showed that membership in GlobaLink was associated with ratification of the FCTC (Wipfli et al., in press).

Much of the current work on diffusion consists of computer simulations or experiments using computer communications. These studies are extremely valuable for building theory and models to understand diffusion. Often they lack individual attributes and behaviors that can be used to more fully understand the behavior change process and test theories explicitly. Further, simulations are valuable to the extent they can mimic real-world issues and the assumptions are calibrated to empirical data. Thus, empirical data are urgently needed to build better agent-based models.

It may be that new diffusion data will become available within the course of research and application of network interventions. Building school- and community-based behavioral change programs that explicitly incorporate the power of social networks is a promising area of research and practice. Moreover, many groups are using network techniques to do community outreach and recruit community members into studies or interventions. Such interventions provide the opportunity to collect network data within the context of administering interventions that have the potential to improve individual and community health.

Finally, there will continue to be research opportunities using ERGM to understand social network properties, dynamics, and behavioral processes within networks. The software and estimation theory for estimating network influence and selection (as well as many other theoretical processes) using stochastic Markov Chain Monte Carlo methods (MCMC) is becoming more widely available so that researchers with appropriate data can now test network hypotheses in ways not previously available. Tests comparing selection and influence as explanations for diffusion effects can be conducted as well as investigations designed to test for behavioral homophily (Boulay & Valente, 2005).

In sum, there are many different future directions for research using social network analysis approaches. The avenues include methodological inquiries on how best to collect network data, algorithms to process it, or how behaviors spread or are spread within it. The increased availability of appropriate computational and statistical tools has meant that researchers are now only limited by their imaginations and perseverance.

The network field took 70 years to become an overnight success. The field has embraced a vision in which many behavioral phenomena can be explained by network techniques. Phenomena as varied as power grids to earthworms have been shown to have similar network configurations (Watts & Strogatz, 1998), yet clearly these are different beings. What does it mean to have a similar architecture yet to be so different? Recent research on the contagiousness of chronic conditions such as obesity (Christakis & Fowler, 2007) and smoking (Christakis & Fowler, 2008) suggests that social network influences are ubiquitous but may be controversial to specify. It is facile to say "more research is needed," but clearly when it comes to network effects, we are just beginning to understand how they influence behavior.

How to Get Started

The intrepid reader may now wonder: How can one get started doing this work? Appendix E contains print versions of two small files that can be copied and read into UCINET. (These may also be accessed on the author's website.) The first is the node list for the network in Figure 1–1, and one can use UCINET to calculate the many network indicators discussed in this book to learn how to do network analysis. The second is an example of an attribute file that can be attached to this network. This second file is included so the reader knows how to construct an attribute file with his or her own data. These small sample datasets can be used to understand and explore network data.

The next step would be to collect some small network data from a group with which the researcher is familiar. Students in my network class often collect data from a club they belong to or a class they teach or are taking. Data are also often collected in small organizations and businesses. The researcher can then enter the data in Excel and make a text file similar to the one in Appendix E. The data can be analyzed and interpreted and reported back to the organization. Perhaps the researcher takes several measures and compares their evolution over time. For more advanced training, researchers can take one of several 1-day or 1-week workshops presented by seasoned network analysts. (Dates of trainings are often posted on the INSNA website at www.insna.org.)

Limitations

Network analysis has its limitations. The sociometric technique is amenable to studies with populations in settings with natural boundaries (organizations, schools, small communities) and lacks some of the strengths of random sample designs. It also tends to quantify, reducing to a number, the complexity of interpersonal communication and relationships (not all ties are the same). Finally, there are issues regarding appropriate statistical tests for nonindependent data as are often used in network studies.

It also seems that network researchers have spent comparatively little time studying what gets transmitted, communicated, or exchanged in the links that connect nodes. Most published network research is conducted using binary indicators for the connections between people with little discussion on what is said or how valued the links might be. More research is clearly needed on why people choose the friends they do and what motivates their communications and exchanges.

One issue many network analysts have wrestled with is whether social network research is a theory or a method applied to different theories (Monge & Contractor, 2003). Although resolution of this issue is unlikely in the near future, it is fair to ask: What is the role of theory in network research? Do networks simply provide a tool to be used to measure concepts suggested by theory or does taking a network perspective change the nature of the theory being investigated? These limitations aside, network analysis offers a promising new area of research to understand the causes, consequences, and implications of social connectedness.

Conclusion

The contributions of network analysis have been delayed for decades because social science disciplines focused on individual attributes (socioeconomic status, ethnicity, gender) as key determinants of behavior. While these factors are certainly important, increasingly it has been recognized that people's social circles and their social capital (or lack thereof) are also key determinants of behavior. The social network approach provides a rigorous yet versatile approach to studying these peer influences.

The social network field has begun to mature as evidenced by this rich body of research findings and its expanded application to intervention design, program monitoring and evaluation, and use as a means to disseminate evidence-based programs. The maturation, however, is not without costs. Increasingly it is difficult for those outside the field to learn the specialized jargon, software, and culture of social network analysis. Nonetheless, the field is open to new discovery and approaches; social network analysts are united by a common method (the focus on relationships rather than attributes) that transcends disciplinary boundaries. The goals of this transdisciplinary perspective are to blend these perspectives and to develop a more complete understanding of the ways systems and people are connected and evolve. To that end, I hope this volume proves valuable to novice and seasoned social network researchers so that behavioral science may increasingly understand the role and function social network influences on behavior.

Appendix A: Glossary

Average path length Average distance connecting nodes in the network (aka characteristic path length)

Bridge Ability of an individual to connect otherwise unconnected individuals or groups (Granovetter, 1973)

Centrality betweenness Degree an individual lies on the shortest path connecting others in the network (Freeman, 1979)

Centrality closeness Degree an individual is near others in the network (Freeman, 1979)

Centrality degree Number of ties an individual sends (out-degree) or receives (in-degree) (Freeman, 1979)

Centrality power Degree an individual can exert control over other members of the network (Bonacich, 1987)

Centralization The extent to which network links are focused on one or few nodes (Freeman, 1979)

Clique Set of individuals who communicate more frequently with one another than with others in the community

Component Set of individuals who are connected with another, but not with others in the community

Connectedness Ability of two individuals to reach one another directly or through intermediaries (Scott, 1991)

Density-personal network Proportion of ties among an individual's nominees (Scott, 1991)

Density-network Proportion of ties in the network (Scott, 1991)

Diameter Length of the longest geodesic path; distance between the two most distally connected nodes in the network

Distance In a network is the number of steps separating nodes

Egocentric Network data collected from respondents about their contacts without interviewing those contacts (Burt, 1983; Marsden, 1987) (Appendix A)

ERGM Exponential random graph models used to test for structural properties of networks such as whether a network has a tendency for transitivity

Flow Measures the capacity of two individuals to transmit information to one another through all paths in the network (Freeman, Borgatti, & White, 1991)

Geodesic Shortest path between two people (Harary, Norman, & Cartwright, 1965)

INSNA International Network for Social Network Analysis (INSNA), the professional association for network analysts (see www.insna.org)

Matrix Array of rows and columns used to store network links. Usually a matrix is referred to as a letter and the number of rows and columns are subscripted. Each element in the matrix is given by its row and column number (Namboodori, 1983)

Multinet Computer program for testing co-evolution of networks and attributes

Name generator The specific network question asked in a survey to generate the network

Network exposure Percentage in an individual's personal network who have some property (Valente, 1995); for example, the percentage of friends who use the Internet

Network Set of relations between members of a community

Network threshold Proportion of adopters in an individual's personal network necessary for an individual to adopt (Valente, 1995, 1996)

Orgnet Software program used for social network analysis http://www.orgnet.com/

ORA Organizational Risk Analyzer; software used for social network analysis (http://www.casos.cs.cmu.edu/project/ora)

P* Methodology for testing structural properties of a network such as whether there is a tendency for transitivity in the network (Wasserman & Faust, 1994)

Pajek Software program used for social network analysis (http://vlado.fmf.uni-lj.si/pub/networks/pajek/)

R Computer language used to program network measures that is open-source and freely available on the Internet

Reach Ability of one node to contact another node through any number of intermediaries (Wasserman & Faust, 1994)

SIENA Simulation Investigation of Empirical Network Analysis; software platform used to estimate actor-oriented co-evolution models (Snijders, 2005)

Snowball sampling Snowball sampling consist of generating an initial sample of individuals and acquiring from this group a list of names that are then in turn interviewed and the ties of these second step individuals may also be interviewed, and so on

Sociometric Network data collected from the entire community (Wasserman & Faust, 1994)

STATNET Comprehensive network analysis software platform written in R

Structural equivalence Degree to which individuals have similar patterns of network ties in the community (status similarity) (Burt, 1987); sometimes referred to as positional equivalence

Tie Link between nodes

Triad Configuration of links between three nodes

Transitivity Tendency for two nodes linked to the same node to also be linked to each other

Triad census Calculate the percent of triads in a network that fall into 16 unique configurations

UCINET University of California at Irvine (UCI) Network Analysis software; a comprehensive network analysis package so named because the authors were at UCI when they created it

Visualizer Software program used for social network analysis (http://www.mdlogix.com/)

Appendix B: Sample Sociometric Survey

ID Number_____

Who are your five BEST FRIENDS in this class?

Write their names on the lines below starting with your best friend in this class. After you write their name, look at the list of names on the roster that has been provided. Match the name to the number and write the number in the boxes. If you cannot think of five people in this class, then leave the extra lines blank.

For example, your best friend's name may be John Angeles. Then you would write his name and then look up his number, which is 1 2 3 and then write that in the boxes. It is written in as an example below.

	FIRST NAME	LAST NAME	ROSTER NUMBER
	John	*Angeles*	*1 2 3*
1			
2			
3			
4			
5			

Who are the five BEST LEADERS in this class?

Think about the five people in this class who would make the best leaders for
working on group projects. Write up to five names on the lines below, starting
with the best leader on the first line. After you write their name, look at the list
of names on the roster that has been provided. Match the name to the number
and write the number in the boxes. If you cannot think of five names in this
class, then leave the extra lines blank. You can name yourself if you want.

	FIRST NAME	LAST NAME	ROSTER NUMBER
1			
2			
3			
4			
5			

Appendix C: Sample Egocentric Survey

Please provide the first names or initials of up to five people you talk to about important matters.

	Name 1	Name 2	Name 3	Name 4	Name 5
a. How do you know _____?	1. Family 2. Friend 3. Neighbor 4. School mate 5. Other _____	1. Family 2. Friend 3. Neighbor 4. School mate 5. Other _____	1. Family 2. Friend 3. Neighbor 4. School mate 5. Other _____	1. Family 2. Friend 3. Neighbor 4. School mate 5. Other _____	1. Family 2. Friend 3. Neighbor 4. School mate 5. Other _____
b. Does _____ live within 5 miles of your home?	No Yes	No Yes	No Yes	No Yes	No Yes
c. Is _____ male or female?	Male Female	Male Female	Male Female	Male Female	Male Female
d. How long have you known _____?	_____ mos _____ yrs	_____ mos _____ yrs	_____ mos _____ yrs	_____ mos _____ yrs	_____ mos _____ yrs
e. How often do you talk to _____?	1. Daily 2. 1x/week 3. 1x/month 4. 1x/year	1. Daily 2. 1x/week 3. 1x/month 4. 1x/year	1. Daily 2. 1x/week 3. 1x/month 4. 1x/year	1. Daily 2. 1x/week 3. 1x/month 4. 1x/year	1. Daily 2. 1x/week 3. 1x/month 4. 1x/year
f. Does _____ smoke?	No Yes	No Yes	No Yes	No Yes	No Yes
g. What do you usually discuss with _____?	1. Family 2. Politics 3. Neighborhood 4. Work 5. Other _____	1. Family 2. Politics 3. Neighborhood 4. Work 5. Other _____	1. Family 2. Politics 3. Neighborhood 4. Work 5. Other _____	1. Family 2. Politics 3. Neighborhood 4. Work 5. Other _____	1. Family 2. Politics 3. Neighborhood 4. Work 5. Other _____

Appendix D: Centrality Scores for Network in Figure 1–1

ID	1	2	3	4	5	6	7	8	9	10	11	12	13	14	15	16
1	3	4	8.33	11.11	12.00	10.68	33.33	29.66	4.11	4.14	51.39	51.74	9.23	0.73	0.10	14.68
2	5	2	13.89	5.56	2.50	15.25	6.94	42.36	0.64	5.56	7.99	69.44	31.78	2.52	0.20	28.71
3	5	1	13.89	2.78	1.50	14.17	4.17	39.35	0.42	5.42	5.21	67.71	8.31	0.66	0.22	30.45
4	5	4	13.89	11.11	10.58	13.85	29.40	38.47	3.81	5.08	47.57	63.54	19.92	1.58	0.24	33.90
5	5	6	13.89	16.67	15.40	8.33	42.78	23.15	5.81	2.56	72.57	31.94	42.03	3.34	0.05	6.97
6	5	5	13.89	13.89	11.33	10.37	31.48	28.81	3.94	3.58	49.31	44.79	3.56	0.28	0.09	12.14
7	5	11	13.89	30.56	16.00	11.68	44.44	32.44	4.39	4.19	54.86	52.43	163.91	13.01	0.23	32.09
8	5	4	13.89	11.11	12.50	12.75	34.72	35.42	4.19	4.67	52.43	58.33	141.27	11.21	0.16	22.43
9	5	5	13.89	13.89	11.33	10.37	31.48	28.81	3.94	3.58	49.31	44.79	3.56	0.28	0.09	12.14
10	4	8	11.11	22.22	16.73	8.00	46.48	22.22	5.92	2.56	73.96	31.94	15.16	1.20	0.06	7.71
11	5	5	13.89	13.89	11.67	10.37	32.41	28.81	4.00	3.58	50.00	44.79	9.24	0.73	0.12	17.37
12	5	6	13.89	16.67	14.76	8.67	41.01	24.07	5.39	2.61	67.36	32.64	16.55	1.31	0.06	7.87
13	5	6	13.89	16.67	12.83	10.37	35.65	28.81	4.14	3.58	51.74	44.79	12.80	1.02	0.12	17.37
14	5	7	13.89	19.44	15.48	8.25	43.00	22.92	5.47	2.53	68.40	31.60	35.41	2.81	0.03	4.82
15	3	5	8.33	13.89	14.31	6.53	39.76	18.15	5.39	2.31	67.36	28.82	7.71	0.61	0.03	3.76
16	5	6	13.89	16.67	14.81	8.25	41.15	22.92	5.42	2.53	67.71	31.60	39.44	3.13	0.03	4.21
17	5	8	13.89	22.22	13.50	13.52	37.50	37.55	4.14	5.03	51.74	62.85	93.88	7.45	0.29	40.84

(Continued)

ID	1	2	3	4	5	6	7	8	9	10	11	12	13	14	15	16
18	5	1	13.89	2.78	1.50	13.25	4.17	36.81	0.42	4.86	5.21	60.76	4.33	0.34	0.18	25.42
19	5	3	13.89	8.33	10.25	13.52	28.47	37.55	3.81	5.03	47.57	62.85	2.08	0.17	0.22	31.74
20	5	1	13.89	2.78	1.00	13.98	2.78	38.84	0.22	5.39	2.78	67.36	1.75	0.14	0.21	29.45
21	5	11	13.89	30.56	15.17	13.52	42.13	37.55	4.25	5.03	53.13	62.85	101.13	8.03	0.36	50.42
22	5	4	13.89	11.11	13.73	8.83	38.14	24.54	5.36	2.64	67.01	32.99	33.83	2.69	0.04	5.13
23	4	1	11.11	2.78	1.00	14.73	2.78	40.93	0.22	5.56	2.78	69.44	8.34	0.66	0.13	18.82
24	5	6	13.89	16.67	13.39	8.25	37.21	22.92	4.78	2.53	59.72	31.60	10.95	0.87	0.03	4.72
25	5	2	13.89	5.56	10.84	8.67	30.12	24.07	4.53	2.61	56.60	32.64	12.93	1.03	0.03	3.82
26	5	2	13.89	5.56	12.27	7.83	34.07	21.76	5.42	2.44	67.71	30.56	20.82	1.65	0.06	8.07
27	5	7	13.89	19.44	12.42	14.92	34.49	41.44	3.94	5.39	49.31	67.36	293.42	23.29	0.31	44.46
28	5	6	13.89	16.67	15.57	8.50	43.24	23.61	5.83	2.58	72.92	32.29	14.59	1.16	0.05	7.21
29	5	6	13.89	16.67	16.92	8.50	46.99	23.61	6.28	2.58	78.47	32.29	250.44	19.88	0.09	11.99
30	5	8	13.89	22.22	12.92	13.52	35.88	37.55	3.97	5.03	49.65	62.85	22.32	1.77	0.30	42.97
31	5	7	13.89	19.44	16.40	8.83	45.56	24.54	5.92	2.64	73.96	32.99	141.83	11.26	0.05	7.65
32	5	7	13.89	19.44	12.83	12.00	35.65	33.33	4.08	4.53	51.04	56.60	29.63	2.35	0.21	30.26
33	5	6	13.89	16.67	11.92	13.52	33.10	37.55	3.92	5.03	48.96	62.85	16.63	1.32	0.26	36.13
34	5	4	13.89	11.11	9.67	10.37	26.85	28.81	3.67	3.58	45.83	44.79	0.00	0.00	0.09	12.14
35	5	0	13.89	0.00	0.00	16.75	0.00	46.53	0.00	6.36	0.00	79.51	0.00	0.00	0.16	22.42
36	5	0	13.89	0.00	0.00	9.17	0.00	25.46	0.00	2.81	0.00	35.07	0.00	0.00	0.03	4.32
37	5	4	13.89	11.11	13.28	8.25	36.88	22.92	4.92	2.53	61.46	31.60	38.21	3.03	0.05	6.84

Key: 1. Out Degree, 2. In Degree, 3. Out Degree Normalized, 4. In Degree Normalized, 5. In Closeness, 6. Out Closeness, 7. In Closeness Normalized, 8. Out Closeness Normalized, 9. Integration, 10. Radiality, 11. Integration Normalized, 12. Radiality Normalized, 13. Betweenness, 14. Betweenness Normalized, 15. Eigenvector, 16. Eigenvector Normalized

Appendix E: Input Files (Network and Attribute) for the Network in Figure 1–1

```
dl n = 37 format = nodelist
labels:
 1   2   3   4   5   6   7   8   9  10
11  12  13  14  15  16  17  18  19  20
21  22  23  24  25  26  27  28  29  30
31  32  33  34  35  36  37

data:
 1   8  32   7
 2  32  21  30  37   7
 3   2  17  21  30  33
 4  19  17  27  21   7
 5  28  29  12  22  10
 6   9  11  34  13   7
 7  13   9   6   8   1
 8   1   7  32  21  17
 9   6   7  11  13  34
10  28  29   5  31
```

```
11   34    9    6    7   13
12   22   28   10   31   29
13    7    6    9   11   34
14   24   16   15   25   31
15   16   24   14
16   15   24   14   37   25
17   33   30   27    8    4
18    7   21    1   17    4
19   32   30   33   21   27
20   17   21   30    4    3
21   30   32   19   33   27
22   12   37   31   14    5
23   17   18   27   26
24   14   15   16   37   31
25   10   14   28   16   24
26   29    5   28   12   10
27    4   13    7   11   29
28    5   10   12   29   31
29   26    5   10   31   28
30   21   33   32   19   27
31   10   15   12   16   14
32   30   21   33    8    1
33   17   21   30   32   27
34   11    9    6    7   13
35   17    2   23   21   20
36   10    5   24   22   12
37   16   14   15   22   24
```

```
Dl  nr = 37  nc = 1
row  labels  embedded
col  labels:
sex

data:
 1   0
 2   0
 3   1
 4   1
 5   2
 6   1
 7   1
 8   1
 9   1
10   2
11   1
12   2
13   1
14   2
15   2
16   2
17   1
18   1
19   1
20   1
21   1
22   0
23   0
24   2
25   2
26   2
27   1
28   2
29   2
30   1
31   2
32   1
33   1
34   1
35   1
36   2
37   2
```

References

Albrecht, T. L., & Adelman, M. B. (1987). *Communicating social support*. Newbury Park, CA: Sage.

Alexander, C., Piazza, M., Mekos, D., & Valente, T. W. (2001). Peer networks and adolescent cigarette smoking: An analysis of the national longitudinal study of adolescent health. *Journal of Adolescent Health, 29*, 22-30.

Allison, P. D. (1984). *Event history analysis*. Newberry Park, CA: Sage.

Aloise-Young, P., Graham, J. W., & Hansen, W. B. (1994). Peer influence on smoking initiation during early adolescence: A comparison of group members and group outsiders. *Journal of Applied Psychology, 79*, 281-287.

Amirkhanian, Y. A., Kelly, J. A., Kabakchieva, E., Kirsanova, A. V., Vassileva, S., Takacs, J., DiFranceisco, W. J., McAuliffe, T. L., Khoursine, R. A., & Mocsonaki, L. (2005). A randomized social network HIV prevention trial with young men who have sex with men in Russia and Bulgaria. *AIDS, 19*, 1897-1905.

Anderson, C. J., Wasserman, S., & Crouch, B. (1999). A P* primer: Logit models for social networks. *Social Networks, 21*, 37-66.

Anderson, R. M., & May, R. M. (1991). *Infectious diseases of humans: Dynamics and control*. New York, NY: Oxford University Press.

Aral, S. O., Hughes, J. P., Stoner, B., Whittington, W., Handsfield, H. H., Anderson, R. M., & Holmes, K. K. (1999). Sexual mixing patterns in the spread of gonococcal and chlamydial infections. *American Journal of Public Health, 89*, 825-833.

Asch, S. E. (1956). Studies of independence and conformity: A minority of one against a unanimous majority. *Psychological Monographs, 70*(9), whole no. 416.

Bailey, N. T. J. (1975). *The mathematical theory of infectious diseases and its applications*. London, UK: Charles Griffen.

Bak, P. (1996). *How nature works: Science of self-organised criticality.* New York, NY: Copernicus Press.

Bandura, A. (1986). *Social foundations of thought and action: A social cognitive theory.* Upper Saddle River, NJ: Prentice Hall.

Banks, D. L., & Carley, K. M. (1997). Models of network evolution. In P. Doreian & F. Stokman (Eds.). *Evolutions of Social Networks.* New York, NY: Routledge.

Barabási, A.-L. (2003). *Linked: The new science of networks.* Cambridge, MA: Perseus.

Barrera, M., Jr. (1986). Distinctions between social support concepts, measures, and models. *American Journal of Community Psychology, 14,* 413-416.

Barrera, M., & Ainlay, S. L. (1983). The structure of social support: A conceptual and empirical analysis. *Journal of Community Psychology, 11,* 133-143.

Bass, F. M. (1969). A new product growth model for consumer durables. *Management Science, 15,* 215-227.

Bauman, K. E., & Ennett, S. T. (1994). Peer influence on adolescent drug use. *American Psychologist, 49,* 820-822.

Bauman, K. E., Faris, R., Ennett, S. T., Hussong, A., & Foshee, V. A. (2007). Adding valued data to social network measures: Does it add to associations with adolescent substance use? *Social Networks, 29,* 1-10.

Beal, G. M., & Bohlen, J. M. (1955). *How farm people accept new ideas.* Ames, IA: Cooperative Extension Service Report 15.

Bearman, P. S., & Moody, J. (2004**).** Suicide and friendships among American adolescents. *American Journal of Public Health, 94,* 89-95.

Bearman, P. S., Moody, J., & Stovel, K. (2004). Chains of affection: The structure of adolescent romantic and sexual networks. *American Journal of Sociology, 110,* 44-91.

Becker, M. H. (1970). Sociometric location and innovativeness: Reformulation and extension of the diffusion model. *American Sociological Review, 35,* 267-282.

Beniger, J. R. (1983). *Trafficking in drug users: Professional exchange networks in the control of deviance.* Cambridge UK: Cambridge University Press.

Berkman, L. F., & Syme, S. L. (1979). Social networks, host resistance, and mortality: A nine-year follow-up study of Alameda County residents. *American Journal of Epidemiology, 109,* 186-204.

Bernard, H. R., Killworth, P., Kronenfeld, D., & Sailer, L. (1984). The problem of informant accuracy: The validity of retrospective data. *Annual Review of Anthropology, 13,* 495-517.

Bernard, H. R., Killworth, P. D., McCarty, C., & Shelley, G. A. (1990). Comparing four different methods for measuring personal social networks. *Social Networks, 12,* 179-215.

Bernard, H. R., Shelly, G. A., & Killworth, P. (1987). How much of a network does the GSS and RSW dredge up? *Social Networks, 9,* 49-61.

Bertrand, J.T. (2004). Diffusion of innovations and HIV/AIDS. *Journal of Health Communicatio*n, *9,* 113-121.

Bettinger, J. A., Adler, N. E., Curriero, F. C., & Ellen, J. E. (2004). Risk perceptions, condom use, and sexually transmitted diseases among adolescent females according to social network position. *Sexually Transmitted Diseases, 31,* 575-579.

Bhatia, S., Mosley, W. H., Faruque, A. S. G., & Chakraborty, J. (1980). The matlab family planning-health services project. *Studies in Family Planning, 11,* 202-212.

Bloor, M., Frankland, J., Langdon, N. P., et al. (1999). A controlled evaluation of an intensive, peer-led, schools-based, anti-smoking programme. *Health Education Journal, 58,* 17-25.

Blythe, J., McGrath, C., & Krackhardt, D. (1996). The effect of graph layout on inference from social network data. *Graph Drawing, 1027*, 40-51.

Bogue, D. J. (1967). *Sociological contributions to family planning research*. Chicago, IL: University of Chicago.

Boissevain, J. (1974). *Friends of friends: Networks, manipulators and coalitions*. Oxford, UK: Blackwell.

Bonacich, P. (1987). Power and centrality: A family of measures. *American Journal of Sociology, 92*, 1170-1182.

Bonacich, P. (1972). Technique for analyzing overlapping memberships. *Sociological Methodology, 4*, 176-185.

Bonacich, P. (2004). The invasion of the physicists. *Social Networks, 26*, 285-288.

Boorman, S. A., & White, H. C. (1976). Social structure from multiple networks. II. Role structures. *American Journal of Sociology, 81*, 1384-1446.

Borgatti, S. P. (2002). *NetDraw: Graph visualization software*. Harvard, MA: Analytic Technologies.

Borgatti, S. (2006). Identifying key players in a social network. *Computational and Mathematical Organization Theory, 12*, 21-34.

Borgatti, S. P., Carley, K., & Krackhardt, D. 2006. Robustness of centrality measures under conditions of imperfect data. *Social Networks 28*, 124-136.

Borgatti, S. P., & Everett, M. G. (1997). Network analysis of 2-mode data. *Social Networks, 19*, 243-269.

Borgatti, S. P., & Everett, M. G. (1999). Models of core/periphery structures. *Social Networks, 21*, 375-395.

Borgatti, S. P., & Everett, M. G. (2006). A graph-theoretic perspective on centrality. *Social Networks, 28*, 466-484.

Borgatti, S. P., Everett, M. G., & Freeman, L. C. (2006). *UCINET VI for Windows: Software for social network analysis*, Lexington, KY: Analytic Technologies.

Borgatti, S. P., Jones, C., & Everett, M. G. (1998). Network measures of social capital. *Connections, 21*(2), 27-36.

Borgatti, S. P., Mehra, A., Brass, D. J., & Labianca, G. (2009). Network analysis in the social sciences. *Science, 323*, 892-895.

Botvin, G. J., Baker, E., Botvin, E. M., Dusenbury, L., Cardwell, J., & Diaz, T. (1993). Factors promoting cigarette smoking among black youth: A causal modeling approach. *Addictive Behaviors, 18*, 397-405.

Boulay, M., & Valente, T. W. (2005). The selection of family planning discussion partners in Nepal. *Journal of Health Communication, 10*, 519-536.

Brandes, U., & Erlebach, T. (2005). *Network analysis: Methodological foundations*. Berlin, Germany: Springer.

Breiger, R. (1974). The duality of persons and groups. *Social Forces, 53*, 181-190.

Broadhead, R. S., Hechathorn, D. D., Weakliem, D. L., Anthony, D. L., Madray, H., Mills, R. J., & Hughes, J. (1998). Harnessing peer networks as an instrument for raids prevention: Results from a peer-driven intervention. *Public Health Reports, 113*(S1), 42-57.

Buller, D., Buller, M. K., Larkey, L., Sennott-Miller, L., Taren, D., Aickin, M., Wentzel, T. M., & Morrill, C. (2000). Implementing a 5-a-day peer health educator program for public sector labor and trades employees. *Health Education & Behavior, 27*, 232-240.

Buller, D. B., Morrill, C., Taren, D., Aickin, M., Sennott-Miller, L., Buller, M. K., Larkey, L., Alatorre, C., & Wentzel, T. M. (1999). Randomized trial testing the effect of a peer education at increasing fruit and vegetable intake. *Journal of the National Cancer Institute, 91,* 1491-1500.

Brown, L. (1981). *Innovation diffusion: A new perspective.* New York, NY: Methuen.

Burk, W. J., Steglich, C. E. G., & Snijders, T. A. B. (2007). Beyond dyadic interdependence: Actor-oriented models for co-evolving social networks and individual behaviors. *International Journal of Behavioral Development, 31,* 397-404.

Burt, R. (1984). Network items and the general social survey. *Social Networks, 6,* 293-339.

Burt, R. (1987). Social contagion and innovation: Cohesion versus structural equivalence. *American Journal of Sociology, 92,* 1287-1335.

Burt, R. S. (1980). Models of network structure. *Annual Review of Sociology, 6,* 79-141.

Burt, R. S. (1992). *Structural holes: The social structure of competition.* Boston, MA: Harvard University Press.

Burt, R. S. (2005). *Brokerage and closure: An introduction to social capital.* New York, NY: Oxford University Press.

Burt, R. S., & Minor, M. J. (1983). *Applied network analysis: A methodological approach.* Thousand Oaks, CA: Sage.

Cairns, R. B., Cairns, B. D., Neckerman, H. J., Gest, S. D., & Gariépy, J. L. (1988). Social networks and aggressive behavior: Peer support or peer rejection? *Developmental Psychology, 24,* 815-823.

Campbell, K. E., & Lee, B. A. (1991). Name generators in surveys of personal networks. *Social Networks, 13,* 203-221.

Carrington, P. J., Scott, J., & Wasserman, S. (2005): *Models and methods in social network analysis.* Boston, MA: Cambridge University Press.

Cassel, J. (1976). The contribution of the social environment to host resistance, *American Journal of Epidemiology, 104,* 107-123.

Christakis, N. A., & Fowler, J. H. (2007). The spread of obesity in a large social network over 32 years. *The New England Journal of Medicine, 357,* 370-379.

Christakis, N. A., & Fowler, J. H. (2008). The collective dynamics of smoking in a large social network. *The New England Journal of Medicine, 358,* 2249-2258.

Christakis, N. A. & Fowler, J. H. (2009). *Connected: The surprising power of our social networks and how they shape our lives.* New York: Little Brown and Company.

Clark-Lempers, D. S., Lempers, J. D., & Ho, C. (1991). Early, middle, and late adolescents' perceptions of their relationships with significant others. *Journal of Adolescent Research, 6,* 296-315.

Cohen, S., & Syme, S. L. (1985). Issues in the study and application of social support. In S. Cohen & S.L. Symes (Eds.) *Social support and health.* San Francisco, CA: Academic Press.

Coleman, J. S. (1990). *Foundations of social theory.* Boston, MA: Harvard University Press.

Coleman, J. S., Katz, E., & Menzel, H. (1966). *Medical innovation: A diffusion study.* New York, NY: Bobbs Merrill.

Coleman, J. S., Menzel, H., & Katz, E. (1957). The diffusion of an innovation among physicians. *Sociometry, 20,* 253-270.

Cornwell, B. (2005). A complement-derived centrality index for disconnected graphs. *Connections, 26,* 70-81.

Coromina, L., & Coender, G. (2006). Reliability and validity of egocentered network data collected via Web: A meta-analysis of multilevel multitrait multimethod studies. *Social Networks, 28,* 209-231.

Costenbader, E., & Valente T.W. (2003). The stability of centrality measures when networks are sampled. *Social Networks, 25,* 283-307.

Crabb, A. R. (1947). *The hybrid-corn makers: Prophets of plenty.* New Brunswick, NJ: Rutgers University Press.

Crane, D. (1972). *Invisible colleges: Diffusion of knowledge in scientific communities.* Chicago, IL: University of Chicago Press.

Cross, R., & Parker, A. (2004). *The hidden power of social networks: Understanding how work really gets done in organizations.* Cambridge, MA: Harvard Business School Press.

Cutrona, C. E., & Suhr, J. A. (1992). Controllability of stressful events and satisfaction with spouse support behaviors. *Communication Research, 19,* 154-174.

Davis, A., Gardner, B. B., & Gardner, M. R. (1941). *Deep South: A social anthropological study of caste and class.* Chicago, IL: The University of Chicago Press.

Degenne, A., & Forsé, M. (1999). *Introducing social networks* (translated by A. Borges). Thousand Oaks, CA: Sage.

de Nooy, W., Mrvar, A., & Batagelj, V. (2005). *Exploratory social network analysis with Pajek.* New York, NY: Cambridge University Press.

Diani, M., & McAdam, D. (Eds.). (2003). *Social movements and networks: Relational approaches to collective action.* New York, NY: Oxford University Press.

Dishion, T. J., McCord, J., & Poulin, F. (1999). When interventions harm: Peer groups and problem behavior. *American Psychologist, 54,* 755-764.

Dodge, K. A., Lansford, J. E., & Dishion, T. J. (2007). *Deviant peer influences in programs for youth.* New York, NY: Guilford Press.

Donato, F., Monarca, S., Chiesa, R., et al. (1994). Smoking among high school students in 10 Italian towns: Patterns and covariates. *International Journal of the Addictions, 29,* 1537-1557.

Donohew, L., Clayton, R. R., Skinner, W. F., & Colon, S. (1999). Peer networks and sensation seeking: Some implications for primary socialization theory, *Substance Use and Misuse, 34,* 1013-1023.

Doreian, P., Batagelj, V., & Ferligoj, A. (2005). *Generalized blockmodeling.* New York, NY: Cambridge University Press.

Doreian, P., & Stokman, F. (Eds.) (1997). *Evolutions of social networks.* New York, NY: Routledge.

Dunbar, R. I. M. (1992). *Neocortex size as a constraint on group size in primates. Journal of Human Evolution, 22,* 469-493.

Dunbar, R. I. M. (1993). Co-evolution of neocortex size, group size, and language in humans. *Behavioral and Brain Sciences, 16,* 681-735.

Dunphy, D. C. (1963). The social structure of urban adolescent peer groups. *Sociometry, 26,* 230-246.

Dutton, W. H., Rogers, E. M., & Jun, S. (1987). Diffusion and social impacts of personal computers. *Communication Research, 14,* 219-250.

Ellen, J., Brown, B., Chung, S., et al. (2005). Impact of sexual networks on risk for gonorrhea and Chlamydia among low-income urban African American adolescents. *Journal of Pediatrics, 146,* 518-522.

Engels, R. C. M. E., Knibbe, R. A., Drop, M. J., & de Haan, Y.T. (1997). Homogeneity of cigarette smoking within peer groups: Influence or selection? *Health Education & Behavior, 24,* 801-811.

Ennett, S. T., & Bauman, K. E. (1993). Peer group structure and adolescent cigarette smoking: A social network analysis. *Journal of Health and Social Behavior, 34,* 226-236.

Ennett, S. T., & Bauman, K. E. (1994). The contribution of influence and selection to adolescent peer group homogeneity: The case of adolescent cigarette smoking. *Journal of Personality and Social Psychology, 67,* 653-663.

Ennett, S. T., Bauman, K. E., Hussong, A., et al. (2006). The peer context of adolescent substance use: Findings from social network analysis. *Journal of Research on Adolescence, 16*(2), 159-186.

Ennett, S. T., Faris, R., Hipp, J., Foshee, V. A., Bauman, K. E., Hussong, A. & Cai, L. (2008). Peer smoking, other peer attributes, and adolescent cigarette smoking: A social network analysis, *Prevention Science, 9*, 88-98.

Entwisle, B., Rindfuss, R. D., Guilkey, D. K., Chamratrithirong, A., Curran, S. R., & Sawangdee, Y. (1996). Community and contraceptive choice in rural Thailand: A case study of Nang Rong. *Demography, 33*, 1-11.

Epstein, J. M. (2006). *Generative social science*. Princeton, NJ: Princeton University Press.

Faust, K. (2008). Triadic configurations in limited choice sociometric networks: Empirical and theoretical results. *Social Networks, 30*, 273-282.

Feiring, C., & Lewis, M. (1991). The transition from middle-childhood to early adolescence: Sex differences in the social network and perceived self-competence. *Sex Roles, 24*, 489-509.

Fernandez, R. M., & Gould, R. V. (1994). A dilemma of state power: Brokerage and influence in the national health policy domain. *American Journal of Sociology, 99*, 1455-1491.

Festinger, L. (1954). A theory of social comparison processes. *Human Relations, 7*, 117-140.

Fishbein, M., & Ajzen, I. (1981). On construct validity: A critique of Miniard and Cohen's paper. *Journal of Experimental Social Psychology, 17*, 340-350.

Fisher, L. A., Bauman, K. E. (1988). Influence and selection in the friend-adolescent relationship: Findings from studies of adolescent smoking and drinking. *Journal of Applied Social Psychology, 18*, 289-314.

Fisher, J. (1988). Possible effects of reference group-based social influence on AIDS-risk behavior and AIDS prevention. *American Psychologist, 43*, 914-920.

Flay, B. R., Hu, F. B., Siddiqui, O., et al. (1994). Differential influence of parental smoking and friends' smoking on adolescent initiation and escalation of smoking. *Journal of Health & Social Behavior, 35*, 248-265.

Freeman, L. (1979). Centrality in social networks: Conceptual clarification. *Social Networks, 1*, 215-239.

Freeman, L. (2000). Visualizing social networks. *Journal of Social Structure, 1*(1), February 4, 2000. www.cmu.edu/joss.

Freeman, L. (2004). *The development of social network analysis: A study in the sociology of science*. Vancouver, BC, Canada: Empirical Press.

Freeman, L. C., Borgatti, S. P., & White, D. R. (1991). Centrality in valued graphs: A measure of betweenness based on network flow. *Social Networks, 13*, 141-154.

Friedkin, N. E. (1998). *A structural theory of social influence*. New York, NY: Cambridge University Press.

Friedman, S. R., Flom, P. L., Kottiri, B. J., Neaigus, A., Sandoval, M., Curtis, R., des Jarlais, D. C., & Zenilman, J. M. (2001). Consistent condom use in the heterosexual relationships of young adults who live in a high-HIV risk neighborhood and do not use 'hard drugs'. *AIDS Care, 13*, 285-296.

Friedman, S. R., Jose, B., Deren, S., Des Jarlais, D. C., & Neaigus, A. (1995). Risk factors for HIV seroconversion among out-of-treatment drug injectors in high- and low-seroprevalence cities. *American Journal of Epidemiology, 142*, 864-874.

Friedman, S. R., Neaigus, A., Jose, B., Curtis, R., Goldstein, M., Ildefonso, G., Rothenberg, R. G., & Des Jarlais, D. C. (1997). Sociometric risk networks and risk for HIV infection. *American Journal of Public Health, 87*, 1289-1296.

Fujimoto, K., Pentz, M. P., & Valente, T. W. (in press). Network structural influences on the adoption of evidenced-based prevention in communities. *Journal of Community Psychology*.

Galaskiewicz, J. (1985). Interorganizational relations. *Annual Review of Sociology, 11,* 281-304.

Gavin, L. A., & Furman, W. (1989). Age differences in adolescents' perceptions of their peer groups. *Developmental Psychology, 25,* 827-834.

Gilmore, J. B. (1998). *In cold pursuit: Medical intelligence investigates the common cold.* New York, NY: Stoddart Publishing.

Girvan, M., & Newman, M. E. J., (2002). Community structure in social and biological networks. *Proceedings of the National Academy of Science, 99*(12), 7821-7826v.

Gladwell, M. (2000). *The tipping point: How little things can make a big difference.* New York, NY: Little, Brown and Company.

Glanz, K., Rimer, B. K., & Lewis, F. M. (Eds.). (2002). *Health behavior and health education: Theory, research, and practice,* 3rd ed. San Francisco, CA: Jossey-Bass.

Goodman, L. A. (1961). Snowball sampling. *Annals of Mathematical Statistics, 32,* 148-170.

Gottlieb, B. H. (1985). Social support and the study of personal relationships. *Journal of Social and Personal Relationships, 2,* 351-375.

Granovetter, M. (1973). The strength of weak ties. *American Journal of Sociology, 78,* 1360-1380.

Granovetter, M. (1974). *Getting a job: A study of contacts and careers.* Cambridge, MA: Harvard University Press.

Granovetter, M. (1978). Threshold models of collective behavior. *American Journal of Sociology, 83,* 1420-1443.

Gross, C. P., Cruz-Correa, M., Canto, M. I., McNeil-Solis, C., Valente, T. W., & Powe, N. R. (2002). The adoption of ablation therapy for Barrett's esophagus: A cohort study of gastroenterologists. *American Journal of Gastroenterology, 97,* 279-286.

Hägerstrand, T. (1967). *Innovation diffusion as a spatial process* (translated by A. Pred). Chicago, IL: University of Chicago Press.

Harary, F., Norman, R., & Cartwright, D. (1965). *Structural models: An introduction to the theory of directed graphs.* New York, NY: Wiley.

Hall, J., & Valente, T.W. (2007). Adolescent smoking networks: The effects of influence and selection on future smoking. *Addictive Behaviors, 32,* 3054-3059.

Hamblin, R. L., Jacobsen, R. B., & Miller, J. L. L. (1973). *A mathematical theory of social change.* New York, NY: John Wiley & Sons.

Hammer, M. (1983). 'Core' and 'extended' *social* networks in relation to health and illness. *Social Science and Medicine, 17,* 405-411.

Harary, F., Norman, R., & Cartwright, D. (1966). *Structural models: An introduction to the theory of directed graphs.* New York, NY: Wiley.

Harrigan, N. (2009). *Exponential random graph (ERG) models and their application to the study of corporate elites. Center for research methods in the social sciences.* Department of Politics and International Relations, University of Oxford.

Harris, J. K., Luke, D. A., Burke, R. C., & Mueller, N. B. (2008). Seeing the forest and the trees: Using network analysis to develop an organizational blueprint of state tobacco control systems. *Social Science & Medicine, 67,* 1669-1678.

Harris, J. K., Luke, D. A., Zuckerman, R. B., & Shelton, S. C. (2009). Forty years of secondhand smoke research: The gap between discovery and delivery. *American Journal of Preventive Medicine, 36,* 538-548.

Havanon, N., Bennett, A., & Knodel, J. (1993). Sexual networking in provincial Thailand. *Studies in Family Planning, 24*, 1-17.

Heckathorn, D. (1997). Respondent-driven sampling: A new approach to the study of hidden populations. *Social Problems, 44*, 174-199.

Heckathorn, D. (2002). Respondent-driven sampling, II: Deriving valid population estimates from chain-referral samples of hidden populations. *Social Problems, 49*, 11-34.

Heider, F. (1958). *The psychology of interpersonal relations.* New York, NY: John Wiley & Sons.

Hoffman, B., Sussman, S., Rohrbach, L., & Valente, T. W. (2006). Peer influence on adolescent smoking: A theoretical review of the literature. *Substance Use & Misuse, 41*, 103-155.

Hoffman, B. R., Monge, P., Chou, C. P., & Valente, T. W. (2007). The roles of perceived peer influence and peer selection on adolescent smoking. *Addictive Behaviors, 32*, 1546-1554.

Holland, P. W., & Leinhardt, S. (1979). *Perspectives on social network research.* New York, NY: Academic Press.

House, J. S. (1981). *Work stress and social support.* Reading, MA: Addison-Wesley.

Huisman, M., & van Duijn, M. A. J. (2005). Software for social network analysis. In P. J. Carrington, J. Scott, & S. Wasserman (Eds.) *Models and methods in social network analysis* (pp. 270-316). Cambridge, UK: Cambridge University Press.

Hummon, N. B., & Carley, K. (1993). Social networks as normal science. *Social Networks, 15*, 71-106.

Ianotti, R. J., & Bush, P. J. (1992). Perceived vs. actual friends' use of alcohol, cigarettes, marijuana, and cocaine: Which has the most influence? *Journal of Youth and Adolescence, 21*, 375-389.

INSNA (2003). International Network for Social Network Analysis. http://www.insna.org.

Israel, B. A., Eng, E., Schulz, A. J., & Parker, E. A. (Eds.) (2005). *Methods in community-based participatory research for health.* San Francisco, CA: Jossey-Bass.

Jasuja, G. K., Chou, C., Bernstein, K., Wang, E., McClure, M., & Pentz, M. (2005). Using structural characteristics of community coalitions to predict progress in adopting evidence-based prevention programs. *Evaluation and Program Planning, 28*, 173-184.

Jenkins, J. E. (2001). Rural adolescent perceptions of alcohol and other drug resistance. *Child Study Journal, 31*, 211-224.

Jenkins. J. E., & Zunguze, S. T. (1998). The relationship of family structure to adolescent drug use, peer affiliation and perception of peer acceptance of drug use. *Adolescence, 33*, 811-823.

Kandel, D. (1985). On processes of peer influences in adolescent drug use: A developmental perspective. *Advances in Alcohol and Substance Abuse, 4*, 139-163.

Katz, E. (1957). The two-step flow of communication: An up-to-date report on a hypothesis. *Public Opinion Quarterly, 21*, 61-78.

Katz, E. (1962). The social itinerary of technical change: Two studies on the diffusion of innovation. *Human Organization, 20*, 70-82.

Katz, E., Levine, M. L., & Hamilton, H. (1963). Traditions of research on the diffusion of innovation. *American Sociological Review, 28*, 237-253.

Kelly, J. A., Lawrence, J. S., St., Diaz, Y. E., et al. (1991). HIV risk behavior reduction following intervention with key opinion leaders of population: an experimental analysis. *American Journal of Public Health, 81*, 168-171.

Kelner, M., & Wellman, B. (1997). Health care and consumer choice: Medical and alternative. *Social Science & Medicine, 45,* 203-212.

Killeya-Jones, L. A., Nakajima, R., & Costanzo, P. R. (2007). Peer standing and substance use in early-adolescent grade-level networks: A short-term longitudinal study. *Preventive Science, 8,* 11-23.

Killworth, P. D., Johnsen, E. C., Bernard, R. H., et al. (1990). Estimating the size of personal networks. *Social Networks, 12,* 289-312.

Killworth, P. D., McCarty, C., Johnsen, E. C., et al. (2006). Investigating the variation of personal network size under unknown error conditions. *Sociological Methods & Research, 35,* 84-112.

Kirke, D. (2004). Chain reactions in adolescents' cigarette, alcohol, and drug use: Similarity through peer influence or the patterning of ties in peer networks. *Social Networks, 26,* 3-28.

Kirke, D. M. (2005). *Teenagers and substance use: Social networks and peer influence.* New York, NY: Palgrave.

King, C. W., Summers, J. O., & Childers, T. L. (1999). Opinion leadership. In W. O. Bearden, R. G. Netemeyer, & M. F. Mobley (Eds.) *Handbook of marketing scales: Multi item measures for marketing and consumer behavior research* (2nd ed., pp.77-80). Newbury Park, CA: Sage.

Klovdahl, A. S. (1985). Social networks and the spread of infectious diseases: The AIDS example. *Social Science and Medicine, 21,* 1203-1216.

Klovdahl, A. S. (1989). Urban social networks: Some methodological problems and possibilities. In M. Kochen (Ed.) *The small world.* Norwood, NJ: Ablex.

Klovdahl, A. S., Gravis, E. A., Yaganehdoost, A., Ross, M. W., Wanger, A., Adams, G. J., & Musser, J. M. (2001). Networks and tuberculosis: An undetected community outbreak involving public places. *Social Science and Medicine, 52,* 681-694.

Klovdahl, A. S., Potterat, J. J., Woodhouse, D., Muth, S. Q., Muth, J., & Darrow, W. W. (1994). Social networks and infectious disease: The Colorado Springs study. *Social Science and Medicine, 38,* 79-88.

Knoke, D., & Kuklinski, J. H. (1982). *Network analysis.* Thousand Oaks, CA: Sage.

Knoke, D., & Yang, S. (2008). *Network analysis.* Thousand Oaks, CA: Sage.

Knowlton, A. R. (2003). Informal HIV caregiving in a vulnerable population: Toward a network resource framework. *Social Science and Medicine, 56,* 1307-1320.

Koehly, L., Goodreau, S., & Morris, M. (2005). Exponential family models for sampled and census network data. *Sociological Methodology, 34,* 241-270.

Kohler, H. P. (1997). Learning in social networks and contraceptive choice. *Demography, 34,* 369-383.

Koschützki, D., Lehmann, K. A., Peeters, L., Richter, S., Tenfelde-Podehl, D., & Zlotowski., O. (2005). Centrality indices. In U. Brandes & T. Erlebach (Eds.) *Network analysis: Methodological foundations.* Berlin, Germany: Springer-Verlag.

Kossinets, G., & Watts, D. J. (2006). Empirical analysis of an evolving social network. *Science, 311,* 88-90.

Krackhardt, D. (1987). QAP partialling as a test of spuriousness. *Social Networks, 9,* 171-186.

Krackhardt, D. (1988). Predicting with networks: A multiple regression approach to analyzing dyadic data. *Social Networks, 10,* 359-381.

Krackhardt, D. (1992). The strength of strong ties: The importance of philos in organizations. In N. Nohria & R. Eccles (Eds.) *Networks and organizations: Structure, form, and action* (pp. 216-239). Boston, MA: Harvard Business School Press.

Krackhardt, D., & Stern, R. N. (1988). Informal networks and organizational crises: An experimental simulation. *Social Psychology Quarterly, 51*, 123-140.

Krebs, V. E. (2002). Mapping networks of terrorists cells. *Connections, 24*(3), 31-34.

Kretzschmar, M., & Morris, M. (1996). Measures of concurrency in the networks and the spread of infectious disease. *Mathematical Biosciences, 133*, 165-195.

Kwait, J., Valente, T. W., & Celentano, D. D. (2001). Interorganizational relationships among HIV/AIDS service organizations in Baltimore: A network analysis. *Journal of Urban Health, 78*, 468-487.

Latkin, C. (1998). Outreach in natural setting: The use of peer leaders for HIV prevention among injecting drug users' networks. *Public Health Reports, 113*(S1), 151-159.

Latkin, C. A., Donnell, D., Metzger, D., Sherman, S., Aramrattna, A., Davis-Vogel, A., Quan, V. M., Gandham, S., Vongchak, T., Perdue, T., & Celentano, D. D. (2009). The efficacy of a network intervention to reduce HIV risk behaviors among drug users and risk partners in Chiang Mai, Thailand and Philadelphia, USA. *Social Science and Medicine, 68*, 740-748.

Laumann, E., Marsden, P., & Prensky, D. (1983). The boundary specification problem in network analysis. In R. Burt & M. Minor (Eds.) *Applied network analysis.* Newberry Park, CA: Sage.

Lewis, K., Kaufman, J., Gonzalez, M., Wimmer, A., & Christakis, N. A. (2008). Tastes, ties, and time: A new (cultural, multiplex, and longitudinal) social network dataset using Facebook.com. *Social Networks, 30*, 330-342.

Liben-Nowell, D., & Kleinberg, J. (2008). Tracing information flow on a global scale using Internet chain-letter data. *Proceedings of the National Academy of Sciences USA, 105*, 4633-4638.

Lin, N. (2001). *Social capital: A theory of social structure and action.* New York, NY: Cambridge University Press.

Lomas, J., Enkin, M., Anderson, G. M., Hanna, W. J., Vayda, E., & Singer, J. (1991). Opinion leaders vs. audit feedback to implement practice guidelines: Delivery after previous cesarean section. *Journal of American Medical Association, 265*, 2202-2207.

Lorrain, F., & White, H. C. (1971). Structural equivalence of individuals in social networks. *Journal of Mathematical Sociology, 1*, 49-80.

Luce, R. D., & Perry, A. D. (1949). A method of matrix analysis of group structure. Psychometrika, 14, 95-116.

Luke, D. A., & Harris, J. (2007). Network analysis in public health: History, methods, and applications. *Annual Review of Public Health, 28*, 69-93.

Luthar, S. S., & D'Avanzo, K. (1999). Contextual factors in substance use: A study of suburban and inner-city adolescents. *Development and Psychopathology, 11*, 845-867.

MacKinnon, D. P., Johnson, C. A., Pentz, M. A., Dwyer, J. H., Hansen, W. B., Flay, B. R., & Wang, E. Y. (1991). Mediating effects in a school-based drug prevention program: First-year effects of the Midwestern Prevention Project. *Health Psychology, 10*, 164-172.

Mahajan, V., & Peterson, R. A. (1985). *Models of innovation diffusion.* Newbury Park, CA: Sage.

Markus, M. L. (1987). Toward a critical mass theory of interactive media: Universal access, interdependence and diffusion. *Communication Research, 14*, 491-511.

Marsden, P. V. (1987). Core discussion networks of Americans. *American Sociological Review, 52*, 122-131.

Marsden, P. V. (1990). Network data and measurement. *Annual Review of Sociology, 16*, 435-463.

Marsden, P. V. (2005). Recent developments in network measurement. In P. J. Carrington, J. Scott, & S. Wasserman (Eds.) *Models and methods in social network analysis* (pp. 8-30). Cambridge, UK: Cambridge University Press.

Marsden, P. V., & Friedkin, N. E. (1993). Network studies of social influence. *Sociological Methods & Research, 22*, 127-151.

Marsden, P. V., & Lin, N. (1982). *Social structure and network analysis.* Thousand Oaks, CA: Sage.

Marsden, P. V., & Podolny, J. (1990). Dynamic analysis of network diffusion processes. In J. Weesie & H. Flap (Eds.) *Social networks through time.* Utrecht, Netherlands: ISOR.

Marwell, G., Oliver, P., & Prahl, R. (1988). Social networks and collective action: A theory of the critical mass. III. *American Journal of Sociology, 94*, 503-534.

McCarty, C., Bernard, H. R., Killworth, P. D., Shelley, G. A., & Johnson, E. C. (1997). Eliciting representative samples of personal networks. *Social Networks, 19*, 303-323.

McGrath, C., Krackhardt D., & Blythe, J. (2002). Visualizing complexity in networks: Seeing both the forest and the trees. *Connections, 25*(1), 30-34.

McPherson, M., Smith-Lovin, L., & Cook, J. M. (2001). Birds of a feather: Homophily in social networks. *Annual Review of Sociology, 27*, 415-444.

McPherson, M., Smith-Lovin, L., & Brashears. M. (2006). Social isolation in America: Changes in core discussion networks over two decades. *American Sociological Review, 71*, 353-375.

Meijer, R. R., Muijtjens, A. M. M., & van der Vleuten, C. P. M. (1994). Nonparametric person-fit research: Some theoretical issues and an empirical example. *Applied Measurement in Education, 9*, 77-89.

Michell, L., & Amos, A. (1997). Girls, pecking order and smoking. *Social Science Medicine, 44*, 1861-1869.

Milgram, S. (1967). The small world problem. *Psychology Today, 22*, 561-67.

Mizruchi, M. (1982). *The structure of the American corporate network: 1904-1974.* Thesis (Ph.D.), State University of New York at Stony Brook.

Mizruchi, M. (1992). *The structure of corporate political action: Interfirm relations and their consequences.* Cambridge, MA: Harvard University Press.

Monge, P. R., & Contractor, N. S. (2003). *Theories of communication networks.* New York, NY: Oxford University Press.

Montgomery, M. R., & Chung, W. (1999). Social networks and the diffusion of fertility control in the Republic of Korea. In R. Leete (Ed.) *Dynamics of values in fertility change.* Oxford, UK: Oxford University Press.

Moore, K .A., Peters, R. H., Hills, H. A., LeVasseur, J. B., Rich, A. R., Hunt, W. M., Young, M. S., & Valente, T. W. (2004). Characteristics of opinion leaders in substance abuse treatment agencies. *American Journal of Drug and Alcohol Abuse, 30*, 187-203.

Moore, S., Shiell, A., Hawe, P., & Haines, V. A. (2005). The privileging of communitarian Ideas: citation practices and the translation of social capital into public health research, *American Journal of Public Health, 95*, 1330-1337.

Moreno, J. L. (1934). *Who shall survive? A new approach to the problem of human interrelations,* Washington, DC: Nervous and Mental Disease Publishing Co.

Morris, M. (1993). Epidemiology and social networks: Modeling structured diffusion. *Sociological Methods and Research, 22*, 99-126.

Morris, M. (1995). Data driven network models for the spread of disease. In D. Mollison (Ed.) *Epidemic models: Their structure and relation to data* (pp. 302-322). Cambridge, UK: Cambridge University Press.

Morris, M. (Ed.) (2004). *Network epidemiology: A handbook for survey design and data collection*. New York, NY: Oxford University Press.

Morris, M., & Kretzschmar, M. (1997). Sexual networks and HIV. *AIDS, 11*, S209-S216.

Moscovici, S. (1976). *Social influence and social change* (translated by C. Sherrard & G. Heinz). New York, NY: Academic Press.

Murray, D. M. (1998). *Design and analysis of group-randomized trial*. New York, NY: Oxford University Press.

Myers, D. J. (2000). The diffusion of collective violence: Infectiousness, susceptibility, and mass media networks. *American Journal of Sociology, 106*, 173-208.

Namboodori, K. (1983). *Matrix algebra*. Beverly Hills, CA: Sage.

Needle, R. H., Coyle, S. L., Genser, S. G., & Trotter, R. (1995). *Social networks, drug abuse, and HIV transmission*. NIDA research monograph #151, Rockville, MD.

Neaigus, A., Friedman, S. R., Curtis, R., Des Jarlais, D. C., Furst, R. T., Jose, B., Mota, P. Stephenson, B., Sufian, M., Ward, T., & Wright, J. W. (1994). The relevance of drug injectors' social and risk networks for understanding and preventing HIV infection. *Social Science & Medicine, 38*, 67-78.

Neaigus, A., Friedman, S. R., Kottiri, B. J., & Des Jarlais, D. C. (2001). HIV risk networks and HIV transmission among injecting drug users. *Evaluation and Program Planning, 24*, 221-226.

Newman, M., Barabási, A. L., & Watts, D. (2006). *The structure and dynamics of networks*. Princeton, NJ: Princeton University Press.

Newman, M. E. J. (2005). A measure of betweenness centrality based on random walks. *Social Networks, 27*, 39-54.

Newman, M. E. J., & Girvan, M. (2004). Finding and evaluating community structure in networks. *Physics Review, E69*, 1-16.

Nohria, N., & Eccles, R. (Eds.) (1992). *Networks and organizations: Structure, form and action*. Cambridge, MA: Harvard University Press.

Obbo, C. (1993). HIV transmission through social and geographic networks in Uganda. *Social Science and Medicine, 36*, 949-955.

Oh, H., Chung, M., & Labianca, G. (2004). Group social capital and group effectiveness: The role of informal socializing ties. *Academy of Management Journal, 47*, 860-875.

Orth-Gomer, K., & and Unden, AL. (1987). The measurement of social support in population surveys, *Social Science and Medicine, 24*, 83-94.

Palmore, J. A. (1967). The Chicago snowball: A study of the flow and diffusion of family planning information. In D. J. Bogue (Ed.) *Sociological contributions to family planning research* (pp. 272-363). Chicago, IL: University of Chicago.

Park, H. J., Chung, K. K., Han, D. S., & Lee, S. B. (1974). *Mothers' clubs and family planning in Korea*. Seoul, Korea: School of Public Health, Seoul National University.

Pearson, M., & West, P. (2005). Drifting smoke rings: Social network analysis and Markov processes in a longitudinal study of friendship groups and risk-taking. *Connections, 26*(2).

Pennings, J. (1980). *Interlocking directorates*. San Francisco, CA: Jossey-Bass.

Peters, R. H., Moore, K. A., Hills, H. A., Young, M. S., LeVasseur, J. B., Rich, A. R., Hunt, W. M., & Valente, T. W. (2005). Use of opinion leaders and intensive training to implement evidence-based co-occurring disorders treatment in the community. *Journal of Addictive Diseases, 24*(S1), 52-74.

Pierce J. P., Choi, W. S., Gilpin, E. A., Farkas, A. J., & Merritt, R. K. (1996). Validation of susceptibility as a predictor of which adolescents take up smoking in the United States. *Health Psychology*, 15, 355-361.

Pitts, F. R. (1979). The Medieval River trade network of Russia revisited. *Social Networks*, *1*, 285-292.

Pool, I. S., & Kochen, M. (1978). Contacts and influence. *Social Networks*, *1*, 5-51.

Potterat, J. J., Rothenberg, R. B., & Muth, S. Q. (1999). Network structural dynamics and HIV transmission. *International Journal of STD/AIDS*, *10*, 182-185.

Provan, K. G., Nakama, L., Veazie, M. A., Teufel-Shone, N. I., & Huddleston, C. (2003). Building community capacity around chronic disease services through a collaborative interorganizational network. *Health Education and Behavior*, *30*, 646-662.

Putnam, R. D. (2000). *Bowling alone: The collapse and revival of American community*. New York, NY: Simon & Schuster.

Rai, A. A., Stanton, B., Wu, Y., Li, X., Galbraith, J., Cottrell, L., Pack, R., Harris, C., D'Alessandri, D., & Burns, J. (2003). Relative influences of perceived parental monitoring and perceived peer involvement on adolescent risk behaviors: An analysis of six cross-sectional data sets. *Journal of Adolescent Health* 33,108-118.

Rice, R. E. (1982). Communication networking in computer-conferencing systems: A longitudinal study of groups, roles, and system structure. In M. Gurgoon (Ed.) *Communication Yearbook, 9*, 315-339.

Rice, R. E., Borgman, C. L., & Reeves, B. (1988). Citation networks of communication journals, 1977-1985: Cliques and positions, citations made and citations received. *Human Communication Research*, *15*, 256-283.

Rice, R. E., Donohew, L., & Clayton, R. (2003). Peer network, sensation seeking, and drug use among junior and senior high school students. *Connections*, *26*(2), 32-58.

Robertson, T. S. (1971). *Innovative behavior and communication*. New York, NY: Holt, Rinehart and Winston.

Robins, G., & Pattison, P. (2005). Interdependencies and social processes: Dependence graphs and generalized dependence structures. In P. J. Carrington, J. Scott, & S. Wasserman (Eds.) *Models and methods in social network analysis*. Cambridge, UK: Cambridge University Press.

Robins, G., Pattison, P., Kalish, Y., & Lusher, D. (2007). An introduction to exponential random graph (p*) models for social networks. *Social Networks*, *29*, 173-191.

Rogers, E. M. (1962). *Diffusion of innovation*. New York, NY: The Free Press.

Rogers, E. M. (2003). *Diffusion of innovations* (5th ed.). New York, NY: The Free Press.

Rogers, E. M., & Cartano, D. G. (1962). Methods of measuring opinion leadership. *Public Opinion Quarterly*, *26*, 435-441.

Rogers, E. M., & Kincaid, D. L. (1981). *Communication networks: A new paradigm for research*. New York, NY: Free Press.

Rosenfield, A. G., Asavasena, W., & Mikhanorn, J (1973). Person-to-person communication in Thailand. *Studies in Family Planning*, *4*, 145-150.

Rothenberg, R., Sterk, C., Toomey, K. E., Potterat, J. J., Johnson, D., Schrader, M., & Hatch, S. (1998). Using social network and ethnographic tools to evaluate a syphilis transmission. *Sexually Transmitted Diseases*, *25*, 154-160.

Ryan, R., & Gross, N. (1943). The diffusion of hybrid seed corn in two Iowa communities. *Rural Sociology*, *8*, 15-24.

Salganik, M. J., & Heckathorn, D. D. (2004). Sampling and estimation in hidden populations using respondent-driven sampling. *Sociological Methodology*. 34, 193-239.

Sarason, I. G., Levine, H. M., Basham, R. B., & Sarason, B. R. (1983). Assessing social support: The social support questionnaire. *Journal of Personality and Social Psychology*, *44*, 127-139.

Schelling, T. (1978). *Micromotives and macrobehavior.* New York, NY: Norton.

Scott, J. (2000). *Network analysis: A handbook* (2nd Ed.). Newbury Park, CA: Sage.

Seary, A. J., & Richards, W. D. (2003). Spectral methods for analyzing and visualizing networks: An introduction. In R. Breiger, K. Carley, & P. Pattison (Eds.) *Dynamic social network modeling and analysis: Workshop summary and papers* (pp. 209-228). Washington, DC: The National Academics Press.

Shaw, M. E. (1971). *Group dynamics.* New York, NY: McGraw-Hill.

Shrum, W., & Cheek, N. H. (1987). Social structure during the school years: Onset of the degrouping process. *American Sociological Review, 52*, 218-223.

Sieving, R., Perry, C., & Williams, C. (2000). Do friendships change behaviors, or do behaviors change friendships? Examining paths of influence in young adolescents' alcohol use. *Journal of Adolescent Health, 26*, 27-35.

Sikkema, K. J., Kelly, J. A., Winett, R. A., et al. (2000). Outcomes of a randomized community-level HIV prevention intervention for women living in 19 low-income housing developments. *American Journal of Public Health, 90*, 57-63.

Snijders, T. A. (2005). Models for longitudinal data. In P. J. Carrington, J. Scott, & S. Wasserman (Eds.) *Models and methods in social network analysis.* Cambridge, UK: Cambridge University Press.

Snijders, T. A. B. (2001). The statistical evaluation of social network dynamics. *Sociological Methodology, 31*, 361-395.

Snijders, T. A. B., Steglich, C. E. G., Schweinberger, M., & Huisman, M. (2007). *Manual for SIENA, version 3.* Groningen, the Netherlands: University of Groningen.

Snijders, T. A. B., & Baerveldt, C. (2003). A multilevel network study of the effects of delinquent behavior on friendship evolution. *Journal of Mathematical Sociology, 27*, 123-151.

Snijders, T. A. B., van de Bunt, G. G., & Steglich, C. (in press). Introduction to stochastic actor-based models for network dynamics. *Social Networks.*

Soumerai, S. B., McLaughlin, T. J., Gurwitz, J. H., et al. (1998). Effect of local medical opinion leaders on quality of care for acute myocardial infarction: A randomized controlled trial. *Journal of the American Medical Association, 279*, 1358-1363.

Stephenson, K., & Zelen, M. (1989). Rethinking centrality: Methods and applications. *Social Networks, 11*, 1-37.

Stoebenau, K., & Valente, T. W. (2003). The role of network analysis in community-based program evaluation: A case study from Highland Madagascar. *International Family Planning Perspectives, 29*, 167-173.

Strang, D., & Tuma, N. B. (1993). Spatial and temporal heterogeneity in diffusion. *American Journal of Sociology, 99*, 614-639.

Sussman, S., Dent, C. W., Mestel-Rauch, J., Johnson, C. A., Hansen, W. B., & Flay, B. R. (1988). Adolescent nonsmokers, triers, and regular smokers' estimates of cigarette smoking prevalence: When do overestimations occur and by whom? *Journal of Applied Social Psychology, 18*, 537-551.

Sussman, S., Dent, C. W., Stacy, A., Sun, P., Craig, S., Simon, T. R., & Burton, D. (1993). Flay, B. R. Project towards no tobacco use: 1-Year behavior outcomes. *American Journal of Public Health, 83*, 1245-1250.

Sussman, S., Stacy, A. W., Dent, C. W., Simon, T. R., Galaif, E. R., Moss, M. A., Craig, S., & Johnson, C. A. (1995). Continuation high schools: Youth at risk for drug abuse. *Journal of Drug Education, 25*, 191-209.

Sussman, S., Sun, P., & Dent, C. W. (2006) A meta-analysis of teen cigarette smoking cessation, *Health Psychology, 25*, 549-557.

Tanjasiri, S. P., & Tran, J. (2008). Community capacity for cancer control collaboration: The Weaving an Islander Network for Cancer Awareness, Research and Training. *Cancer Detection and Prevention, 32,* S37-S40.

Tanjasiri, S. P., Tran, J., Palmer, P. H., & Valente, T. W. (2007). Network analysis of a collaboration for Pacific Islander Cancer Control. *Journal of Health Care for Poor and Underserved, 18,* 184-196.

Travers, J., & Milgram, S. (1969). An experimental study of the small world problem. *Sociometry 32,* 425-443.

Treboux, D., & Busch- Rossnagel, N. A. (1990). Social network influences on adolescent sexual attitudes and behavior. *Journal of Adolescent Research, 5,* 175-189.

Trotter, R. T., II, Bowen, A. M., & Potter, J. M., Jr. (1995). *Network models for HIV outreach and prevention programs for drug users.* Department of Anthropology, Northern Arizona University, Flagstaff.

Turner, R. J., & Marino, F. (1994). Social support and social structure: A descriptive epidemiology. *Journal of Health and Social Behavior, 35,* 193-212.

Tutzaer, F. (2007). Entropy as a measure of centrality in networks characterized by path-transfer flow. *Social Networks, 29,* 249-265.

Unger, J. B., & Chen, X. (1999). The role of social networks and media receptivity in predicting age of smoking initiation: A proportional hazards model of risk and protective factors, *Addictive Behaviors, 3,* 371-381.

Unger, J. B., Chou, C. P., Palmer, P. H., Ritt-Olson, A., Gallagher, P., Cen, S., Lichtman, K., Azen, S., & Johnson, C. A. (2004). Project Flavor: 1-Year outcomes of a multicultural, school-based tobacco prevention curriculum for adolescents. *American Journal of Public Health, 94,* 263-265.

Urberg, K. A., Degirmencioglu, S. M., & Pilgrim, C. (1997). Close friend and group influence on adolescent cigarette smoking and alcohol use. *Developmental Psychology, 33,* 834-844.

Uzzi, B. (1997) Social structure and competition in interfirm networks: The paradox of embeddedness. *Administrative Science Quarterly, 42,* 417-418.

Valente, T. W. (1993). Diffusion of innovations and policy decision-making. *Journal of Communication, 43,* 30-41.

Valente, T. W. (1995). *Network models of the diffusion of innovations.* Cresskill, NJ: Hampton Press.

Valente, T. W. (1996). Social network thresholds in the diffusion of innovations. *Social Networks, 18,* 69-89.

Valente, T. W. (2002). *Evaluating health promotion programs.* New York, NY: Oxford University Press.

Valente, T. W. (2005). Models and methods for innovation diffusion. In P. J. Carrington, J. Scott, & S. Wasserman (Eds.) *Models and methods in social network analysis.* Cambridge, UK: Cambridge University Press.

Valente, T. W. (2007). Communication network analysis. In M. D. Slater, A. Hayes, & L. B. Snyder (Eds.) *The Sage handbook of advanced data analysis methods for communication research* (pp. 247-273). Thousand Oaks, CA: Sage.

Valente, T. W., Chou, C. P., & Pentz, M. A. (2007a). Community coalition networks as systems: Effects of network change on adoption of evidence-based prevention. *American Journal of Public Health, 97,* 880-886.

Valente, T.W., Coronges, K., Lakon, C., & Costenbader, E. (2008a). How correlated are centrality measures? *Connections, 28*(1), 16-26.

Valente, T. W., Coronges, K., Stevens, G., & Cousineau, M. (2008b). Collaboration and competition in a children's health initiative coalition: A network analysis. *Evaluation & Program Planning, 31*, 392-402.

Valente, T. W., & Davis, R. L. (1999). Accelerating the diffusion of innovations using opinion leaders. *The Annals of the American Academy of the Political and Social Sciences, 566*, 55-67.

Valente, T. W., & Foreman, R. K. (1998). Integration and radiality: Measuring the extent of an individual's connectedness and reachability in a network. *Social Networks, 20*, 89-109.

Valente, T. W., & Fosados, R. (2006). Diffusion of innovations and network segmentation: The part played by people in the promotion of health. *Journal of Sexually Transmitted Diseases, 33*, S23-S31.

Valente, T. W., & Fujimoto, K. (submitted). Bridges: Locating critical connectors in a network. Submitted to *Social Networks*.

Valente, T. W., Fujimoto, K., Chou, C. P., & Spruijt-Metz, D. (2009). Friendship affiliations and adiposity: A social network analysis of adolescent friendships and weight status. *Journal of Adolescent Health.*, 45, 202-204.

Valente, T. W., Fujimoto, K., Palmer, P., & Tanjasiri, S. P. (In press). A network assessment of community-based participatory action: Linking communities and universities to reduce cancer disparities. American Journal of Public Health.

Valente, T. W., Hoffman, B. R., Ritt-Olson, A., Lichtman, K., & Johnson, C. A. (2003). The effects of a social network method for group assignment strategies on peer led tobacco prevention programs in schools. *American Journal of Public Health, 93*, 1837-1843.

Valente, T. W., Kim, Y. M., Lettenmaier, C., Glass, W., & Dibba, Y (1994). Radio promotion of family planning in Gambia. *International Family Planning Perspectives, 20*, 96-100.

Valente, T. W., Mouttapa, M., & Gallaher, M. (2004). Social network analysis for understanding substance abuse: A transdisciplinary perspective. *Substance Use & Misuse, 39*, 1685-1712.

Valente, T. W., Paredes, P., & Poppe, P. R. (1998). Matching the message to the process: The relative ordering of knowledge, attitudes and practices in behavior change research. *Human Communication Research, 24*, 366-385.

Valente, T. W., & Pumpuang, P. (2007). Identifying opinion leaders to promote behavior change. *Health Education & Behavior, 34*, 881-896.

Valente, T. W., & Rogers, E. M. (1995). The origins and development of the diffusion of innovations paradigm as an example of scientific growth. *Science Communication: An Interdisciplinary Social Science Journal, 16*, 238-269.

Valente, T. W., & Saba, W. (1998). Mass media and interpersonal influence in a reproductive health communication campaign in Bolivia. *Communication Research, 25*, 96-124.

Valente, T. W., Sussman, S., Unger, J., Ritt-Olson, A., Okamoto, J., & Stacey, A. (2007b). Peer acceleration: Effects of a network tailored substance abuse prevention program among high risk adolescents. *Addiction, 102*, 1804-1815.

Valente, T. W., Unger, J., & Johnson, A. C. (2005). Do popular students smoke? The association between popularity and smoking among middle school students. *Journal of Adolescent Health*, 37, 323-329.

Valente, T. W., Unger, J., Ritt-Olson, A., Cen, S. Y., & Johnson, A. C. (2006). The inter-action of curriculum and implementation method on 1 year smoking outcomes. *Health Education Research: Theory & Practice, 21*, 315-324.

Valente, T. W., & Vlahov, D. (2001). Selective risk taking among needle exchange partic-ipants in Baltimore: Implications for supplemental interventions. *American Journal of Public Health, 91*, 406-411.

Valente, T. W., Watkins, S., Jato, M. N., Van der Straten, A., & Tsitsol, L. M. (1997). Social network associations with contraceptive use among Cameroonian women in voluntary associations. *Social Science and Medicine, 45*, 677-687.

Valente, T. W., Zogg, J., Christensen, S., Richardson, J., Kovacs, A., & Operskalski, E. (2009). Using social networks to recruit an HIV vaccine preparedness cohort. *JAIDS*.

Van den Bulte, C., & Lillien, G. L. (2001). Medical innovation revisited: Social contagion versus marketing effort. *American Journal of Sociology, 106*, 1409-1435.

Van den Bulte, C., & Wuyts, S. (2007). *Social networks and marketing*. Cambridge, MA: Marketing Science Institute.

Vaux, A. (1988). *Social support: Theory, research, and intervention*. New York, NY: Praeger.

Vega, W. A., Apospori, E., Gil, A. G., et al. (1996). A replication and elaboration of the self esteem-enhancement model. *Psychiatry: Interpersonal Biological Processes, 59*, 128-144.

Wallace, R. (1994). A fractal model of HIV transmission on complex socio-geographic networks. Part 2: Spread from a ghettoized "core group" into a "general popula-tion." *Environment and Planning* A, *26*(5), 767-778.

Wallerstein, N. B., & Duran, B. (2006). Using community-based participatory research to address health disparities. *Health Promotion Practice, 7*, 312-323.

Wang, M. Q., Fitzhugh, E. C., Eddy, J. M., et al. (1997). Social influences on adolescents' smoking progress: a longitudinal analysis. *American Journal of Health Behavior, 21*, 111-117.

Wasserman, S., & Faust, K. (1994). *Social networks analysis: Methods and applications*. Cambridge, UK: Cambridge University Press.

Watts, D. (1999). *Small worlds: The dynamics of networks between order and random-ness*. Princeton, NJ: Princeton University Press.

Watts, D. J., & Strogatz, S. H. (1998). Collective dynamics of 'small-world' networks. *Nature, 393*, 409-410.

Wellman, B., & Berkowitz, S. D. (1988). (Eds.) *Social structures: A network approach*. Cambridge, UK: Cambridge University Press.

Wiist, W. H., & Snider, G. (1991). Peer education in friendship cliques: Prevention of adolescent smoking. *Health Education Research, 6*(1), 101-108.

Wipfli, H., Fujimoto, K., & Valente, T. W. (in press). Global tobacco control diffusion: The case of the framework convention on tobacco control. *American Journal of Public Health*.

White, H. C., Boorman, S. A., & Breiger, R. L. (1976). Social structure from mul-tiple networks. I. Blockmodels of roles and positions. *The American Journal of Sociology, 81*(4), 730-780.

White, K., & Watkins, S. C. (2000). Accuracy, stability and reciprocity in informal conversational networks in rural Kenya. *Social Networks, 22,* 337-356.

Wickizer, T. M., Korff, M. V., Cheadle, A., Maeser, J., Wagner, E. H., Pearson, D., Beery, W., & Psaty, B. M. (1993). Activating communities for health promotion: A process evaluation method. *American Journal of Public Health, 83,* 561-567.

Windle, M. (2000). Parental, sibling, and peer influences on adolescent substance use and alcohol problems. *Applied Developmental Science, 4,* 98-110.

Young, P. H. (2006) *The spread of innovations through social learning.* Washington, DC: Brookings Institute, working paper.

Author Index

Adelman, M. B., 36
Ainlay, S. L., 37
Ajzen, I., 33, 34
Albrecht, T. L., 36
Alexander, C., 8, 16, 30, 31, 35, 67, 96, 188
Allison, P. D., 184
Aloise-Young, P., 30
Amirkhanian, Y. A., 204
Amos, A., 32
Anderson, C. J., 153
Anderson, R. M., 37
Aral, S. O., 36, 37
Asch, S. E., 33

Baerveldt, C., 169
Bailey, N. T. J., 172
Bak, P., 19
Bandura, A., 321
Banks, D. L., 12
Barabási, A. L., 11, 22
Barrera, M., 37
Bass, F. M., 172

Bauman, K. E., 31, 32, 73
Beal, G. M., 173
Bearman, P. S., 8
Becker, M. H., 16, 180
Beniger, I. R., 39
Berkman, L. F., 36
Berkowitz, S. D., 7
Bernard, H. R., 50, 65, 234
Bertrand, J. T., 178
Bettinger, J. A., 37
Bhatia, S., 38
Bloor, M., 201
Blythe, J., 53
Bogue, D. J., 45
Bohlen, J. M., 173
Boissevain, J., 7
Bonacich, P., 28, 56, 93, 240
Boorman, S. A., 56
Borgatti, S. P., 4, 12, 16, 17, 21, 56, 81, 90, 93, 116, 117, 131, 141, 145, 168, 202, 207, 240
Botvin, G. J., 30, 31
Boulay, M., 236

Brandes, U., 21, 88
Breiger, R., 43, 48, 49, 50, 56
Broadhead, R. S., 205
Brown, L., 172
Buller, D. B., 18, 204
Burk, W. J., 151, 163
Burt, R. S., 7, 43, 44, 56, 62, 69–70,
  122–124, 133, 182, 183, 185, 240
Busch-Rossnagel, N. A., 37
Bush, P. J., 34, 73, 234

Cairns, R. B., 27
Campbell, K. E., 44, 234
Carley, K. M., 12, 50, 115
Carrington, P. J., 7
Cartano, D. G., 96, 197
Cassel, J., 36
Cheek, N. H., 35
Chen, X., 31
Christakis, N. A., 7, 8, 50,
  188, 222, 237
Chung, W., 38
Clark-Lempers, D. S., 35
Coender, G., 234
Cohen, S., 36
Coleman, J. S., 12, 39, 179, 193
Contractor, N. S., 7, 153, 238
Cornwell, B., 93
Coromina, L., 234
Costenbader, E., 21, 89, 91
Coyle, S. L., 7
Crabb, A. R., 175
Crane, D., 174
Cross, R., 18
Cutrona, C. E., 37

D'Avanzo, K., 35
Davis, A., 43, 48, 50
Davis, R., 8, 16, 19, 204
de Nooy, W., 254
Degenne, A., 7
Diani, M., 7
Dishion, T. J., 214
Dodge, K. A., 214
Donato, F., 31
Donohew, L., 32
Doreian, P., 12, 115
Dunbar, R. I. M., 129, 232
Dunphy, D. C., 35

Duran, B., 166
Dutton, W. H., 50

Eccles, R., 7
Ellen, J., 95
Engels, R., 32
Ennett, S. T., 8, 31, 32
Entwisle, B., 8
Epstein, J. M., 19
Erlebach, T., 21, 88
Everett, M. G., 16, 17, 81, 141

Faust, K., 7, 94, 133, 138
Feiring, C., 35
Fernandez, R. M., 133
Festinger, L., 133
Fishbein, M., 33, 34
Fisher, J., 32, 37
Flay, B. R., 30
Forsé, M., 7
Fowler, J. H., 7, 8, 50, 188, 222, 237
Foreman, R. K., 182
Freeman, L. C., 16, 26, 30, 54, 56,
  81–83, 87, 88, 93, 99, 139, 239–240
Friedkin, N. E., 7, 185
Friedman, S. R., 8, 31, 37, 178
Fujimoto, K., 112, 143, 190, 210
Furman, W., 35

Galaskiewicz, J., 39
Gavin, L. A., 35
Gilmore, J. B., 110
Girvan, M., 105–107, 117, 120, 203
Gladwell, M., 177, 184
Glanz, K., 172
Goodman, L. A., 43
Gottlieb, B. H., 36
Gould, R. V., 133
Granovetter, M., 13, 18, 38, 66, 133,
  181–182, 191, 209, 210, 211, 239
Gross, C. P., 173, 174, 188
Gross, N., 8

Hägerstrand, T., 172
Hall, J., 33, 189
Hamblin, R., 184
Hammer, M., 36
Harary, F., 7
Harrigan, N., 151, 160

Harris, J., 7, 8, 36, 50
Havanon, N., 37
Heckathorn, D. D., 45, 205
Heider, F., 133
Hoffman, B., 15, 30
Holland, P. W., 132, 133, 152
House, J. S., 36, 37
Huisman, M., 8, 21, 51, 93
Hummon, N. B., 50, 115

Ianotti, R. J., 34, 73, 234
Israel, B. A., 166

Jasuja, G. K., 134
Jenkins. J. E., 31, 35

Kandel, D., 32
Katz, E., 172, 173, 193
Kelly, J. A., 38
Kelner, M., 38
Killeya-Jones, L. A., 213
Killworth, P. D., 129
Kincaid, D. L., 7, 16, 38, 46, 95, 179
King, C. W., 216
Kirke, D., 30
Kleinberg, J., 10
Klovdahl, A. S., 36, 37, 43, 45, 46
Knoke, D., 7, 27
Knowlton, A., 36
Kochen, M., 9
Koehly, L., 161
Kohler, H. P., 36
Koschützki, D., 21
Kossinets, G., 50, 181
Krackhardt, D., 53, 107, 110, 145
Krebs, V. E., 18
Kretzschmar, M., 68
Kuklinski, J. H., 7, 27
Kwait, J., 8, 36

Latkin, C. A., 37, 200, 205
Laumann, E., 47
Lee, B. A., 44, 234
Leinhardt, S., 132, 133, 152
Lewis, K., 50
Lewis, M., 35
Liben-Nowell, D., 10
Lillien, G. L., 188
Lin, N., 7, 12

Lomas, J., 19, 36, 39, 199, 201
Lorrain, F., 115
Luce, R. D., 138
Luke, D. A., 7
Luthar, S. S., 35

MacKinnon, D. P., 34
Mahajan, V., 173, 184
Marino, F., 36
Markus, M. L., 184
Marsden, P. V., 7, 21, 43, 44, 51, 63,
    185, 240
Marwell, G., 184
May, R. M., 37
McAdam, D., 7
McCarty, C., 44
McGrath, C., 53, 54
McPherson, M., 12, 44
Meijer, R. R., 31
Michell, L., 32
Milgram, S., 9–10
Minor, M. J., 7
Mizruchi, M., 43, 48
Monge, P. R., 7, 238
Montgomery, M. R., 38
Moody, J., 8
Moore, K. A., 200
Moore, S., 12
Moreno, J. L., 26
Morris, M., 8, 37, 68, 172
Moscovici, S., 101
Murray, D. M., 30, 42
Myers, D. J., 190

Neaigus, A., 8, 37
Needle, R. H., 6, 37
Newman, M. E. J., 21, 88, 100,
    105–107, 117, 120, 203
Noria, N., 7

Obbo, C., 37
Oh, H., 111
Orth-Gomer, K., 36

Palmore, J. A., 43
Park, H. J., 38
Parker, A., 18
Pattison, P., 160, 161
Pearson, M., 31, 32

Pennings, J., 48
Perry, A. D., 138
Peters, R. H., 200
Peterson, R. A., 173, 184
Pierce, J., 6
Pitts, F. R., 95
Podolny, J., 185
Pool, I. S., 9
Potterat, J. J., 178
Provan, K. G., 8, 39
Pumpuang, P., 16, 98, 197
Putnam, R. D., 12

Rai, A. A., 31
Rice, R. E., 34, 50, 73, 234
Richards, W. D., 93
Robertson, T. S., 172
Robins, G., 157, 160, 162
Rogers, E. M., 7, 14, 16, 29, 38, 46, 95,
    96, 172, 173, 179, 197
Rosenfield, A. G., 38
Rothenberg, R., 8, 37
Ryan, R., 173, 174

Saba, 44, 184, 193
Salganik, M. J., 45, 206
Sarason, I. G., 36, 43
Schelling, T., 183
Scott, J., 7, 27, 101
Seary, A. J., 93
Shaw, M. E., 95
Shrum, W., 35
Sieving, R., 31
Sikkema, K. J., 200
Snider, G., 203, 204
Snijders, T. A. B., 151, 160, 161, 162,
    163, 169, 171
Soumerai, S. B., 36, 200
Stephenson, K., 56, 93
Stern, R. N., 107
Stoebenau, K., 36
Stokman, F., 12
Strang, D., 190
Strogatz, S. H., 22, 137, 183, 237
Suhr, J. A., 37
Sussman, S., 34, 35, 36, 215
Syme, S. L., 36

Tanjasiri, S. P., 166
Tran, J., 166

Travers, J., 10
Treboux, D., 37
Trotter, R. T., 38
Tuma, N. B., 190
Turner, R. J., 36
Tutzaer, F., 93

Unden, A. L., 36
Unger, J. B., 31, 204
Urberg, K. A., 30, 31, 33
Uzzi, B., 111

Valente, T. W., 6, 7, 8, 14, 15, 16, 17,
    18, 19, 21, 23, 29, 33, 34, 36, 38, 42,
    43, 44, 46, 51, 58, 66 72, 73, 75, 85,
    89, 91, 92, 93, 96, 98, 109, 110, 111,
    125, 131, 134, 141, 142, 143, 161, 162,
    166, 168, 170, 172, 173, 174, 175,
    182, 184, 187, 188, 189, 191, 193, 197,
    198, 204, 206, 210, 214, 215, 234,
    236, 240
Van den Bulte, C., 7, 62, 96, 188
van Duijn, M. A. J., 8, 21, 51, 93, 157
Vaux, A., 36
Vega, W. A., 35
Vlahov, D., 66, 234

Wallace, R., 37
Wallerstein, N. B., 166
Wang, M. Q., 31
Wasserman, S., 7, 94, 138, 153
Watkins, S. C., 21
Watts, D. J., 9, 22, 50, 137,
    181, 183, 237
Wellman, Barry, 7
Wellman, Beverly, 38
West, P., 31, 32
White, H. C., 56, 115
White, K., 21
Wickizer, T. M., 36, 39
Wiist, W. H., 203, 204
Windle, M., 31
Wipfli, H., 190, 236
Wuyts, S., 7

Yang, S., 7
Young, P. H., 173

Zelen, M., 56, 93
Zunguze, S. T., 31

Subject Index

Accuracy (of perception), 34
Acute myocardial
    infarction (AMI), 200
Actor-oriented model, 163
Adoption, 62, 174
Adjacency Matrix, 126
Affiliation Network, 144
Agent based models (ing), 19–21,
    224–233
AIDS, 27, 36
Alcohol, 31
Algorithms, 21
Alter, 62
Alternative high school, 215
Archival sources, 50
Asymmetric, 55, 82, 88, 92–93, 119,
    123, 130–133, 231
Attributes, 3–4, 5, 7, 58, 73, 83,
    119–120, 125, 145, 152, 154,
    156, 159, 163–164, 170, 190, 196,
    212–213, 222, 223, 233
    attribute effect in SIENA, 165
Average Path Length, 134, 135, 239

Balance, 132–133, 165
Barnes, J., 27
Bavelas, A., 81
Behaviors, 3, 6, 8, 14, 22–25, 31, 32,
    72, 108, 124–125, 143, 152, 172
Behavioral science, 30
Betweenness, *see* Centrality
    betweenness
Bibliometrics, 50
Blockmodeling, 115–117, 119
BMI (Body-Mass Index), 161
Brazilian farmers
    data, 15, 126, 187, 188
Bridge, 45, 208–212, 239
Boissevain, J., 27
Bonacich, P., 27
Boorman, S. A., 27
Bott, E., 27
Breiger, R., 27
Brokerage, 133

Carley, K., 27
Cartwright, D., 27

Census (sampling), 43, 48
Centrality, 16–17, 21, 56, 81–99
  betweenness, 56, 87, 88, 239
  closeness, 56, 83–84, 239
  degree, 56, 82, 83, 84, 88, 239
Centralization, 94, 112, 138–139, 239
Characteristic Path Length, *see* average
  path length
Chain length, 10
Clique, 103–104, 239
Closeness, *see* centrality
Clustering, 137, 183
Co-occurring disorders, 200
Coalitions, 111, 134, 141
Cohesion, 135–136
Collective action, 7
Collaboration, 8, 36, 142
Community health, 38–39
Community based participatory
  research (CBPR), 166
Compatibility (of innovations), 180
Complete network, 46
Composition measures (for ego-centric
  data), 63
Component, 100–101, 239
CONCOR, 121–122, 125
Concurrency, 68
Connectedness, 56, 239
Contact tracing, 205
Contraception, 8, 34, 65–66, 72–73,
  95, 193
Conformable (as in matrices), 49, 144
Constraint, 56, 69, 183
Contagion, *see* diffusion
  of innovations
Correlation (among
  centrality measures), 91
Core-periphery, 102, 140–144
Critical mass index, 191

Data collection, 41–42
Data management, 41, 43–44, 57
Decision-making, 194
Degeneration (in model estimation), 160
Degree, 82, 84, 165
  see also centrality
Density, 129–130, 239
  effective density, 130
  optimal levels, 18, 110–112

personal network density, 69–70, 137,
  239
Dependence graph (or network), 159
Deviancy training, 214
Diabetes screening, 180
Diffusion of innovations, 14–16, 110,
  140, 172–195, 225–231
Diameter, 86, 134–135, 239
Distance, 9, 16, 83, 85, 86, 122–123,
  207, 211, 240
  in disconnected networks, 85–86
Disconnected networks, 86
Duality, *see* two-mode
Dyad/dyadic, 51, 58, 70–72

E-I index, 107
Edge, 93
Eigenvector centrality, 89–90, 92, 93
Efficiency, 17–18
Ego-centric, 7, 42, 44–45, 51, 61–77,
  220, 239
  measures, 63
Email, 109
Euclidean distance, 123
Event history analysis, 186
Expansiveness, 82
Exponential random graph model
  (ERGM), 151, 156–161, 161, 240
Exposure, Network, 61, 65–66, 73, 126,
  184–188, 189–190, 240

Facebook, 50, 109, 175, 215
Family planning, 15, 36, 38
Festinger, L., 27
Flow, 240
Fruits and vegetables, 204
Funneling (questions), 55

Granovetter, M., 27
General social survey (GSS), 44, 50–51,
  62–63
Geodesic, 240
Girvan-Newman, 105–108, 117
Group, 100–113, 114
  for interventions, 202–203

Hawaii meetings, 27
Health service delivery, 8, 39
Heider, F., 27

Hierarchical network, 120
HIV, 8, 37, 67, 200, 204
HIV vaccine, 76
History (of Network Analysis), 26–30
Homans, G., 27
Homophily, 12–13, 30–31, 178
Hybrid seed, 174–175

Iatrogenic effects, 214
Identity (social), 100–101
Incidence matrix, *see* affiliation network
In-degree, *see* centrality degree
Infection (estimating in diffusion), 190
Influence, 61, 66, 69, 73, 97–98, 108,
    177–178
    see also social influence
Injection Drug Users (IDUs), 8, 37, 200
INSNA (International Network
    for Social Network Analysis,
    http://www.insna.org), 27, 240
Interventions, 18, 196–218
Isolates, 4, 5
Image Matrix, 115–120
Imaginary network, 45
Inter-organizational Relations, 36, 39
Integration/Radiality, 85, 178, 179
IQV (Index of Qualitative Variation), 63

Jobs, 13
Jointness, *see* two-mode

K-core, 102–103
K-plex, 103
Keyplayer, 201–202
Korean family planning data, 15, 187,
    188, 192

Lifespan approaches, 35
Limitations (to network analysis),
    237–238
Link (deletion or addition), 208–209
    estimation, 153
Link centrality, 93, 106
Link list, 51, 71
LinkedIn, 50, 215
Local network, 44

Malaria, 37
MAN (distribution), 132

Manchester Anthropologists, 27
Marketing, 7
Markov Chain Monte Carlo
    (MCMC), 157
Matches, 122
Mathematical models
    (of diffusion), 174
Matrix, 240
Maximum pseudo-likelihood estimation
    (MPLE), 154
Measles immunization, 180
Medical Innovation data, 179, 187,
    188, 192
Michigan, University of, 27
Micro/macro, 115
Missing data, 89
Mitchell, J. C., 27
Modularity, 106
Multi-level models, 154
Mutuality, 130–132
Myspace, 50, 215

Name generator, 43, 44, 62, 65, 74, 234
N-clique, 103
Net Draw, 168, 240
Network evolution, 163–166
Network level, 128–147
Network relations, 55
Newman-Girvan algorithm, *see*
    Girvan-Newman
Node list, 51
Norms, 33–35

Obesity, 161
Objective function (in SIENA), 163, 164
Opinion leaders, 95–98, 140, 177–178,
    179–180, 184, 197–198
    characteristics, 98
Organizational behavior, 7
ORA (Organization Risk Analyzer), 52,
    240
Orgnet, 240
Out-degree
    see also centrality
Overestimation, 34

Pajek, 52, 240
Partial network, 45
Perceptions, 34, 72, 73, 75

Peripheral, 147
Personal networks, 61–77, 136
Personal network density, 56
Pharmaceutical example, 216–217
Physicians, 8, 38–39, 217
PNET, 163
Population measures, 64
Positional equivalence, 56
Positions, 114–126
  for interventions, 203
Potential bridges, 208
Popularity, 96

Q (modularity), 106–107
QAP (Quadratic Assignment
  Procedure), 145–146
Questionnaires, 43

R, 52, 58, 240
Radial, 69
Random effects (regression), 154
Random network, 20
Random sampling, 6, 28–30, 41–42
Rate function (in SIENA), 164
RDS (respondent driven sampling),
  75, 205
Reach, 56, 240
Reciprocity, 130–132, 165
Reduced form network, 115
Relational measures, 55–56
Relationships, 3–4
Research questions, 233–234
Reshape (data), 59
Respondent driven sampling, *see* RDS
Roles, 27, 43, 44, 114, 119, 181
  see also social roles

SAS, 28, 50, 52, 71
Sabidussi, G., 81
Scale Free Network, 11–12
Selection, 14, 32, 108
Sequenced data, 45–46, 74
SIENA, 163–166, 240
Simulation, 19
  in ERGM, 157
  see also agent based models
Size, 65, 129
Small world, 9–11
Small world network, 9

Smoking, 8, 29–30, 32–33, 96, 152,
  204–205
Snowball sampling, 42, 74, 240
Social capital, 12–13, 24, 61, 109
Social consequences, 35
Social influence, 7, 66, 147, 234
Social Learning Theory, 31–32
Social networks (journal), 115
Social roles, 43
Social support, 36–37
Sociograms, 53
Sociometric, 42, 240
SPSS, 28, 50, 52, 71
STATA, 28, 50, 52, 71
STATNet, 52, 58, 163, 240
STDs /STIs (Sexually transmitted
  diseases/infections), 36, 75, 205
Strength of weak ties, 133, 181–182, 211
Structural equivalence, 122–123, 240
Structural holes, 133, 182–183
Substance use, 30–31, 111, 213
Suicide, 8
Surveys, 43
survey samples, 241–243
Susceptibility (estimating in
  diffusion), 190
Susceptibility to smoking, 6
Symmetry, 55
Syringe sharing, 67

TB, 37
Terrorist networks, 18
Texting, 109
Theory, 30, 117, 132, 164, 196–197, 220
Thresholds, 16, 61, 73, 184, 231–232, 240
Tie strength, 66–68, 73, 131, 182, 234
Tipping point, 184
Tobacco use, *see* smoking
Transitivity, 132–134, 165, 240
Transpose (a matrix), 48–49, 144
Triad census, 133, 240
Triads, 132–134, 137
Trust, 97, 109, 110
Two-mode, 43, 48, 144–146
Two-step flow hypothesis, 45, 177–178,
  193

UCINET, 28, 51, 52, 54, 93, 103–105,
  116–118, 122, 202, 237, 240

Vaccine recruitment, 206
Variance measures (for egocentric data), 63–64
VBAC (Vaginal Birth After C-section), 39, 199
Virtual network, 45
Visualizer, 52, 240

Weak ties, 65, 66
    see also strength of weak ties
Weight matrix, 185
Weighting (ties), 55, 73
Wellman, B., 27
WINCART, 166–170

Printed and bound by CPI Group (UK) Ltd, Croydon, CR0 4YY